Delivering
Mental Health
in Primary Care

Delivering Mental Health in Primary Care

An evidence-based approach

Edited by Alan Cohen

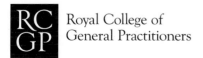

Royal College of
General Practitioners

The Royal College of General Practitioners was founded in 1952 with this object:
'To encourage, foster and maintain the highest possible standards in general practice and for that purpose to take or join with others in taking steps consistent with the charitable nature of that object which may assist towards the same.'

Among its responsibilities under its Royal Charter the College is entitled to:
'Diffuse information on all matters affecting general practice and issue such publications as may assist the object of the College.'

British Library Cataloguing-in-Publication Data
A catalogue record for this book is available from the British Library

© Royal College of General Practitioners 2008
Published by the Royal College of General Practitioners 2008
14 Princes Gate, Hyde Park, London SW7 1PU

Disclaimer
This publication is intended for the use of medical practitioners in the UK and not for patients. The authors, editors and publisher have taken care to ensure that the information contained in this book is correct to the best of their knowledge, at the time of publication. Whilst efforts have been made to ensure the accuracy of the information presented, particularly that related to the prescription of drugs, the authors, editors and publisher cannot accept liability for information that is subsequently shown to be wrong. Readers are advised to check that the information, especially that related to drug usage, complies with information contained in the *British National Formulary*, or equivalent, or manufacturers' datasheets, and that it complies with the latest legislation and standards of practice.

Designed and typeset by Robert Updegraff
Printed by Cromwell Press
Indexed by Carol Ball

ISBN: 978-0-85084-314-9

I cannot think of any need in childhood as strong as the need for a father's protection.

Sigmund Freud, *Civilization and Its Discontents*

By the time a man realizes that maybe his father was right, he usually has a son who thinks he's wrong.

Charles Wadsworth

For Norman and John.

Contents

Notes on authors

Dr Alan Cohen FRCGP was a GP principal for 20 years in Mitcham, South London. In that time the practice developed from a three-partner practice with 6000 patients to a five-partner training and teaching practice working from new cost-rent premises with 10,000 patients. For seven years Dr Cohen was the only trainer in the practice, and made links with the local medical school and the FSHA (Family Health Service Authority) (as was). He was chair of the Medical Audit Advisory Group (MAAG), and later chair of the Primary Care Group.

In April 2004, he left the practice as a principal to join Kensington and Chelsea Primary Care Trust (PCT) as Clinical Director. From 2005 he was appointed as Senior Primary Care Adviser to the Care Services Improvement Partnership (CSIP). The CSIP is part of the Department of Health and is responsible for service improvement and policy development for the 'care services', i.e. mental health, older people and children's health, people with learning and/or physical disabilities, and social care.

Dr Cohen also works as Senior Fellow at the Sainsbury Centre for Mental Health, a national mental health charitable trust, and chaired the London Development Centre for Mental Health, one of the eight regional development centres of the National Institute of Mental Health in England (NIMHE) up until 2006.

Dr Cohen maintains his clinical skills working as a GP consultant in a practice in Wimbledon. He undertakes clinical work, including routine sessions, and also provides advice to other clinicians in the team on managing patients with complex mental health problems.

Dr Les Ashton is a part-time GP working in a Leicester-based primary care service solely for asylum seekers. He is a Programme Director for the East Midlands Deanery, GP appraisal Lead for Leicester City PCT and, for the last two years, has been a Balint group facilitator. He has a special interest in primary care mental health and in particular the role of education and training in its development. He has been involved with developments for the CSIP, New Ways of Working and Trailblazer programmes. Currently, he is the Curriculum Lead for Primary Care Mental Health and Education (PRIMHE) and is leading on both a new master's programme for practitioners with a special interest (PwSIs) in mental health and also an educational programme to support the newly launched Improving Access to Psychological Therapies (IAPT) initiative.

Nicola Bent is the Associate Director for Implementation Systems for the National Institute for Health and Clinical Excellence (NICE), with responsibility for managing the Institute's activities relating to the strategic development of the implementation systems for, and monitoring uptake of, NICE guidance. This role involves the development of a programme of work to evaluate the uptake of NICE guidance, overseeing an educational strategy, working on spreading best practice and integrating NICE guidance into health-related software packages. Nicola is a registered member of the Royal Pharmaceutical Society of Great Britain and has a wealth of experience, having worked in all areas of the pharmaceutical profession, both in primary and secondary care. She spent two years developing a successful Implementation Strategy involving major collaborative engagement between four Primary Care Trusts, three Acute Trusts and a Mental Health Partnership NHS trust within the Bristol Health community prior to her role at NICE.

Dr Angela Burnett is a GP at the Sanctuary Practice in Hackney, East London, which was originally established to provide a dedicated service for asylum seekers and refugees, and which now caters for a wider practice population, including homeless people. She is also a Senior Clinician at the Medical Foundation for the Care of Victims of Torture. She provides training on the health care of refugees and torture survivors, and has assisted in the development of health services throughout the UK. Previously she has worked in Zambia, providing health care for people affected by HIV/AIDS and their families, and researching collaboration between traditional healers and formal health workers. She has also worked in Macedonia, evaluating a professional development programme for doctors, and in Ethiopia with Oxfam, with people affected by drought and famine. With the Refugee Education and Training Advisory Service (RETAS) she provided mentoring support for refugee doctors, in order to assist them to work in the UK. She has written on the health of refugees and survivors of torture, including a series in the *British Medical Journal*, several book chapters, guidelines and a resource pack for health workers.

Dr Dick Churchill FRCGP is a part-time GP in Nottingham and Associate Clinical Professor in the Division of Primary Care at the University of Nottingham Medical School. He has both clinical and research interests in the health of children and young people, and in mental health issues. He is a member of the RCGP Adolescent Task Group and a spokesperson for the College on child health.

Prof. Chris Drinkwater CBE FRCGP FFPHM was an inner-city GP in Newcastle for 23 years. He is now Emeritus Professor of Primary Care Development at Northumbria University in Newcastle. He is the President and the Public Health Lead for the NHS Alliance, company secretary of the West End Health Resource Centre (a prototype Healthy Living Centre) and a member of the North East Sports Board. In 2004 he chaired the National Task Group on Primary Care for the 'Choosing Health' consultation. He is currently a member of the NICE Programme Development Group that is producing guidelines for Community Engagement and Community Development. His research and publications cover a wide range of subjects, and he has recently co-authored *Involving Patients and the Public: how to do it better* (Radcliffe, 2003) and edited *Primary Care in Urban Disadvantaged Communities* (Radcliffe, 2003).

Dr Brian Fisher MBE has been a GP in Southeast London for 25 years and is a member of one of four Practice-Based Commissioning (PBC) clusters in Lewisham. A member of the Professional Executive Committee in Lewisham PCT with a particular responsibility for older adults, public and user involvement, and mental health, he is also Chair of the Managing Demand Project, which improves the experience of referral for patients, consultants and GPs. Dr Fisher was on the Working Group for Copying Letters to Patients and has helped to write a document for the NHS Alliance on enabling patient forums to work productively with PCTs. He has a longstanding interest in user involvement and has championed patient record access. He also helped to write the NHS Alliance publication *Effective Practice-Based Commissioning: engaging with local people* (2006), which outlines approaches to Patient and Public Involvement (PPI) for PBC.

Denise Fisher initially trained as a mental health nurse in Liverpool. She has worked in hospital, community and primary care settings with adults and older people with mental health problems. She first began working in primary mental health care in 1990 (in Berkshire) and in 1998 established a mental health primary care service in Northeast Yorkshire, working closely with the Sainsbury Centre for Mental Health. This service was one of the first mental health services awarded NHS Beacon status in 1999. In 2004 she moved to John Moores University, Liverpool, where she is currently Programme Director for the Postgraduate Certificate in Primary Mental Health Care and remains committed to improving services for common mental health problems.

Liben Gebremikael, a refugee from Ethiopia, has extensive professional experience in working with refugees by providing direct social and therapeutic services as a social worker and bilingual counsellor with various agencies. He has co-facilitated a therapeutic group for unaccompanied refugees from mixed Ethiopian and Eritrean heritage with the Medical Foundation for the Care of Victims of Torture. As the Coordinator of the Woodpath Project – Refugee Resource, he was involved in the establishment of a partnership project for young unaccompanied refugees and asylum seekers in Oxford. He has also served as a member and Chair of the Management Committee of the Ethiopian Health Support Association in London.

Dr Clare Gerada MBE MRCPsych FRCGP has been a GP for 14 years in a large inner-city practice, where she set up and continues to run the CLAS (Consultancy Liaison Addiction Service) Team. Prior to this she was a psychiatrist, having trained at the

Maudsley Hospital, and developed an interest in community management of substance misuse. She is the Director and Lead for the RCGP Substance Misuse Unit and was the previous Senior Policy Officer for drugs and alcohol. She was responsible, amongst other things, for pulling together the 1999 National Clinical Guidelines for Substance Misuse. She is currently the Director of the National Clinical Governance Support Team. She is Chair of the RCGP's Medical Ethics Committee.

Dr Hilary Guite MRCGP FFPH is Consultant in Public Health for the Greenwich Teaching Primary Care Trust (TPCT) and Associate of the London Development Centre for Mental Health. Dr Guite qualified as a doctor in 1981, initially working in medical oncology and later training in general practice in London's East End. This gave her an insight into the impact of socio-demographic deprivation on people's physical and mental wellbeing. She retrained in Public Health Medicine, completing this in 1994. She now works part time for Greenwich TPCT on a range of public mental health topics including the impact of the physical environment on mental health, equity audits for community mental health teams and the development of primary care mental health.

Dr John Hague is a GP in Ipswich, where he has worked for 20 years, and a Mental Health Adviser to Suffolk PCT. He also works as an independent consultant for the Sainsbury Centre for Mental Health. At present he is working on the Expert Reference group for the Improving Access to Psychological Therapies (IAPT) programme, and leading on a county-wide mental health PBC project. With Alan Cohen and Swaran Singh he co-wrote *The Primary Care Guide to Managing Severe Mental Illness* (Sainsbury Centre for Mental Health, 2004) and with Alan Cohen he co-wrote *The Neglected Majority* (Sainsbury Centre for Mental Health, 2005), a book about intermediate mental health care.

Gillian Leng is an Executive Director at NICE with responsibility for the implementation programme. Previously she worked as the Guidelines Programme Director at NICE, and before that at Bedfordshire Health Authority as a consultant in public health medicine with responsibility for clinical governance and implementing National Service Frameworks. She is also an editor of the Cochrane Review Group on peripheral vascular diseases and an Honorary Senior Lecturer at University College London. Her research interests include the evaluation of factors that promote guidance implementation and stimulate behaviour change.

Dr Helen Lester is Professor of Primary Care at the National Primary Care Research and Development Centre, University of Manchester, and Honorary Professor of Primary Care Mental Health at the University of Birmingham. She has been a GP in inner-city Birmingham since 1990.

Dr Andrew McCulloch has been Chief Executive of the Mental Health Foundation for five years. He was formerly Director of Policy at the Sainsbury Centre for Mental Health for six years and a senior civil servant in the Department of Health for 16 years, where he was responsible for mental health and learning disabilities policy from 1992 to 1996. He has particular interests in policy development, partnership working, models of care, human resources and public mental health. He has spoken and published widely on these issues. Dr McCulloch has also been the non-executive Director of an NHS Trust, the Chair of Mental Health Media and has served on numerous advisory committees and policy inquiries. His PhD is in the psychology of old age.

Dr Ian McPherson FBPsS is Programme Director for the National Institute of Mental Health in England (NIMHE) within the CSIP. A clinical psychologist by professional background, Dr McPherson worked as a practitioner, researcher and trainer before moving into service development and management. He has had nine years' experience as Director of Mental Health for two large NHS trusts before taking up his post with NIMHE. He has a longstanding clinical and research interest in mental health in primary care, and is lead CSIP Director for the IAPT programme.

Stephen Pilling is joint Director of the National Collaborating Centre for Mental Health (NCCMH), which is responsible for developing the NICE Mental Health Clinical Practice Guideline, and is a partnership between the Royal College of Psychiatrists and the British Psychological Society. He is also the Director of the British Psychological Society's Centre for Outcomes Research and Effectiveness (CORE) based in the Sub-department of Clinical Health Psychology, University College London, where his focus is on health service research. He also works as Consultant Clinical Psychologist for Camden and Islington Mental Health and Social Care Trust.

Katy Price is the Guidelines Development Manager at the NCCMH. This role involves working with colleagues at the NCCMH, NICE and other organisations to support implementation of NICE Mental Health Guidelines in the NHS. She leads on implementation activities including organising conferences, developing information leaflets for service users and carers, and producing training materials for professionals. Together with NCCMH colleagues, she also works with NICE to assist in the development of its guideline-specific implementation tools. These include slide presentations, costing tools and implementation advice.

Mike Scanlan is currently a Nurse Consultant in Primary Care Mental Health. His professional areas of interest are around social prescribing, relapse prevention and new ways of working within mental health. He delivers mental health training for the Changing Minds Centre for Mental Health Education and Service Development. Mike has worked with older persons, young offenders, as a CPN and as a Mental Health

Senior Lecturer at the University of Northampton. Mike has published on a wide variety of topics including maternal mental health, antipsychotic side effects and post-traumatic stress disorder (PTSD). He has recently led the development of a distance learning course aimed at primary care practitioners.

Dr David Shiers has been a GP in North Staffordshire since 1980 and is a carer of a daughter with schizophrenia. Dr Shiers is currently GP Adviser to the West Midlands CSIP and for the last three years has been on a GP career break to co-lead (with Jo Smith) the NIMHE/Rethink National Early Intervention Programme.

Prof. Andre Tyleé FRCGP MRCPsych directs the Section of Primary Care Mental Health at the Institute of Psychiatry, King's College London. He is currently Principal Investigator on five randomised clinical trials (THREAD, RESPOND, SWITCH, QUEST and UPBEAT) of depression management in primary care, and three qualitative studies on patients and professional views on depression. He collaborates on several of these studies with departments of general practice in Manchester, Liverpool, Sunderland and Southampton. UPBEAT is part of a five-year NIHR Programme to improve care for patients with coronary heart disease and depression. He is on the working group for the NIHR Biomedical Research Centre at South London and the Maudsley Trust. His clinical work involves running a secondary care outreach physical health service for the High Support Rehabilitation Team at the South London and Maudsley Trust. He was a GP in Sutton, Surrey, for 21 years and is a member of the Mental Health Task Force of the RCGP and a co-founder of PRIMHE.

Paul Walters MRCPsych is an MRC Research Fellow in the Section of Primary Care Mental Health at the Institute of Psychiatry in London, and an Honorary Consultant Psychiatrist. His research interests include co-morbidity between physical health problems and common mental health problems, and the primary–secondary care interface in relation to mental health service provision.

Dr Mark Williamson studied at the Royal Free Hospital School of Medicine and became a GP and medical educationalist before working in Health Authorities and PCTs as a Medical Adviser and Medical Director. His passion in support of prison and offender health links to his interests in social exclusion, mental health and substance misuse care. He is now a Senior Medical Adviser at the Department of Health and the Chair of the RCGP's Secure Environments Group. He is also a Regional Adviser to the National Programme for IT in the NHS and is a practising general practitioner at HMP Hull and the Quays social exclusion practice in Hull.

Abbreviations

A&E	accident and emergency
ACCT	Assessment, Care in Custody and Teamwork
ADHD	attention deficit hyperactivity disorder
AMHP	approved mental health professional
AN	anorexia nervosa
ASW	approved social worker
AUDIT	Alcohol Use Disorder Identification Test
BA	behavioural activation
BDD	body dysmorphic disorder
BDI	Beck Depression Inventory
BMA	British Medical Association
BMI	body mass index
BNF	*British National Formulary*
CAB	Citizens Advice Bureau
CAMHS	Child and Adolescent Mental Health Services
CARAT	Counselling, Assessment, Referral, Advice and Throughcare
CBT	cognitive behavioural therapy
CCAWI	Centre for Clinical and Academic Workforce Innovation
cCBT	computerised cognitive behavioural therapy
CCP	Cheltenham Community Projects
CD	community development
CDW	Community Development Workers
CHD	coronary heart disease
CHI	Commission for Health Improvement
CI	confidence interval
CMHT	Community Mental Health Team
CORE	Centre for Outcomes Research and Effectiveness
CPA	Care Programme Approach
CPC	Association of Counsellors and Psychotherapists in Primary Care
CPD	continuing personal development
CPK	creatine phosphokinase
CPN	community psychiatric nurse
CSIP	Care Services Improvement Partnership
CSI-R	revised Clinical Interview Schedule
DES	Directly Enhanced Service

DNA	did not attend
DRC	Disability Rights Commission
DSM-IV	*Diagnostic and Statistical Manual of Mental Disorders*, fourth edition
DUP	Duration of Untreated Psychosis
DWP	Department of Work and Pensions
EI	Early Intervention
EIS	Early Intervention Services
EMDR	eye movement desensitisation and reprocessing
EPDS	Edinburgh Postnatal Depression Scale
ERP	exposure and response prevention
ESC	Essential Shared Capabilities
EtHSA	Ethiopian Health Support Association
FEP	first-episode psychoses
FSHA	Family Health Service Authority
GABA	gamma-aminobutyric acid
GAD	generalised anxiety disorder
GHC	General Health Questionnaire
GMHW	graduate mental health worker
GPC	General Practitioners Committee
GPwSI	general practitioner with a special interest
GRIP	Gloucestershire Recovery in Psychosis
HADS	Hospital Anxiety and Depression Scale
HDL	high-density lipoprotein
HEIs	higher education institutes
HKD	hyperkinetic disorder
HoNOS	Health of the Nation Outcome Scale
IAPT	Improving Access to Psychological Therapies
ICD-10	*The ICD-10 Classification of Mental and Behavioural Disorders*
ICHPPC	International Classification of Health Problems in Primary Care
IHD	ischaemic heart disease
IICP	Integrated Inclusive Care Programme
ITP	innovative training placements
JCPTGP	Joint Committee for Postgraduate Training in General Practice
KSF	Knowledge and Skills Framework
LCDP	Lewisham Community Development Partnership
LES	Locally Enhanced Service
LINK	Local Involvement Networks
MAOIs	monoamine oxidase inhibitors
ME	myalgic encephalomyelitis
MHHE	Mental Health in Higher Education
MHRA	Medicines and Healthcare products Regulatory Agency

MMSE	Mini-Mental State Examination
NASS	National Asylum Support Service
NCCMH	National Collaborating Centre for Mental Health
NEIT	Northumberland Early Interventions Team
NES	National Enhanced Service
nGMS	new General Medical Services
NIAMH	Northern Ireland Association for Mental Health
NICE	National Institute for Health and Clinical Excellence
NIMHE	National Institute for Mental Health in England
NOS	National Occupational Standards
NPfIT	The National Programme for Information Technology
NSAIDs	non-steroidal anti-inflammatory drugs
NSC	National Screening Committee
NSF	National Service Framework
NTORS	National Treatment Outcome Research Study
NWCs	National Workforce Competencies
NWP	NHS National Workforce Projects
OCD	obsessive-compulsive disorder
ONS	Office of National Statistics
OR	odds ratio
PAT	Patients as Teachers
PBC	Practice-Based Commissioning
PbR	Payment by Results
PCA	Patient-Centred Audit
PCO	primary care organisation
PCP	primary care professional
PCT	Primary Care Trust
PD	panic disorder
PDP	personal development plan
PEC	Professional Executive Committee
PHCT	primary healthcare team
PHCW	primary healthcare worker
PHQ	Patient Health Questionnaire
PHQ-9	Patient Health Questionnaire-9
PMEQ	Patient Mental Health Experience Questionnaire
PMETB	Postgraduate Medical Education and Training Board
PPI	Patient and Public Involvement
PREP	Prevention and Relationship Enhancement Programme
PRIME-MD	Primary Care Evaluation of Mental Disorders
PRIMHE	Primary Care Mental Health and Education
PSC	Paediatric Symptom Checklist

PSE	Present State Examination
PSPD	People with a Severe and dangerous Personality Disorder
PTSD	post-traumatic stress disorder
PwSI	practitioner with a special interest
QOF	Quality and Outcomes Framework
RCGP	Royal College of General Practitioners
RCO	refugee community organisation
RETAS	Refugee Education and Training Advisory Service
SAD-Q	Severity of Alcohol Dependence Questionnaire
SCT	Supervised Community Treatment
SDC	Scottish Development Centre for Mental Health
SDO	Service Delivery and Organisation Programme
SDQ	Strengths and Difficulties Questionnaire
SEMI	severe and enduring mental illness
SfH	Skills for Health
SHA	Strategic Health Authority
SIGN	Scottish Intercollegiate Guideline Network
SMI	severe mental illness
SMR	standardised mortality rate
SNRIs	selective noradrenergic reuptake inhibitors
SSRIs	selective serotonin reuptake inhibitors
STI	sexually transmitted infection
TAG	Threshold Assessment Grid
TCAs	tricyclic antidepressants
TPCT	Teaching Primary Care Trust
TSH	thyroid-stimulating hormone
VTS	vocational training schemes
WHO	World Health Organization

Introduction

Alan Cohen

The clinical perspective

Consider the following case history. A 53-year-old man presents to his GP with rectal bleeding and frequent bowel movements. He has a history of ulcerative colitis. The GP elicits that the exacerbation of the ulcerative colitis coincided with a stressful time of the patient's life, with some symptoms of depression, and sleeplessness. These symptoms coincided with anxieties about the health of his parents, and he was moving house. The GP arranged for some haematological investigations, treated him appropriately, and he was reviewed four weeks later.

Really rather boring as a case history, as it describes a fairly routine consultation, with a routine patient, handled in an entirely routine but appropriate fashion. It nevertheless demonstrates what every primary care clinician knows: the physical health of the individual is closely linked to his or her mental health, and to his or her social circumstances. In the above example, the exacerbation of the colitis was related to a complex set of relationships with his parents (mental health) and moving house (social circumstances). The GP caring for this patient does not need to be a mental health specialist to understand the relationship between the various external stressors and the exacerbation of the colitis.

The prevention, identification and management of all mental health conditions are the responsibility of primary care. In the above example, the mental health condition itself may not be a severe and enduring mental illness, like schizophrenia, but it is of significance to the patient. It is closely related to the exacerbation of the colitis, which is having a profound effect on the health and welfare of the patient. Although the GP is managing the colitis, he is also reviewing the patient, sometimes called 'watchful waiting'. This GP is clearly interested in the mental welfare of his patient. The GP will continue to see the patient and continue to assess, amongst other things, if there is a developing mental illness, such as depression. The GP is fulfilling his role of identification and management of a mental health condition.

The background

I was going to start this introduction with: 'GPs are not interested in mental health – at least that is what I am told by numerous psychiatrists, mental health nurses and mental health managers.' But I thought it would be better to describe what GPs and primary care clinicians do so well – manage the whole person. I do not believe that GPs are 'not interested' in mental health – whatever that means. GPs know only too well that there is a close relationship between the physical health of the individual and his or her mental health and social wellbeing. There were 280 million consultations in primary care last year, of which a third had a significant mental health component. To believe that GPs are not interested in that third of their caseload is frankly unbelievable. It is unbelievable because all the evidence points to the contrary. That evidence is what this book is about: it presents the case for the role of primary care in the management of people with mental health problems. This book will describe how people with mental health problems can be identified, how disorders can be classified, and how individuals can be managed appropriately. It will also look at particular groups of people such as children, or those in prison, who have special needs in relation to their mental disorder. The training needs of primary care staff, and issues specific to mental health, such as use of the Mental Health Act are also discussed.

Delivering Mental Health in Primary Care is not an academic treatise of the latest research on mental health in primary care. The Royal College of Psychiatrists has commissioned such a book from eminent professors of general practice. It is written, mostly, by practising general practitioners and primary care clinicians, to provide practical, up-to-date information on how to best manage a group of patients with complex needs. The book is intended to be easy to read, with practical examples of how care can be provided in the primary care setting. It will also meet the educational needs of the new specialty training curriculum recently published by the RCGP.

This book provides an overview of the development of mental health policy, as well as describing how some of the changes in primary care, such as the 2004 General Medical Services (GMS) contract and Practice-Based Commissioning, can have an impact on mental health services.

The last five years or so have seen a number of important changes in primary care mental health, which are described in detail in the various chapters of the book. It is worthwhile summarising several of these, as together they describe the way that primary care mental health services have changed recently, and perhaps provides a view of the direction in which services are likely to develop.

The Layard proposal

In 2004, at a policy seminar for the Prime Minister, Lord Layard presented information about the relationship between mental illness and unemployment. Whilst there has been much written since then, some of the 'headlines' are worth repeating:

- there are now more people on incapacity benefit due to mental health problems (850,000) than the total numbers of unemployed people on Jobseeker's Allowance

- 90 per cent of those who are on incapacity benefit with a mental health problem are not known to specialist mental health teams, and do not suffer from a severe and enduring mental health problem

- the corollary is that this group of people are managed entirely in primary care

- effective interventions exist for the management of these people (see below – NICE guidelines), but access to services such as cognitive behavioural therapy (CBT) is poor and uneven throughout the UK.

Lord Layard proposed the development of teams of clinicians that would sit between standard primary care services and specialist mental health services, to provide care to this group of people. This intermediate care team would be staffed predominantly with experienced psychologists, the funding for which would be generated by savings made in unemployment benefits, reduced supported housing costs, and improved physical health. A Department of Health programme – Improving Access to Psychological Therapies (IAPT) – has two pilots (in Doncaster and Newham, London), which are being rigorously evaluated to test this proposal. This national programme demonstrates the central importance that primary care plays in managing people with common mental health problems, that effective interventions exist but are not universally available, and that improved management will have cost benefits to the economy as a whole.

NICE guidelines

In December 2004 the National Institute for Health and Clinical Excellence (NICE) published guidelines for the management of depression and for anxiety. NICE guidelines review the currently available evidence and, based on that evidence, publish recommendations for practice. The guidelines included both primary and specialist mental healthcare services, and described a 'stepped-care approach' to the management of depression. The depression guidelines in particular recommended different interventions dependent on the severity of the disorder, and recommended that medication was not usually advisable for people with mild depression. The stepped-care approach and all the consequences of that approach – of assessment of severity, a graded response that did not necessarily include medication – allowed GPs to develop a structured approach to this common condition, where previously there had been none. The guideline 'released' GPs from the bind that they had previously been in – having identified that a person suffered from depression, the only intervention available was medication. It was not surprising that the approach to common mental health conditions in primary care was difficult, when the only intervention offered to virtually all patients was something probably inappropriate, and not what most people wanted. To add to the difficulty, it was the mental health professionals, nurses, managers and psychiatrists who were telling primary care staff that they should manage people with common mental health problems differently by referring, for example, for CBT. Yet access to CBT and other psychological services were blocked, as specialist mental health services prioritised people with severe mental illness. Now with the NICE guidelines recommending a structured approach, it was reasonable for primary care clinicians to expect these other services to be made available by the commissioners of healthcare services – the Primary Care Trusts (PCTs).

Practice-Based Commissioning

The abolition of GP Fund Holding in 1999/2000 and the subsequent introduction of Practice–Based Commissioning (PBC) in 2004/5 are part of the continuing reform of the NHS. The introduction of PBC provides the opportunity for GPs to commission services that are needed by their local population. For example, since CBT has a strong evidence base, is recommended by NICE guidelines, and is what many patients want (rather than medication), it is not unreasonable to consider whether or not CBT may be commissioned in the future through a PBC route.

GMS contract

The 2004 GMS contract was part of a wider system reform within the NHS. The contract itself was 'ground breaking' in a number of different ways, but not least in the development of a Quality and Outcomes Framework – the holy grail of GP contract negotiations. For the first time it had been possible to agree a number of evidence-based, process or outcome statements of good practice that could be used to generate incentives for primary care practices. These statements were grouped into clinical domains such as diabetes or ischaemic heart disease. Whilst the 2004 contract had, what most agreed, an ill-considered, single domain on people with a severe mental illness, the 2006 review corrected some of the errors and included a new domain on depression. The new domain for depression took the evidence and recommendations provided by the NICE guidelines and converted them into indicators. Taken together, the NICE guidelines and the GMS contract have provided the most powerful implementation of research findings into daily practice ever seen.

Primary care mental health is stronger now than it has ever been. The changes described above are contributing towards a real change in the way that people with mental health problems can be managed in primary care – how primary care can support not only their mental health needs but also their physical health needs, and contribute to supporting their social care needs. Supporting all these areas allows an individual to become a fully participating member of society – for that can be one definition of a healthy individual. A healthy individual is an individual who is not just 'not ill' but positively well – physically well, mentally well and socially well.

Consider depression:

- according to the WHO, depression is going to be the second most common long-term condition in the world by 2020
- the GMS contract makes the link between mental health and physical health in depression
- the NICE guidelines for depression provide the recommendations and the supporting evidence to indicate the most effective therapeutic interventions
- PBC provides a route to deliver these new interventions
- The IAPT programme makes the link between mental illness and unemployment and housing.

Individually each of these elements is important – together they form a set of interventions that will improve the health of the population and make people healthier. That has to be a good reason to read this book!

1 | The new GMS contract and mental health

Alan Cohen

What this chapter contributes:

a review of where mental health fits in the General Medical Services (GMS) contract

advice on completing the mental health elements of the Quality and Outcomes
   Framework (QOF) Enhanced Services for Depression.

In April 2004 a new contract was introduced for general practitioners and primary
care practices.[1,2] It is known as the nGMS contract and is quite different from previous
contracts between the independent providers of GMS and the Department of Health. It
differs in a number of important ways.

First, the contract is with a practice providing GMS, and not an individual general
practitioner. This allows providers other than individual GPs to be commissioned to
provide a service. Other providers can include private for-profit organisations, voluntary-sector organisations, other trusts, and even the primary care organisation (PCO)
itself. All these variations and opportunities are designed so that there is a wider range
of services made available to the population – encouraging choice, and hence driving
up quality. There is also the added benefit that a Primary Care Trust (PCT) can commission a bespoke service to meet the needs of a particular group of people for whom
'usual' GMS is not sufficient or appropriate. Examples of these groups of people may be
refugees, a prison population, or homeless and roofless people.

Second, the nGMS contract is different because it is able to define what is considered to
be essential services – the level of care to be provided by all general practitioners – and
it has an incentive scheme for the delivery of evidence-based, high-quality, essential
care, called the Quality and Outcomes Framework (QOF). Since the contract is able to
describe what is considered to be an essential service, it is therefore also able to
describe what might be considered 'extra' to essential services, either as an additional
service or as an enhanced service.

Essential services to be provided by all practices have been defined as:

- management of patients who are ill or believe themselves to be ill, with conditions from which recovery is generally expected, for the duration of that condition, including relevant health promotion advice and referral as appropriate, reflecting patient choice wherever practicable

- general management of patients who are terminally ill

- management of chronic disease in the manner determined by the practice, in discussion with the patient.

Additional services are those that cover:

- cervical screening

- contraceptive services

- vaccinations and immunisations

- child health surveillance

- maternity services – excluding intrapartum care (which will be an enhanced service)[3]

- minor surgery procedures of curettage, cautery, cryocautery of warts and verrucae, and other skin lesions.

The QOF provides an incentive scheme to deliver high-quality, evidence-based, essential care. The basis underlying the incentive scheme is that points are achieved by the practice for delivering high-quality clinical care or high-quality administration and organisation within the practice.

A total of 1050 points are available, of which 550 are related to clinical areas, and 500 are related to the administration and organisation of the practice. Each point has a value, and this rises year on year as a consequence of negotiation between the British Medical Association (BMA) and the Department of Health. When the contract was first introduced in 2004, there were ten clinical indicators, one of which was described as 'mental health'. The distribution of the points to these ten areas is shown in Table 1.1.

The negotiators, in setting out the contract, made clear that the QOF would over time need to be reviewed, to take into account changing priorities, and to acknowledge emerging evidence in the way that particular conditions were managed. The negotiators should be congratulated for their perspicacity in recognising the need for constant review of this aspect of the contract.

When the contract was first published there was inevitably criticism about aspects of the contract, and there was considerable criticism from the mental health community that 'mental health' services were not featured prominently – the number of points

Table 1.1: Distribution of points to the ten clinical indicators

Clinical domain	Points awarded
Coronary heart disease	121
Stroke and transient ischaemic attack	31
Cancer	12
Diabetes	99
Hypertension	105
Hypothyroidism	8
Mental health	41
Asthma	72
COPD	45
Epilepsy	16
Clinical maximum	550

allocated to mental health did not reflect the workload associated with these conditions, nor the importance that mental health played in people's lives.

The review undertaken by the negotiators in 2005 enabled some changes to be made to the QOF that reflected some of the concerns identified above. The review[2] introduced significant change to the current mental health domain, and also introduced new domains for depression, dementia and learning disability.

Mental health domain

Table 1.2 shows how the mental health domain had changed from 2004 to 2006.

Overview

The major changes to the mental health domain are a greater specificity in who should be included and who should not, a reduction in the emphasis on lithium, new indicators that encourage the application of a care plan, and the planned follow-up of people who might otherwise have defaulted from care.

Registers

An interesting change in the 2006 indicator (MH8) from the 2004 indicator (MH1) is the omission of the phrase 'agreed to regular follow-up'. This phrase always seemed a little odd and inconsistent both with other parts of the QOF and more widely with current policy.

- Other long-term conditions domains, such as diabetes or hypertension, did not give people the choice of whether or not they wished to be placed on a register. If

Table 1.2: Changes to the mental health domain, 2004 to 2006

Pts	Domain 2004	Pts	Domain 2006
Indicator			
MH1 7	The practice can produce a register of people with severe long-term mental health problems who require and have agreed to regular follow-up	MH8 4	The practice can produce a register of people with schizophrenia, bipolar disorder and other psychoses
Ongoing care			
MH2 23	The percentage of patients with severe long-term mental health problems with a review recorded in the preceding 15 months. This review includes a check on the accuracy of prescribed medication, a review of physical health and a review of coordination arrangements with secondary care	MH9 23	The percentage of patients with schizophrenia, bipolar affective disorder and other psychoses with a review recorded in the preceding 15 months. In the review there should be evidence that the patient has been offered routine health promotion and prevention advice appropriate to his or her age, gender and health status
MH3 3	The percentage of patients on lithium therapy with a record of lithium levels checked within the previous six months		
MH4 3	The percentage of patients on lithium therapy with a record of serum creatinine and TSH in the preceding 15 months	MH4 1	The percentage of patients on lithium therapy with a record of serum creatinine and TSH in the preceding 15 months
MH5 5	The percentage of patients on lithium therapy with a record of lithium levels in the therapeutic range within the previous six months	MH5 2	The percentage of patients on lithium therapy with a record of lithium levels in the therapeutic range within the previous six months
		MH6 6	The percentage of patients on the register who have a comprehensive care plan documented in the records agreed between individuals, their family and/or carers as appropriate
		MH7 3	The percentage of patients with schizophrenia, bipolar affective disorder and other psychoses who do not attend the practice for their annual review who are identified and followed up by the practice team within 14 days of non-attendance

informed choice is appropriate and 'good practice' then it should apply to all conditions and not just mental health problems.

* What happens to people who wished not to be placed on a register? Would they be offered the same standard of care as that offered to those who did elect to be on it?

* If mental health services are to be 'mainstreamed' – the phrase used to indicate that mental health services are managed in the same way that all other services are, so that stigma and discrimination are reduced – then it flies in the face of current policy for people with long-term mental health problems to be treated differently.

* It is in the nature of severe mental illness for people to be paranoid; thus an individual refusing to allow his or her name to be entered onto a register may reflect the severity of the disorder, and not a rational, informed choice. Perversely, allowing people this choice in mental health may result in those in most need of active follow-up and care to be the least likely to receive it.

That the negotiators were able to acknowledge that the phrase 'agreed to follow-up' was inappropriate and inconsistent is warmly welcomed.

Indicator MH8

As the guidance from the NHS Employers makes clear, the changes to this indicator specify which diagnoses are to be included in the register. The intention is that people with schizophrenia and bipolar affective disorder are to be included, as well as the much smaller number with an as yet unspecified form of psychosis. People with chronic depression, personality disorder, etc. are excluded, as are children (unless they have one of the above conditions), and older people with dementia (for which there is a separate domain). Software houses will deliver the appropriate search engines to ensure that registers are created, providing the correct diagnoses are entered clinically.

The Read codes to use for the register are either 9H8 or 9H6. Code 9H7 designates that the individual has been excluded from the register. These codes are unchanged from the 2004 QOF.

Indicator MH9

There is increasing evidence that the physical health of people with a severe mental illness is poor. There have been a number of recent publications in this area, but the most recent and most detailed is the outcome of the Disability Rights Commission Formal Inquiry. This document summarises evidence from around the world, and has many references. In the following section, all the statistics about mortality and morbidity are taken from this report. The interested reader who requires further details of specific references is directed to the report. The details can be found at www.equalityhumanrights.com/en/publications andresources/Pages/legacypublications.aspx#Closing%20the%20gap%20-%20the%20DRC's %20formal%20investigation%20into%20health%20inequalities.[4]

It is appropriate to review annually the physical health of people on the mental health register. The type of review that needs to be undertaken is dependent on the personal circumstances of the individual, but consideration should be given to the following interventions:

1. *Cardiovascular disease.* The standardised mortality rate (SMR) for cardiovascular disease in people with schizophrenia and bipolar disorder is 400. Although figures vary, between 65–90 per cent of people with schizophrenia and 30–45 per cent of people with bipolar disorder smoke. Atypical antipsychotic medication, such as risperidone and olanzapine, cause prolongation of the QT interval, and as such arrhythmias may be more common. All of these facts indicate that screening for cardiovascular disease is appropriate, such as checking blood pressure, pulse and cholesterol levels.

2. *Chronic obstructive pulmonary disease (COPD).* The SMR for respiratory disease in people with schizophrenia and bipolar disorder is 400. Although figures vary, between 65 per cent and 90 per cent of people with schizophrenia smoke, and 30–45 per cent of people with bipolar disorder smoke. Advice on smoking cessation is appropriate, as well as an assessment of the presence of COPD, by checking peak flow rates, and where appropriate assessing reversibility of any airway narrowing.

3. *Diabetes and glucose intolerance.* Diabetes is five times as common in people with schizophrenia and bipolar disorder as those without. There are a number of causes of this, one of which is the use of newer atypical antipsychotic medication. However, the first reports of the association between diabetes and schizophrenia were published in the 1920s, before even chlorpromazine was introduced. It is appropriate to screen for diabetes, using either fasting blood glucose or urine analysis, and to record annually the BMI.

4. *Other health promotion advice.* Cervical screening does not occur as frequently in this group as others, although there is no increase in mortality from cervical cancer. Dietary advice may be appropriate, as well as other specific 'illness prevention' advice. In some groups of people who suffer from schizophrenia and bipolar disorder, and who have had a particularly chaotic early phase of their illness, the prevalence of HIV and hepatitis C may be very high. Figures from the USA record rates of 20 times as high of hepatitis C, and 10 times as high of HIV, although the studies have not yet been repeated in the UK. Therefore depending on personal circumstances it may be appropriate to consider counselling and testing for these conditions.

5. *Drug and alcohol use.* The use of street drugs and/or alcohol is common in the early chaotic phases of the disorders. Around 70 per cent of all acute admissions to mental health beds in London are due to the combined use of street drugs and/or alcohol, with the existing diagnosis of schizophrenia or bipolar disorder. Assessment of the use of drugs and alcohol as part of the annual review is appropriate.

All the interventions that have been undertaken should be recorded in the patient's electronic record, using the standard code for these interventions. The interventions can often be undertaken by a practice nurse, or other suitably qualified professional.

The date of the annual review should be recorded, even though this is done automatically by the practice software. The codes to be used for the annual review are:

6A6 ...
8BM0.

Indicators MH4 and MH5

There are no major changes to the rationale or recording related to these indicators. Relatively few patients are taking lithium, but for those who are it is important that there is clarity as to:

1. who is prescribing the medication

2. who is responsible for monitoring the medication

3. how frequently the patient is required to have appropriate blood tests that monitor renal and thyroid function.

Indicator MH6

Up to 50 per cent of patients with a severe mental illness, including those on the MH register (MH8), are managed entirely in primary care. People with schizophrenia and bipolar disorders have complex disorders that affect not only their mental health, but also their physical health (see MH9) and their social functioning, including employment and accommodation opportunities. A care plan provides the opportunity to review what the needs of the patient may be, and who is best able to provide that care. The GP in this case acts not as the person who is going to provide all the interventions him or herself, but as the person who will coordinate the care that is needed. The Care Programme Approach (CPA) for those people who are in contact with specialist mental health services sets out the same principles, and can be used by the practice as evidence of a comprehensive care plan.

For those people who are not in contact with specialist mental health services, there are two alternatives. Either, with the agreement of the patient, they should be referred to specialist mental health services, where a CPA will be generated. Alternatively, a practice-based 'Patient-Centred Audit' (PCA) should be developed, which addresses the needs of the individual and who should deliver those needs. The principles of either CPA or PCA are exactly the same: an assessment of need, an agreement as to who can fulfil that need, and a review date (to complete the audit cycle). CPA or PCA documents need the agreement of the patient (and/or his or her carer when appropriate) and should cover the following areas:

- physical health needs
  - see above

- social care needs
  - accommodation
  - employment/meaningful occupation

- psychological needs
  - talking therapies
  - medication including adherence to drug regimes

- identifying relapse
  - what are the 'early warning signs'?
  - what is the patient's wishes in case of relapse (medication, need for sectioning, etc.).

CPA documentation always includes the name and contact details of the key worker – who is the first point of contact for patients who are in the care of specialist mental health teams. For individuals who elect to remain under the care of their GP, and with whom a PCA plan is agreed, the equivalence of the key worker is the GP. It should be made clear that this does not mean that the GP is the key worker, or has the training to become a key worker, or is taking on the responsibility of a key worker. It means that the GP and the practice is the first point of contact for that patient as and when necessary.

Care plans need to be reviewed at least annually, when both the physical health needs and broader psychological and social needs can be assessed.

The codes used to describe the presence of a care plan (CPA or PCA) are:

8CR7
8CM2.

Indicator MH7

The practice will need to develop a system to:

1. identify people on the mental health register – MH8

2. invite them for at least an annual review – MH9

3. record the date of that appointment

4. record that the patient did not attend

5. record that the patient was followed up in some way.

The code to use for non attendance for the annual review is 9N4t.

Follow-up can be undertaken by any member of the practice team; follow-up can be either a telephone call or a visit, depending on circumstances.

The number of non-attendances is, in itself, not a 'QOF scoring' indicator; the points are earned by the follow-up within 14 days of the non-attendance. Thus, the experience with other clinical areas is that 'did-not-attend' (DNA) rates are significantly reduced if patients are sent reminders before the appointment that they need to attend. Some practices have become very experienced and innovative in doing this, e.g. they have started using text messages to mobile phones to remind people to attend appointments. Such a system may be very effective for people in this target group.

Depression

This is a new domain and has two indicators, which are shown on Table 1.3.

Table 1.3: Diagnosis and initial management	
Indicator	**Points**
DEP1 The percentage of patients on the diabetes register and/or the CHD register for whom case finding for depression has been undertaken on one occasion during the previous 15 months using two standard screening questions	8
DEP2 In those patients with a new diagnosis of depression, recorded between the preceding 1 April to 31 March, the percentage of patients who have had an assessment of severity at the outset of treatment using an assessment tool validated for use in primary care	25

DEP1

Background

This indicator for depression is derived from the NICE guidance[5] that recommends case finding for people at increased risk of depression. Although other groups apart from those suffering from diabetes and ischaemic heart disease are also at increased risk of depression, the evidence is strongest in these two disease areas, and they also represent the most accessible database/register from which the target population can be identified.

Some practices will decide that this should not preclude other target populations being identified and these too being searched for people who are likely to suffer from depression.

The anticipation is that practices will already be reviewing people with diabetes and ischaemic heart disease, as part of the relevant clinical domains. Therefore there should not be a need to call individuals specifically for this part of the depression domain, but that it should be undertaken as part of the routine health care provided to these groups.

The two standard questions referred into the indicator are together called the PHQ-2, and they are a screening tool for depression. They do not 100 per cent guarantee that an individual scoring positively on the PHQ-2 will definitely have depression – just that it is very likely.

Process

As part of the preparation for starting to use this questionnaire, there should be an agreement within the practice on the following issues:

1. Who should administer the questionnaire? Most practices use their practice nurses or nurse practitioners to manage the routine care associated with people with diabetes and ischaemic heart disease. It is therefore appropriate that it is these nurses who administer the questionnaire.

2. Those who administer the PHQ-2 should know what to do with people who score positively or negatively.

    a. An appropriate response for a POSITIVE SCREEN would be to refer the individual to the GP, for a fuller assessment. Some practices may choose to refer for a fuller assessment to the practice counsellor, or in-house mental health professional, if there is one. Whatever process is agreed, the referral should be recorded appropriately, and an explanation provided to the individual.

    b. An appropriate response for a NEGATIVE/NORMAL SCREEN would be to have recorded the screening questionnaire (see below), and the outcome.

3. There should be an agreement on which Read codes are used to record the appropriate data.

The code for recording the administration of the PHQ-2 is 6896.

4. The two questions that make up the PHQ-2 are shown on Table 1.4.

Table 1.4: PHQ-2				
Over the last 2 weeks, *how often have you been bothered by the following problems? (Use '✔' to indicate your answer)*	Not at all	Several days	More than half the days	Nearly every day
1. Little interest or pleasure in doing things	0	1	2	3
2. Feeling down, depressed or hopeless	0	1	2	3

The score of 3 or above represents a positive screen, and the individual should be referred for a fuller assessment, as agreed above.

DEP2

Background

This indicator is derived from the NICE guidelines for depression,[5] which recommend a stepped-care approach to its management. Further information on the management of depression is provided in Chapters 6 and 20. The stepped-care approach is shown in Figure 1.1.

Figure 1.1: The stepped-care approach

Who is responsible for care?		What do they do?
Acute wards	Risk to life	Medication, inpatient care
Mental health specialists	Treatment resistance and frequent recurrences	Medication, complex psychological interventions
PCMHW, GP, GPwSI, counsellor, social worker, psychologist	Moderate or severe disorders	Medication, brief psychological interventions, support groups
GP, practice nurse, practice counsellor	Mild disorders	Active review: self-help, computerised CBT, exercise
Primary care team	Recognition	Watchful waiting, assessment

Source: adapted from NICE (2004).[5]

The significance of this stepped-care approach is that different management strategies are appropriate for different severities of depression. For example, it is usually not appropriate to use medication for somebody with mild depression.

The different levels of severity of depression described in the stepped-care model relate to the clinical criteria for diagnosis described in the *International Classification of Diagnosis*, tenth revision (ICD-10). It recognises three levels of depression severity: mild, moderate and severe depression.

Hence any questionnaire that is used to assess severity should categorise the severity into one of those three levels, so that there is a clear link between severity of depression and the management plan agreed with the patient.

Three questionnaires have been approved by the negotiators of the contract as appropriate to use to assess the severity of the depression. It should be made clear that the QOF indicator is encouraging the use of questionnaires to assess the *severity* of the depression. The *clinical diagnosis* of depression lies with the clinical acumen of the clinician.

Whilst the QOF indicator is an incentive to use the questionnaire at the beginning of treatment, the questionnaires have also been validated for use as a monitoring tool, and the questionnaires may be repeated to assess the progress of the patient.

The three questionnaires approved by the negotiators for use in this indicator are the Beck II, HADS and PHQ-9. Further details on these questionnaires are found in Chapter 5.

Process

The indicator presupposes that a diagnosis of depression has been made. This diagnosis can be made by a GP, mental health professional working in the practice, or another suitably qualified professional.

The questionnaire to assess severity can be administered either in the waiting room or during the consultation.

The consultation should record that one of the three questionnaires had been administered.

The codes for administering each questionnaire are shown on Table 1.5.

Table 1.5: Questionnaires and Read codes

Questionnaire	Read code
PHQ-9	388f
Beck II	388g
HADS	388P

The outcome of the questionnaire should be recorded as to the severity of the depression. It is recommended that the Eu[X] codes are used, because these map directly to the ICD-10 diagnostic categories, shown on Table 1.6.

Table 1.6: ICD-10 diagnostic categories and Read codes

Diagnostic severity of depression	Read code
Mild depression	Eu[X]32.0
Moderate depression	Eu[X]32.1
Severe depression	Eu[X]32.2

The indicator does *not* assess whether or not an appropriate/NICE guideline intervention has been offered.

The indicator does not apply to people with other conditions such as generalised anxiety disorder or panic disorder, but does apply to the less clearly defined condition 'mixed anxiety and depression'.

What does a practice need to do?

For DEP1:

- identify who normally manages people with diabetes or CHD

- ensure that the practice has a plan so that the professional who administers the screening questions knows what to do with people who have either a positive or negative result

- ensure that at each annual check for people with these conditions, the PHQ-2 is administered

- ensure that the clinical record is annotated appropriately with the code 6896

- record the outcome of the screening question

- where appropriate refer those with a positive screening result to the GP or a mental health professional for further assessment.

For DEP2:

In preparation:

- the practice needs to agree which questionnaire to use:
  – PHQ-9
  – Beck II
  – HADS.

For each patient for whom a diagnosis of depression has been made:

- administer one of three questionnaires that assess severity of depression

- record the administration of that questionnaire with 388f (PHQ-9), 388g (Beck II) or 388P (HADS)

- record the outcome of that questionnaire in terms of severity of depression:
  – mild depression – Eu[X]32.0
  – moderate depression – Eu[X]32.1
  – severe depression – Eu[X]32.2.

Enhanced services

Background

The contract also acknowledged that some services provided by some GPs are 'above and beyond' that provided by most primary care services. These enhanced services were defined in the 2004 contract as:

- essential or additional services delivered to a higher specified standard, for example extended minor surgery

- services not provided through essential or additional services. These might include more specialised services undertaken by GPs or nurses with special interests and allied health professionals, and other services at the primary–secondary care interface. They may also include services addressing specific local health needs or requirements, and innovative services that are being piloted and evaluated.

Enhanced services are to be commissioned by primary care organisations, and three types of enhanced services are described:

1. under national direction with national specifications and benchmark pricing that all PCTs must commission to cover their relevant population – a Directly Enhanced Service (DES)

2. with national minimum specifications and benchmark pricing, but not directed – a National Enhanced Service (NES)

3. developed locally – a Locally Enhanced Service (LES).

In the 2004 contract an NES specification was proposed for depression. This NES pre-dated the NICE guidelines for depression, and was based on the 1994 Defeat Depression campaign. This service was felt by many to be outdated, unhelpful and expensive to implement. There were few places in the UK that implemented the NES.

Implementation was further complicated by the debate as to when a service was considered 'essential' and when it became an 'enhanced' service. Some GPs made the point that they were already providing, as part of essential services, the care that was described in the NES. Not surprisingly, they wished to be paid for what was now considered to be an enhanced service. This debate could have been very destructive, but following the publication of the NICE guidelines it became much clearer as to what constituted an enhanced level of care. It also became clearer that it was possible to develop an amended enhanced service for depression that met local needs, by a PCT creating a locally specific LES. This also allowed a PCT to price the new service at a level that fitted the local financial environment, which for many PCTs was difficult.

The NICE guidelines described a stepped-care approach to the management of depression. This is covered in more detail in the chapter on depression (Chapter 6), and is mentioned above, when discussing the depression clinical domain in the QOF.

The National Institute for Mental Health in England (NIMHE) has produced a very detailed paper on the implications of the stepped-care model, which is useful to consult.[5] The Sainsbury Centre for Mental Health has also produced a workbook, called *The Neglected Majority*,[3] which describes setting up and developing an intermediate care team that fits the concept of an enhanced service.

Where does an enhanced level of care fit? Both papers take the view that the two bottom tiers of the stepped-care programme (illustrated in Figure 1.1) describe the essential services in managing depression. They both also take the view that the responsibility of specialist mental health services is to provide care for the much smaller number of people represented in the top two layers. It is the middle layer, which provides care for people with moderate or severe depression, that constitutes an enhanced level of care. The second indicator in the clinical domain for depression incentivises GPs to assess rigorously the severity of the depression, because the interventions are different. As a consequence of this severity assessment, it becomes clear why the organisation of who provides the different levels of care is so important. The bottom two tiers are provided by primary care essential services, the third tier provides the enhanced level of care, and the top two tiers are provided by specialist mental health services.

Whilst the above is a rational and logical approach to implementing a structured approach to the management of depression, by using different elements of the nGMS contract it remains a fact that few PCTs have actually implemented the intermediate level of care. There are a number of reasons for this:

1. depression management is not a priority for developmental resources – it does not figure as a national 'must do', i.e. the type of priority that receives national monitoring or that makes the headlines in the national press

2. the availability of appropriately trained psychologists and other professionals to deliver the cognitive behavioural therapy that forms a significant part of the intermediate or enhanced care is lacking. There are not enough trained professionals to deliver the service, so that, even if it was commissioned by a PCT, there would not be an easy way to deliver the service.

Since there are neither the professionals nor the central priority to deliver the CBT, it is not surprising to find that few PCTs have commissioned such a service. Indeed in Ipswich, where an the intermediate care team was pioneered, and which formed the basis of the work in *The Neglected Majority*,[3] the service was decommissioned following curtailment of costs.

What are the features of an enhanced service? The underlying principles of an enhanced service for depression, or other common mental health problem, are based on the concept of the benefits of a multidisciplinary team approach. This team approach delivers 'whole person' care, for people who have complex problems that cover physical, mental and social areas of functioning. The characteristics of the team are that it includes a medical specialist (psychiatrist and/or general practitioner with a special interest [GPwSI]) and a mental health professional who actively follows up the patient (who is called in some studies a case manager), as well as expertise and support from a variety of other health and social care agencies such as employment, social care, education and housing. Other members of the team include social workers, occupational therapists, primary care mental health workers, graduate workers, counsellors, counselling psychologists, psychologists, community psychiatric nurses, etc. The membership of the team varies from area to area, and depends on what facilities, and resources, are available locally. The importance is that each team acknowledges that it cannot 'just' manage the mental health component but needs to acknowledge the broader social impact of common and enduring mental illness, and that each team has a case manager that actively follows up individual patients.

Von Korff and Goldberg[6] reviewed how services for people with depression could be improved. The BMJ editorial made a plea for an 'enhanced' level of care, although the term was used here in its routine use – rather than its specific nGMS terminology – since it predated the GP contract by three years. The editorial went on to summarise the characteristics of successful programmes of enhanced care for depression and notes that such a programme should have the following elements:

- responsibility for active follow-up is taken by a case manager

- adherence to treatment and patient outcomes are monitored

- treatment plans are adjusted when patients do not improve

- the case manager and the primary care physician are able to consult and refer to a psychiatrist when necessary.

Since the primary care physician, the case manager and the specialist mental health professionals collaborate closely to deliver care, this is called a 'collaborative' care model. It is confusing because there is a quite separate programme of service improvement led by the National Primary Care Development Team that utilises a collaborative methodology to develop small measurable changes to service delivery. The distinction is important!

Using these principles it is possible to design a service specification for an enhanced service for depression, or other common and enduring mental health problem, that can be applied locally, using local resources, whilst still retaining the essential features of a successful service.

1. Service outline

Who is the service for? The service is available for those patients who have a moderate or severe depression, or other common mental health condition.

Criterion 1

Those who have had a mental health disorder for six months or longer, and for whom the GP has offered at least one available intervention in line with NICE guidelines.

or

Criterion 2

Those who have had a mental health disorder for at least three months, and for whom the GP has offered at least one available intervention in line with NICE guidelines and whose employment or accommodation is at risk because of their mental health disorder.

or

Criterion 3

Those who have had a mental health disorder for at least three months, and for whom the GP has offered at least one available intervention in line with NICE guidelines and whose physical health is at risk because of their mental health disorder.

These criteria are the minimum reasons for access to this service; it may be that if a patient who has been unwell longer than six months (for example in criterion 1) is improving, then a referral will not be necessary. Equally, there will be clinical situations where an earlier referral may be appropriate, and these guidelines should not be used as a rule that inhibits normal good clinical practice.

2. Assessment of need

The provider can demonstrate that he or she has undertaken an assessment of the patient, so that a formulation describing the patient's physical, social and mental needs is illustrated clearly. These needs are described in a Patient-Centred Audit (PCA).

A PCA is a document that provides a structured approach to the management of a patient with depression. The information that should be recorded in the PCA is:

- diagnosis

- relevant past history including if the patient has had a depressive illness previously, and the outcome of that episode

- any co-morbid conditions

- the presence of any alcohol or drug misuse

- severity of the mental health disorder, and on what basis the severity has been assessed; the QOF depression indicators, as part of essential care, form the basis of this part of the specification

- risk assessment, including an assessment of the suicidality of the patient

- treatment interventions agreed with the patient

- referrals made – see above

- frequency of reassessment

- investigations made

- at each consultation an assessment of the progress of the patient, using validated tools such as PHQ-9, HADS or Beck II questionnaires.

These data can be leached from current electronic records by using software templates for each of the existing programmes in primary care use. The intention is to be able to provide a structured approach to care, such that no significant areas of care are omitted, care can be audited, and proactive follow-up offered.

> Scrutiny: the provider can offer for examination a randomly selected example of PCAs. The commissioning body may examine these PCAs, and relate them to interventions offered and any outcome audits undertaken by the provider.

3. Provision of care

Apply a multidisciplinary approach for people with depression that cannot be managed with confidence in primary care (middle tier – see Figure 1.1).

The management of moderate depression requires the use of several interventions, which together are more effective than each intervention on its own – 'the whole is greater than the sum of the parts'. The multidisciplinary approach to managing depression should therefore include access to the following specialists:

- health professionals:
  - doctor, either a GPwSI or psychiatrist
  - psychologist
  - counsellor/talking therapist (either funded by the practice, PCT or voluntary sector)
  - graduate mental health worker (if funded by the PCT)

- social care professionals
  - social worker
  - benefits adviser/citizens advice bureau (CAB)
  - housing adviser
  - employment adviser, such as Jobcentre Plus
  - substance misuse worker.

The provider should be able to access at least three professionals from each of the categories, so that there is a multidisciplinary team providing care for these patients. The provider will be expected to demonstrate how the team will work, by demonstrating shared goals of treatment, shared records, and audit/evaluation of the team's activities.

The provider will also be expected to demonstrate which professional takes on the role of case manager, and how active follow-up is implemented.

> Scrutiny: the provider can demonstrate that it functions as an effective multidisciplinary team.

4. Undertake appropriate training

It is appropriate that those members of the provider team responsible for caring for people with depression, or other common mental health problems, are sufficiently trained to undertake the enhanced level of care. However, there does not yet exist a core curriculum with national validation of the skills required to deliver such a service. The primary care programme of NIMHE is currently undertaking such a development, but until it is complete it is advised that each of the professionals involved should provide an annual update on learning regarding their involvement in the LES. It is also appropriate that all clerical and reception staff receive training on the nature and presentation of common mental health problems, to be delivered by the clinical staff. Records of such training should be kept, and repeated at least at annual intervals.

> Scrutiny: each clinician can demonstrate attendance at approved training courses, and can demonstrate that the clerical and reception staff have received training on the nature and presentation of common mental health problems, as part of their personal development plan (PDP).

5. Make referrals and inquiries as clinically indicated

As part of the work of the multidisciplinary process of care, patients will need to be referred to a variety of professionals. Full records will need to be kept of referrals, which will include:

- routine epidemiological data
- the reason for referral
- a review of the clinical history
- a review of medication prescribed (if any) for this episode of illness
- medication that has been successful in the past when used for depression
- other regular medication and known sensitivities
- information on the social and family background of the patient.

> Scrutiny: the practice will be able to provide an analysis of referrals, demonstrating that full records are being kept.

6. Feedback from the users of the service

The primary care programme of NIMHE has developed a questionnaire to fit this need. Alternatively, each practice can use its own system for assessing patient feedback on the service provided.

> Scrutiny: the practice will demonstrate that it has undertaken a survey of patients included in the enhanced care programme, and that changes in service have been discussed with either the PCT or a Non-Executive Director (NED) at the PCT, and where appropriate changes implemented.

7. Review and audit

The practice will undertake review and audit of the care being provided. Issues that may be addressed include the effectiveness of treatment (what proportion of patients improve and become symptom free), any particular local needs, e.g. asylum seekers, or an analysis of antidepressant medication prescribing. The number of audits should be increased after 12 months, to two per year.

> Scrutiny: the practice can provide one audit annually of the care provided to people included in the enhanced care programme.

References

1. Department of Health. *Investing in General Practice: the new General Medical Services contract* London: BMA and NHS Confederation, 2004.

2. British Medical Association. *Revisions to the GMS Contract, 2006/07: delivering investment in general practice* London: BMA and NHS Employers, 2006.

3. Hague J and Cohen A. *The Neglected Majority* London: The Sainsbury Centre for Mental Health, 2005.

4. Disability Rights Commission. *Bridging the Gap*, 2006, www.equalityhumanrights.com/en/publicationsandresources/Pages/legacypublications.aspx#Closing%20the%20gap%20-%20the%20DRC's%20formal %20investigation%20into%20health%20inequalities [accessed November 2007].

5. National Institute for Mental Health in England. *Improving Primary Care Mental Health Services* Leeds: NIMHE, 2006.

6. Von Korff M and Goldberg D. Improving outcomes in depression *British Medical Journal* 2001; **323**: 948–9.

Further reading

Court C. Report urges better psychological care *British Medical Journal* 1995; **310**: 1027.

Department of Health. *The New NHS* London: DoH, 1998.

Department of Health. *The NHS Plan* London: DoH, 1999.

Department of Health. *Guidance on Commissioning Arrangements for Specialised Services* London: DoH, 2003.

Department of Health. *The NHS Improvement Plan* London: DoH, 2004.

Ford C. *The Somatizing Disorders: illness as a way of life* New York: Elsevier, 1983.

DSM-IV. *Diagnostic and statistical manual of mental disorders* (4th edn), pp. 445–69 and 844–9 Washington: American Psychiatric Press, 1994.

2 | Practice-Based Commissioning

Alan Cohen

What this chapter contributes:

a context for Practice-Based Commissioning (PBC), against the changes that are
occurring in the NHS

some of the opportunities that PBC can provide to the commissioning of services
for people with mental health problems.

The Labour Party, following its election victory in 1997, implemented major changes in
the NHS. These changes included the development of Primary Care Groups, which
later became Primary Care Trusts (PCTs), and the abolition of Fund Holding – a
scheme that gave general medical practices actual budgets to commission services on
behalf of their patients. However, in 1998, the same year that Fund Holding was abol-
ished, the government made clear in *The New NHS*[1] its desire to see practices offered
indicative budgets to commission a full range of services. *The NHS Improvement Plan*[2]
stated that practices would be able to have an indicative budget from April 2005 to
commission, if they wished, a full range of services. The guidance published in October
2004[3] gave details of what the scheme will allow practices and PCTs to do.

There have been other major changes to the NHS since 1997, but they have all been
directed at providing a high-quality service whilst giving the users of the service a
choice as to what is appropriate for their own needs. One of the major stumbling
blocks to introducing choice was in fact lessons learnt from the GP Fund Holding
scheme. Different providers could provide the same service for different costs; thus a
hip replacement or a cataract operation in London might cost more than the same
operation in the North West. As a result a patient would be referred to where the service
was cheapest, or where the contract was placed, rather than being offered a choice of
which provider had, for example, the shortest waiting list, or was most convenient for
the patient. Information as to the outcome of that surgery, or other aspects of the
process or outcome of the service, was unavailable. The consequence was that patients

had no choice, and that services were variable throughout the country – the so-called 'post code' healthcare service. Users of the service had no way of knowing the quality of the service delivered, nor a choice of where to go for that service.

These problems have been addressed by the government in the period from 1998 (the abolition of Fund Holding) through to 2004 with the introduction of Practice-Based Commissioning (PBC). They have been addressed by ensuring: first, the quality of the service; second, that cost was not an issue in choice; and, third, that the information was available so that an informed choice could be made.

Quality

Quality of care was assured through the introduction of National Service Frameworks (NSFs) to ensure that services were of a uniform high standard. The National Institute for Health and Clinical Evidence (NICE) published guidance on managing clinical conditions, based on the latest research, as well as describing when new interventions should be made available to the NHS. The Commission for Health Improvement (CHI) visited provider and commissioning trusts to ensure that the frameworks and clinical guidelines were being adhered to, so that a feedback cycle was established: NSFs and NICE set the quality agenda, trusts implemented those national clinical policies, and the implementation was reviewed by CHI, later to become the Health Care Commission.

Cost

Cost of the service was addressed more recently by the introduction of a scheme called Payment by Results. This is a system whereby a procedure or spell of treatment has a national tariff or cost. This tariff or cost is applied equally throughout the country so that a dermatology outpatient spell of care will cost £240 in London and in the North West. The intention is that cost should not figure in the process of the users of the service choosing where or what service they feel to be most appropriate for their own circumstances.

Information

Accurate information is required to support this major redesign of the underlying principles of the NHS. The government has invested heavily in a national information technology system called *NPfIT* – The National Programme for Information Technology (later to become *Connecting for Health)* – that will deliver the systems, and hence the information, to allow these developments to be implemented successfully. As part of the process of providing better information, not only to the commissioning clinician but also to the public as well, the Choose-and-Book system has been introduced to allow patients real-time opportunities to select the outpatient appointment location and time of their choice

This, then, is the background to the development of PBC – it has not been introduced as a whim, but as part of a continuing long-term strategy to give users of the NHS the ability to choose where and how they access a high-quality, up-to-date service anywhere in the country.

Practice-Based Commissioning and Mental Health Services

The guidance on Practice-Based Commissioning makes clear that all services can be commissioned by a practice except those services identified in *Guidance on Commissioning Arrangements for Specialised Services*.[4] This guidance lists services that should be commissioned by consortia of PCTs, as they are highly complex and low volume, and are frequently high-cost services. They are usually termed 'tertiary services', as patients are referred for these specialist services by secondary care clinicians.

For mental health the list of services is:

- tertiary eating disorder services

- neuropsychiatry

- forensic mental health services

- specialised mental health services for deaf people

- specialised addiction services

- specialist psychological therapies for inpatients and specialist outpatient services

- gender identity services

- perinatal psychiatry services (mother and baby units)

- complex and/or treatment-resistant services

- Asperger's syndrome.

All other services are considered to be secondary care services and are capable of being commissioned by practices with their indicative budgets. This will include community mental health teams, psychological therapies, other talking therapies, and the more specialised community teams such as assertive outreach and early-onset teams.

The implementation of choice is dependent on a consistent high-quality service, that cost is not an issue, and that the user has the information to make an informed choice.

Quality

The first published NSF[5] was in mental health, and it has without doubt gone a long way to improving the quality of the service, and ensuring a consistently high level of care. This chapter is not the place to assess whether or not these aspirations have been successfully implemented, and since the 10-year plan of the NSF is only halfway through such an assessment might be considered premature. NICE[6] has published a number of documents on mental health, such as guidelines on the management of schizophrenia, depression and anxiety, and CHI (and its successors) has reviewed all mental health trusts and PCTs. Certainly the government has gone a long way to ensuring that there is a consistently high level of care in mental health services. There will always be the opportunity, and desire, to improve the service, but without doubt there has been progress over the last five years.

Payment by Results

The same cannot be said of the second principle – that of ensuring that cost is not an issue in patient choice. Payment by Results sets a national tariff for spells of care. When that spell of care is clearly defined by diagnosis, need, duration and intervention, allocating a cost is (relatively) straightforward. There can be an agreement between different trusts that they are comparing like with like. A person needing a hip replacement in London is likely to be very similar in diagnosis, need, duration and intervention required to a person in Dorset. However, the introduction of Payment by Results in April 2005 excludes mental health services because it has not yet been possible to allocate national tariffs to care provided by mental health trusts.

Creating a national tariff for mental health care is the subject of a national Department of Health working group, which is having some success in what is a very difficult area. Some of the difficulties encountered when developing a tariff for mental health include:[7]

- mental health service users have diverse needs; the course of illness even for the same initial diagnosis is often very variable

- patients frequently have other, coexisting conditions that may complicate treatment and add to costs independently of their mental health diagnosis

- mental health problems are often long term and episodic or intermittent

- services are frequently supplied by more than one agency, creating complex 'care pathways'

- professionals often make quite different decisions about which treatments or interventions are most effective for which patients

- care is often provided in different settings

- informal care is very important; for many service users the costs of support by the statutory services may be determined as much by the availability of family and social support as by the diagnosis and severity of their illness.

The principles behind a national tariff are not unique to the UK – other countries in the world use similar ideas to fund their health care. Unfortunately the USA, New Zealand and Australia have all failed to develop an activity-based, funding-based-on-case-mix system for mental healthcare providers. There is not a single place in the world that has such a fully implemented system in place – which certainly makes the UK plans aspirational!

Games to play

There are some interesting lessons to be learnt from other countries, and other specialities, that can be applied to mental health services and commissioning by national tariff.[7]

Skimming

If there is one price for one intervention, it is in the interest of the provider to take the 'easy to treat' patients in any therapeutic group – and leave the more severe for others to manage. They are effectively 'skimming the cream', which can, especially in mental health, leave the most vulnerable at risk. Similar arguments apply to most chronic conditions, and attempts are being made to develop a tariff for 'a year of care' as a way of managing this particular behaviour.

Quicker and sicker

If there is one price for an intervention, there are incentives to either reduce quality (as it costs more) or to reduce duration of stay (as it costs more). The changes to the Mental Health Act, with the introduction of Supervised Community Treatment, raise the fear that providers may elect for supervised community treatment, not because it is in the patient's best interest, but because it reduces costs for beleaguered mental health trusts.

Creep

In this case, there may be two tariffs for different severities of a condition – e.g. depression. It is in the provider's interest for patients with a milder disorder to be categorised to a more severe diagnostic group; because the costs associated are higher, the patient can be treated more cheaply, and discharged more quickly.

Cost spiralling

It is in the interest of the provider to increase activity within a tariff, so that, for example, waiting lists are reduced, or that expertise and skills are increased. The danger is that this increase in activity is unmonitored and uncontrolled so that expenditure from the purchaser's perspective is endangered. The Hammersmith Hospital in West London provided a perfect example of this in the year 2004/5, where it was able to reduce its waiting list very dramatically through service redesign processes. The consequence was that capacity went up, but resources from the commissioning PCTs were unable to keep pace with the activity, so the hospital was 'rewarded' by having to close wards.

The fact that Payment by Results in the UK has not set a national tariff for mental health spells of care – and judging by international experience will find this difficult to do – means that practices will find it extremely difficult to commission mental health services. The situation as proposed is no different from the Fund Holding scheme of the 1990s, when practices could commission some mental health services, and the result was a shift in emphasis away from those with a severe and enduring mental illness, towards providing talking therapies for those with a common mental health problem.

This shift was seen by many in the mental health field as a retrograde step that fragmented the service, and set up a multi-tiered service. There is nothing in the current guidance that will not prevent this happening again. Indeed it could be worse, because in the Fund Holding era practices could not commission services from the Community Mental Health Teams (CMHTs), but only invest in talking therapies. With the current guidance on PBC there is the opportunity to commission all secondary care from a mental health trust. This could significantly fragment services, and put an untenable strain on primary/secondary care relationships.

Information technology

Finally the information infrastructure to support PBC of mental health services is not in place. Despite the enormous resources being invested in NPfIT, and then Connecting for Health, the programme for mental health trusts is lagging well behind acute trusts. The information that is required to both commission services from a practice, and to be able to offer users of the service a meaningful choice, is not in place.

Commissioning mental health services

The foregoing describes some of the difficulties that may be encountered when commissioning specialist mental health services through PBC. However, there are other opportunities that exist to commission a mental health service that would provide some real benefits for both patients and for primary care services.

The chapter on common mental health disorders describes, amongst other conditions, people with somatisation disorder. The reader is directed to Chapter 6 for more details.

Psychiatrists and psychologists have developed a number of ways of describing and defining different aspects of people who present to their doctor with medically unexplained symptoms. Some of the definitions used are described below:

Definitions

Somatisation: the tendency to experience, conceptualise and communicate mental states and distress as physical symptoms or altered bodily function.

Somatoform disorder

This is the presence of physical symptoms that suggest but which are not fully explained by a general medical condition, the direct effects of drugs or a mental disorder. The symptoms must cause clinically significant distress, or impairment in social, occupational or other areas of functioning. In contrast to factitious disorders and malingering, the physical symptoms are not intentional.

Somatisation disorder

This is a rare and extreme version of somatoform disorder where the patient over many years seeks medical attention for many physical symptoms with no evidence of organ pathology. The diagnosis of the disorder requires the presence of 14 of 37 potential symptoms for women and 12 for men (see Table 2.1 on p. 37).

Somatisation syndrome

This is a partial version of somatoform disorder, in which the patient has fewer symptoms (four for men, six for women).

Hypochondriasis

This is a preoccupation with fears of having, or the idea that one has, a serious disease. The preoccupation must last at least six months, persist despite appropriate medical evaluation and reassurance, and cause clinically significant distress or impairment in social, occupational or other important areas of functioning.

Factitious disorder

This is the intentional production of false or grossly exaggerated symptoms for reasons that are not obvious. It is presumed that there is a psychic need to assume the sick role and to receive care. Patients often present their history with flair or gross exaggeration (pseudologia fantastica) and receive multiple hospitalisations (Munchausen's syndrome). When there are external incentives for the behaviour (e.g. financial gain) malingering should be diagnosed.

Neurasthenia

This is 'tired nerves' or 'nervous exhaustion', now defined as complaints of increased fatigue after mental effort, or bodily weakness after minimal physical effort, combined with unpleasant physical symptoms (dizziness, headaches), worry, irritability and sleep disturbance. The modern neurasthenic will more likely be diagnosed with chronic fatigue syndrome, depression or anxiety.

Sick role

When disease occurs in a previously well individual, that person is granted certain privileges (exemption from work and other responsibilities, and the offer of care by family and significant others), but at the same time is expected to accede to certain obligations (to seek appropriate help and to accept the treatment offered in order to get well as soon as possible). Some people seek the privileges of the sick role without accepting the obligations; whether this is malingering or chronic somatisation disorder depends on the degree of conscious, voluntary control the person has over his or her illness behaviour.

Illness behaviour

This is the way an individual in the 'sick role' perceives, evaluates and acts upon symptoms. There is considerable variation in this behaviour. One person may be stoical, another dramatic. One may communicate distress verbally, another physically.

Abnormal illness behaviour

This is inappropriate or maladaptive attempts to be granted the benefits of the sick role without meeting the necessary obligations.

In DSM-IV,[8] the diagnosis of somatisation requires complaints of at least 14 symptoms (for women) and 12 symptoms (for men) from the 37 listed in Table 2.1.

However, in general practice it is frequently difficult to use (and recognise) these very specific distinctions. Singh, an Australian professor of psychiatry in Melbourne, described three groups of people who have some form of somatic symptoms:[9]

1. high level of functional symptoms (= somatisation syndrome)

2. hypochondriasis or 'illness worry'

3. somatic manifestation of anxiety and depression.

Table 2.1: Symptoms in the diagnosis of somatisation

Abdominal pain	Painful menstruation
Joint pain	Pain in extremities
Back pain	Pain in genital area
Chest pain	Pain on urination
Nausea	Other pain (not headaches)
Vomiting spells	Severe vomiting throughout pregnancy or causing hospitalisation during pregnancy
Bloating ('gassy')	Shortness of breath
Difficulty swallowing	Trouble walking
Diarrhoea	Dizziness
Intolerance of a variety of foods	Urinary retention or difficulty urinating
Deafness	Loss of consciousness or fainting
Muscle weakness	Sexual indifference
Loss of voice	Paralysis
Blindness	Double vision
Blurred vision	Memory loss
Palpitations	Belief that he or she has been sickly
Seizures or convulsions	Pain during intercourse
Menstrual irregularity for a good part of life	Excessive menstrual bleeding
Lack of pleasure during intercourse	

Singh also makes the point that each group can occur acutely, intermittently or chronically, and that somatisation may coexist with other long-term conditions.

Wessley, in a lecture at the Royal Society of Medicine in 1999, said 'As in so much of psychiatry, and depression as well, this is an area where psychiatrists make up classifications for patients that we rarely see. Patients are seen by neurologists, cardiologists, and GPs, and it is not really for us to say how they should be classified.' Wessley eloquently makes the point that the complex mixture of physical and psychological symptoms (and frequently social problems as well) are best dealt with by a generalist physician.

How many patients?

Given that there are different degrees of severity, and different ways of describing the disorders associated with somatic symptoms, it is not surprising that there is little consistent information about the frequency with which clinicians encounter the problem.

The most recent study of the prevalence of somatoform disorders in primary care was undertaken by Margot de Waal and colleagues.[10] They used DSM-IV criteria (see p. 36) for diagnosis of somatoform disorder for people attending eight general practices in the Netherlands between 2000 and 2001. The authors found an estimated prevalence of 16.1 per cent in a Dutch population consulting their general practitioner. The prevalence of anxiety disorders was 5.5 per cent and the prevalence of depression was 4.1 per cent in the same population.

Kirmayer and Robbins[11] estimated that 25 per cent of people attending their GP had symptoms of somatoform disorder. Since both depression and anxiety have physical symptoms as part of the clinical syndrome, these figures are close to those described by de Waal *et al.*[10]

Whilst few GPs would disagree that many of the people attending the surgery have somatic symptoms, their subsequent management is frequently difficult. Many individuals are referred on to specialist acute services for further investigation of their physical symptoms.

A paper by Nimnuan *et al.*[12] assessed 500 sequential patients attending a number of acute outpatient clinics at King's College in London.

Table 2.2: Referrals to specialist services

Clinic	Prevalence
Chest	59%
Cardiology	56%
Gastroenterology	60%
Rheumatology	58%
Neurology	55%
Gynaecology	57%

This does not imply that the referrals were in any way 'inappropriate', but that it is difficult to separate out which symptoms have a true physical basis, and which may be related to psychological distress. It may also be the case that access to the investigations needed to exclude a physical cause for a symptom is only possible by referral to an acute trust.

The increasing trend towards the practice of defensive medicine, and to refer a patient if he or she asks for a second opinion, also explains in part the large proportion of referrals for which no physical cause is found.

Identifying people with somatoform disorders – screening questionnaires

Wessley (see p. 37) made the point that psychologists and psychiatrists are good at classifying disorders. A number of different psychiatrists and psychologists have evolved questionnaires that attempt to identify those with somatoform disorder, based on the way that the same psychiatrists have classified the disorder.

The questionnaires are usually designed as research tools, but some have been developed with the requirement that they work in primary care. However, whilst a questionnaire might be validated and tested for use in primary care, it may be an entirely different matter that the questionnaire is used on a regular basis by a general practitioner or practice nurse. Experience suggests that GPs, and less so practice nurses, are unwilling to use questionnaires regularly. The PHQ-2 recommended as part of the depression QOF may be the first questionnaire to be used widely in primary care mental health.

There are some questionnaires that may be of value in screening for somatoform disorder.

The Patient Health Questionnaire (PHQ) is designed to identify people in general practice who may have any of the common mental health conditions encountered in primary care. As such it has different elements, designed to elicit the characteristic criteria that make up the ICD-10 diagnosis. Thus PHQ-9 is designed to diagnose people with depression, and the GAD-7 is designed to diagnose people with generalised anxiety disorders. The PHQ-15 is designed to diagnose the presence of somatoform disorders, and as the name suggests is a 15-item self-complete questionnaire. Thirteen items relate to concerns about physical health and two questions relate to mood.[13]

Other questionnaires include the Very Short Health Anxiety Inventory, developed by Salkovskis, the Health Attitude Survey developed by Noyes *et al.*, a screening index commissioned by Schwartz and colleagues, the Othmer and DeSouza test, the SPHERE questionnaire from Australia, and the 7- or 14-item Whitely scale. There is no shortage of valid questionnaires.[14–19]

Identifying people with somatoform disorders – other techniques

It may be possible to use other techniques to increase the accuracy of diagnosis of people with somatoform disorder.

Improved information technology means that it is possible to identify people who have been admitted or referred to an acute trust. It is also possible to identify those who have been referred or admitted more than once in a set period, usually 12 months. This set of data – those who have been admitted more than twice in 12 months – is usually called the 'frequent flyers', and there has been recent interest in the characteristics of this group, as they are extensive consumers of NHS resources.

Using the same principles it is possible to identify those who have been referred more than once in a 12-month period to an acute outpatient clinic. As with the frequent flyers, the list of people referred more than once will reveal that there are a decreasing number of individuals who are referred more and more frequently. Starting with the very small number of people who have been referred the most, analysis of the notes will indicate if a cause was found for their symptoms. By working through the list eventually all those referred more than twice can be scrutinised, and those for whom no cause found can be identified. It is this group that should be offered a screening questionnaire to assess the presence of somatoform disorder.

Identifying people with somatoform disorders – a general practice perspective

The following is a quote from a North East London GP, who has considered practical ways of identifying people with somatoform disorder. The basis for the criteria for identification is principally pharmacological, but, like so many other areas of the country, there is little opportunity for other interventions.

As a general practitioner, I have always had a particular interest in mental health problems manifesting themselves as medically unexplained symptoms. Over my seven years as a principal in general practice, I have become somewhat frustrated by my inability to help patients with strange symptom sets that have defied treatment, investigation and ultimately any definitive resolution.

In the course of a typical consulting day I expect to see at least two to three patients presenting with medically unexplained symptoms. This makes me feel confused, disempowered and rather helpless. I have tended, in the past, to 'tactically' resolve these consultations by collusion which, in practical terms, means offering another referral, review of treatment or investigation. 'Biting the bullet' and being candid about how I feel with the patient has borne fruit but usually ends up with recrimination, denial and rejection by the latter.

Recent changes in my own career have, however, led me to realise that this is a problem which must be tackled. Through my work as clinical mental health lead for my Primary Care Trust, I have realised, through numerous discussions with peers and colleagues, that my experience of the needs and challenges of this group of patients is very common. In my role as case-reviewer, I have also undertaken tasks usually delegated to others – notes summarisation for either the nGMS GP contract or in preparation for Deanery training accreditation. Looking through these notes I picked up several key characteristics which helped me to 'profile' those with medically unexplained symptoms. I also realised that these patients had often experienced a fairly prodigious 'career' through secondary care, with no resolution or improvement in symptoms – there is an appreciable financial imperative for Primary Care Trusts to manage somatisation disorder effectively.

To estimate the true volume of the client group in my own practice, I devised a calculation based on this experience, which can be used in other practices.

Identifying the 'prescribing profile'

The basis of the technique is similar to one that was used locally (and probably commonly elsewhere) to generate the Seriously Mentally Ill Registers for nGMS – it is based on identifying repeat prescribing. I looked at which categories of drugs tended to appear, and identified the following features in those with medically unexplained symptoms:

1. Antidepressant medication had been prescribed by a variety of practitioners spanning primary and secondary care, to almost every one of these patients. Some of this was a genuine attempt to broach and pay homage to the subject of underlying mental health problems. Most, however, and I am as guilty of this as anybody, were presented to the patient as a panacea for their symptoms with no mention of their mental health as a factor.

2. Most patients had also been prescribed at least one symptomatic treatment. These included 'painkillers' – largely non-steroidal anti-inflammatory drugs (NSAIDs, or aspirin-like drugs used for pain and inflammation), opiates (codeine- or morphine-like drugs) or combination preparations, usually a combination of paracetamol with an opiate (e.g. co-proxamol), in isolation or mixed with each other. Hypnotics (sleeping tablets), especially benzodiazepines, were very common. Finally, many drugs for abdominal discomfort (largely antispasmodics such as mebeverine and hyoscine butyl bromide, but also drugs for sickness or nausea such as prochlorperazine) were also present.

Gathering the data and the calculation

The aim of producing this 'prescribing profile' is to use it to produce a workable list of patients – a quasi-disease register. The practice computer software can be used to identify the number of patients who fulfil these criteria. The following is a step-by-step guide to creating this list. Slightly more advanced, but still fairly easy, is generating a list of names. In essence:

1. identify those patients with repeat prescriptions for antidepressant medication

2. from this group, identify those with active or recent repeats of EITHER

    a. hypnotics (sleeping tablets)

    b. symptomatic GI treatments (drugs for abdominal discomfort)

    c. analgesics (painkillers) (NSAIDs or opiates or combinations)

3. identify which of these patients is receiving palliative care for a terminal illness and delete them from the list

4. multiply the final number (i.e. the number of patients on antidepressants, minus the number not on symptomatic medications, minus the number on palliative care) by £955[20] to estimate the cost of these patients' care to a practice.

The general practice approach to identification is remarkably pragmatic when compared with the very structured approach undertaken by psychiatrists. In part this is a recognition of the different settings in which the identification is being undertaken – one is predominantly a research assessment, and the other a North London practice.

Managing people with somatoform disorder

The literature is reasonably clear that cognitive behavioural therapy (CBT) is effective for people with somatoform disorder. Probably the best review is provided by Raine *et al.*[21] However, the lack of availability of CBT in primary care is a particular problem, and, unless this can be rectified, there is little reason to try and identify this group if there is no access to an effective intervention.

Where the unexplained physical symptoms are a part of depression or anxiety, then those conditions should be treated as recommended in the appropriate NICE guidelines.

A difficulty remains that, for many GPs who are faced with referring a patient to an acute outpatient clinic, the idea that they should, instead of dictating a referral letter, ask the patient to complete a questionnaire, and then offer them a course of CBT for which he or she will have to wait between six and 12 months, is frankly ludicrous.

What is possible, and seems to be acceptable and practical practice, is to use the IT systems in place within the practice to identify those who have been referred more than twice in 12 months, and who have had no cause found for their symptoms. This provides a practice list or register (similar to many other electronic registers in primary care) of people at risk.

The notes are flagged (electronically or otherwise) so that when a further referral is being considered, as part of the process of assessment, a screening tool is used to determine the presence of somatoform disorder. Those few individuals who have been referred several times, who have had no cause found for their symptoms, and who have scored positively on a validated screening questionnaire, are offered two interventions:

- referral to an experienced therapist who can discuss with them what they feel about their symptoms, what they think their symptoms represent, what they think might be happening to their body, etc. For those for whom it is appropriate, the individuals are either offered a CBT course of treatment appropriate to managing their somatic symptoms, or CBT tailored to an underlying depressive or anxiety disorder.

- the GP undertakes to see patients on a regular basis to monitor the progress of their physical symptoms. This provides reassurance that the physical symptoms are being taken seriously, and allows referral to an acute outpatient clinic if the symptom complex changes.

A study has been commissioned from the University of Nottingham to develop a commissioning tool for early identification of people with medically unexplained symptoms. The study is due to be completed in March 2008.

Long-term conditions

People with long-term conditions have similar problems – they rarely have 'just' a long-term condition, but also are more likely to suffer from depression and or anxiety. There is substantial evidence (see references used to support the QOF Depression Indicator 1) that depression is more common in people with diabetes, and that in those individuals the diabetes is less well controlled, the use of health resources is greater, and the outcomes worse, than people with diabetes who are not depressed. Evidence (see the references used to support the QOF Depression Indicator 1) that people with ischaemic heart disease who are depressed also have poorer outcomes, and use healthcare resources more than people who are not depressed with ischaemic heart disease, is also well established. Indeed it was this body of evidence that supported the introduction of the first indicator in the depression clinical domain of the QOF.

There is a good case to make that, by providing effective treatment for people with co-morbid mental health conditions as well as a long-term condition, health service utilisation can be reduced, and outcomes improved.

Resourcing the extra service

Whilst the management plan described above is a rational and practical approach for people with somatoform disorder, there remains an underlying problem – the lack of resources to employ professionals who are trained to deliver CBT, and an absolute lack of numbers of professionals who are qualified to deliver CBT.

The Labour Party manifesto in 2005 stated:

> Almost a third of people attending GP surgeries have mental health problems and mental health occupies approximately one third of a GP's time. So we will continue to invest in and improve our services for people with mental health problems at primary and secondary levels, including behavioural as well as drug therapies.

This political commitment has been translated into Department of Health policy to deliver a large increase in the number of professionals who can provide this behavioural therapy. Estimates of the numbers that are going to be trained vary between 7000–10,000 new professionals, but the clear intention is that providing a large number of new professionals is a priority, and providing them within a reasonable time scale is equally important.

So far as providing care for people with somatoform disorder is concerned, it is important that there will be increasing availability of the necessary professionals to deliver the appropriate talking therapy.

Whilst the extra new staff will be awaited with enthusiasm, it should not be forgotten that there are individuals with the appropriate skills who are not currently employed within the NHS. It is not clear exactly how many such trained professionals exist in the country, and if their skills are up to date, but as a potential resource using private psychologists or other professionals should not be ignored.

Practice-Based Commissioning provides a route for this service to be redesigned and resourced from primary care. The economic impact of somatoform disorder has been estimated by a number of authors over the years, in both the USA and the UK. US studies have estimated the costs at around $1000–$2000, and the most recent UK figure was £1000.[20] The UK studies estimated the costs prior to the introduction of Practice-Based Commissioning and the development of the national tariff. Using these more recent innovations in commissioning, it is possible to make a much more sensitive economic assessment of the costs of providing alternative services for people with somatoform disorder.

In October 2007 the Secretary of State for Health announced funding for the Improving Access to Psychological Therapies programme for three years – £30m in year 1, £100m in year 2, and £170m in year 3, starting in April 2008. This specific new resource is intended to treat 900,000 people, and to train and appoint 3600 new therapists. It is hoped that a second three-year programme will be put in place in 2011, to complete the programme of allowing all who need therapy to receive it, within a time scale that is appropriate to their needs.

An example

The costs of a full-time professional able to deliver CBT safely is about £40,000 (including on-costs).

Such an individual, working for 46 weeks a year, five days per week, and providing four clinical sessions each day (allowing the remaining time in the day for other professional activities), would provide a course of ten sessions of CBT to just under 100 people.

Using pre-national tariff figures, the potential savings in avoided referrals to acute trusts would be around £100,000.

Other benefits would be reduced waiting times at acute trusts. There are also potential savings in reduction of GP prescribing of psychotropic medication, and analgesic medication, although there is little evidence at present to know the quantum of that saving.

Identifying the resource

One of the lessons from Fund Holding was the divisive nature of the argument that meant the allocation for 'mental health' was either for counselling and therapy in primary care, or used to commission a service for people with severe mental illness. It became an entirely unhealthy argument of taking money from one service to fund the other – and professionals and users of the service left to debate which was 'more worthy' of funding.

Practice-Based Commissioning can be used to commission more therapists who can deliver effective interventions for people with somatisation disorder, or with long-term conditions. This service can be funded through reduced activity in the acute sector, not by withdrawing funds from mental health trusts. The acute sector wins as well because the reduced activity shortens waiting lists. There is the potential for a win–win–win situation; moreover the patient receives an evidence-based treatment that was previously not available.

Linking to other developments

The DoH priority to improve access to psychological therapies (as part of the government's manifesto commitment) is working towards the creation of new psychological treatment centres. These would have psychologists and other professionals working as part of a multidisciplinary team to deliver high-quality CBT to patients referred from primary care. The opportunity for PBC to support this development and supplement the resources, by commissioning a service for people with somatoform disorder, should not be missed. The overlap in people who have somatoform disorder and those who are being targeted by this policy initiative is great. PBC offers the real opportunity to redesign services for people who have been unable to access the most appropriate treatment in the past. We must make use of that opportunity.

References

1. Department of Health. *The New NHS* London: DH, 1998.

2. Department of Health. *The NHS Improvement Plan* London: DH, 2004.

3. Department of Health. www.dh.gov.uk/en/Publicationsandstatistics/Publications/Publications PolicyAndGuidance/DH_4127155 [accessed November 2007].

4. Department of Health. *Guidance on Commissioning Arrangements for Specialised Services* London: DH, 2003.

5. Department of Health. *National Service Framework for Mental Health* London: DH, 1999

6. www.nice.org.uk [accessed November 2007].

7. *Payment by Results: what does it mean for mental health? Policy Paper* 4 London: Sainsbury Centre for Mental Health, 2005.

8. *DSM-IV. Diagnostic and statistical manual of mental disorders* (fourth edn) Washington: American Psychiatric Press, 1994, pp. 445–69 and 844–9.

9. Singh B. Managing somatoform disorders *Medical Journal of Australia* 1998; **168(11)**: 572–7, www.mja.com.au/public/mentalhealth/articles/singh/singh.html [accessed November 2007].

10. de Waal M, Arnold IA, Eekhof JA, van Hemert AM. Somatoform disorders in general practice: prevalence, functional impairment and co-morbidity in anxiety and depressive disorders *British Journal of Psychiatry* 2004; **184**: 470–6.

11. Kirmayer LJ, Robbins LN. Three forms of somatisation in primary care *Journal of Nervous and Mental Disease* 1991; **179**: 647–55.

12. Nimnuan C, Hotopf M, Wessely S. Medically unexplained symptoms: an epidemiological study in seven specialities *Journal of Psychosomatic Research* 2001; **51(1)**: 361–7.

13. Spitzer R, Kroenke K, Williams JB. Validation and utilization of a self report version of PRIME-MD *Journal of the American Medical Association* 1999; **282**: 1737–44.

14. World Health Organization. *ICD-10 Classification of Mental and Behavioral Disorders*, p. 162, Geneva: WHO, 1992.

15. Othmer E, DeSouza C. A screening test for somatization disorder *American Journal of Psychiatry* 1985; **142(10)**: 1146–9.

16. Ellen SR, Norman TR, Burrows GD. 3. Assessment of anxiety and depression in primary care *Medical Journal of Australia* 1997; **167**: 328–33.

17. Bass C, Benjamin S. The management of chronic somatisation *British Journal of Psychiatry* 1993; **162**: 472–80.

18. King BH. Hypothesis: involvement of the serotonergic system in the clinical expression of mono symptomatic hypochondriasis *Pharmacopsychiatry* 1990; **23**: 85–9.

19. Wesner RB, Noyes R. Imipramine: an effective treatment for illness phobia *Journal of Affective Disorders* 1991; **22**: 43–8.

20. Reid S, Wesseley S, Crayford T, Hotopf M. Medically unexplained symptoms in frequent attenders of secondary health care: retrospective cohort study *British Medical Journal* 2001; **322**: 767–70.

21. Raine R, Haines A, Sensky T. Systematic review of mental health interventions for patients with common somatic complaints: can research evidence from secondary care be extrapolated to primary care? *British Medical Journal* 2002; **325**: 1082–93

Further reading

Australian Bureau of Statistics. *Mental Health and Wellbeing Profile of Adults* Canberra: ABS, 1998.

Cannon RO. The sensitive heart: a syndrome of abnormal cardiac pain perception *Journal of the American Medical Association* 1995; 273: 883–7.

Clarke D, Smith C. Disorders of somatic function or perception. In: S Bloch, BS Singh (eds). *Foundations of Clinical Psychiatry* Melbourne: Melbourne University Press, 1994.

Escobar JI. Transcultural aspects of dissociative and somatoform disorders *Psychiatric Clinics of North America* 1995; 18: 555–69.

Guthrie EG. Psychotherapy of somatization disorders *Current Opinion in Psychiatry* 1996; 9: 182–7.

Janca A, Isaac M, Bennett LA, Tacchini G. Somatoform disorders in different cultures – a mail questionnaire survey *Social Psychiatry and Psychiatric Epidemiology* 1995; 30: 44–8.

Kashner TM, Rost K, Cohen B. Enhancing the health of somatisation disorder patients *Psychosomatics* 1995; 36: 462–70.

Kenyon FE. Hypochondriacal states *British Journal of Psychiatry* 1976; 129: 1–14.

Kirmayer LJ. Culture, affect and somatization *Transcultural Psychiatric Research Review* 1984; 21: 159–88.

Kleinman A. *Rethinking Psychiatry from Cultural Category to Personal Experience* New York: The Free Press, 1988.

Klimes I, Mayou RA, Pearce MJ. Psychological treatment for atypical non-cardiac chest pain: a controlled evaluation *Psychological Medicine* 1990; 20: 605–11.

Krishnan KRR. Monoamine oxidase inhibitors. In: A Schatzberg, CB Nemeroff (eds). *The APA Textbook of Psychopharmacology*, pp. 183–91, Washington: American Psychiatric Association, 1995.

Mezzich JE, Kleinman A, Fabrega H, Parron DL. *Culture and Psychiatric Diagnosis* Washington: American Psychiatric Association, 1996.

Pilowsky I. *Abnormal Illness Behaviour* Chichester: John Wiley & Sons, 1997.

Reid S, Wessely S, Crayford T, Hotopf M. Frequent attenders with medically unexplained symptoms: service use and costs in secondary care *British Journal of Psychiatry* 2002; 180: 248–53.

Robins LN, Reiger DA (eds). *Psychiatric Disorders in America: the epidemiologic catchment area study* New York: The Free Press, 1991.

Stimmel GL, Escobar JI. Antidepressants in chronic pain: a review of efficacy *Pharmacotherapy* 1986; 6: 262–7.

Tollefson GB. SSRIs. In: A Schatzberg, CB Nemeroff (eds). *The American Psychiatric Association Textbook of Psychopharmacology*, pp. 171–85, Washington: APA, 1995.

Ustun TB, Sartorius N. *Mental Illness in General Health Care: an international study* Chichester: John Wiley & Sons, 1995.

Wool CA, Barsky AJ. Do women somatise more than men? *Psychosomatics* 1994; 35: 445–52.

References for diabetes and ischaemic heart disease co-morbidity

Anderson CS, Linto J, Stewart-Wynne EG. A population-based assessment of the impact and burden of caregiving for long-term stroke survivors *Stroke* 1995; 26: 843–9.

Anderson RJ, Freedland KE, Clouse RE, *et al.* The prevalence of co-morbid depression in adults with diabetes: a meta-analysis *Diabetes Care* 2001; 24: 1069–78.

Audit Commission. *Forget Me Not: mental health services for older people* London: Audit Commission, 2000.

Berkman LF, Leo-Summers L, Horwitz RI. Emotional support and survival after myocardial infarction: a prospective population-based study of the elderly *Annals of Internal Medicine* 1992; **117**: 1003–9.

Bridges KW, Goldberg DP. Somatic presentation of DSM-III psychiatric disorders in primary care *Journal of Psychosomatic Research* 1985; **29**: 563–9.

Carney RM, Freedland KE. Psychological distress as a risk factor for stroke-related mortality – editorial *Stroke* 2002; **33**: 5–6.

Department of Health. *National Service Framework for Mental Health: modern standards and service models* London: DH, 1999, www.dh.gov.uk/assetRoot/04/01/45/01/04014501.pdf [accessed November 2007].

Department of Health. *The NHS Plan: a plan for investment, a plan for reform* London: DH, 2000.

Department of Health. *Practice Based Commissioning: promoting clinical engagement* London: DH, 2004.

Department of Health. *Commissioning a Patient-Led NHS: delivering the NHS improvement plan* London: DH, 2005.

Department of Health. *Our Health, Our Care, Our Say: a new direction for community services* London: DH, 2006, www.dh.gov.uk/en/Publicationsandstatistics/Publications/PublicationsPolicyAndGuidance/DH_4127453 [accessed November 2007].

Egede LE. Effects of depression on work loss and disability bed days in individuals with diabetes *Diabetes Care* 2004; **27(7)**: 1751–3.

Egede LE, Zheng D, Simpson K. Co-morbid depression is associated with increased health care use and expenditures in individuals with diabetes *Diabetes Care* 2002; **25**: 464–70.

Frasure-Smith N, Lespérance F, Gravel G, *et al*. Social support, depression and mortality during the first year after myocardial infarction *Circulation* 2000; **101**: 1919–24.

Frasure-Smith N, Lespérance F, Talajic M. Depression and 18 month prognosis after myocardial infarction *Circulation* 1995; **91**: 999–1005.

Gask L, Lee J, Donnan S, *et al*. The impact of total purchasing and extended fundholding on mental health services: baseline aims and objectives of sites *Journal of Mental Health* 2000; **9**: 421–8.

Gibody S. What is the evidence on effectiveness of capacity building of the primary health care professional in the detection, management and outcome of depression? 2004, www.euro.who.int/HEN/Syntheses/capdepr/20041208_2 [accessed November 2007].

Goldney RD, Phillips PJ, Fisher LJ, *et al*. Diabetes, depression, and quality of life: a population study *Diabetes Care* 2004; **27(5)**: 1066–70.

Hankey GJ. Informal care giving for disabled stroke survivors: training the care giver benefits the patient, the care giver and the community *British Medical Journal* 2004; **328**: 1085–6.

Herrmann N, Black SE, Lawrence J, *et al*. The Sunnybrook Stroke Study: a prospective study of depressive symptoms and functional outcome *Stroke* 1998; **29**: 618–24.

Hippisley-Cox J, Fielding K, Pringle M. Depression as a risk factor for ischaemic heart disease in men: population based case-control study *British Medical Journal* 1998; **316**: 1714–19.

House A, Knapp P, Bamford J, *et al*. Mortality at 12 and 24 months after stroke may be associated with depressive symptoms at 1 Month *Stroke* 32: **2001**; 696–701.

Howard L, Wessely S, Leese M, *et al*. Are investigations anxiolytic or anxiogenic? A randomised controlled trial of neuro-imaging to provide reassurance in chronic daily headache *Journal of Neurology, Neurosurgery & Psychiatry* 2005; **76(11)**: 1558–64.

Kalra L, Evans A, Perez I, et *al*. Training care givers of stroke patients: randomised controlled trial *British Medical Journal* 2004; **328**: 1099–101.

Karlsson H, Lehtinen V, Joukamaa M. Psychiatric morbidity among frequent attender patients in primary care *General Hospital Psychiatry* 1995; 17: 19–25.

Katon WJ. Clinical and health services relationships between major depression, depressive symptoms, and general medical illness *Biological Psychiatry* 2003; 54(3): 216–26.

Kroenke K. Psychological medicine: integrating psychological care into general medical practice (Editorial) *British Medical Journal* 2002; 324: 1536–7.

Layard R. *Mental Health: Britain's biggest social problem*, 2004, www.cabinetoffice.gov.uk/upload/assets/www.cabinetoffice.gov.uk/strategy/mh_layard.pdf [accessed November 2007]

Layard R. *Happiness: lessons from a new science* London and New York: Penguin, 2005.

Linden W, Stossel C, Maurice J. Psychological interventions for patients with coronary heart disease: a meta-analysis *Archives of Internal Medicine* 1996; 156: 745–52.

Livingston G, Manela M, Katona C. Depression and other psychiatric morbidity in carers of elderly people living at home *British Medical Journal* 1996; 312: 153–6.

Lustman PJ, Anderson RJ, Freedland KE, *et al*. Depression and poor glycemic control: a meta-analytic review of the literature *Diabetes Care* 2000; 23(7): 934–42.

McLaughlin T, Geissler EC, Wan GJ. Co-morbidities and associated treatment charges in patients with anxiety disorders *Pharmacotherapy* 2003; 23(10): 1251–6.

May M, McCarron P, Stansfield S, *et al*. Does psychological distress predict the risk of ischemic stroke and transient ischemic attack? The Caerphilly Study *Stroke* 2002; 33: 7–12.

Morrison, V, Pollard B, Johnston M, *et al*. Anxiety and depression 3 years following stroke: demographic, clinical and psychological predictors *Journal of Psychosomatic Research* 2005; 59: 209–13.

Musselman L, Betan E, Larsen H, *et al*. Relationship of depression to Types 1 & 2: epidemiology, biology and treatment *Biological Psychiatry* 2003; 54: 317–29.

Nannetti L, Paci M, Pasquini J. Motor and functional recovery in patients with post stroke depression *Disability and Rehabilitation* 2005; 27(4): 170–5.

National Institute for Clinical Excellence. *Clinical Guideline 23, Depression: management of depression in primary and secondary care* London: NICE, 2004, www.nice.org.uk/CG023NICEguideline [accessed November 2007].

National Institute for Mental Health in England (NIMHE) Northwest Development Centre. *Primary Care PCGMHWs: a practical guide*, 2003, www.northwest.csip.org.uk/work/service-and-workforce-improvement/primary-care.html [accessed November 2007].

Nemeroff CB, Mussleman DL. Are platelets the link between depression and ischaemic heart disease? *American Heart Journal 2000*; **140(Suppl. 4)**: 57–62.

NIMH. *Depression and Stroke* National Institutes of Health, US Department of Health and Human Services NIH Publication No. 02-5006, 2002, http://health.nih.gov/result.asp/183/16 [accessed November 2007].

Nolan M, Grant G, Keady J. *Understanding Family Care* Buckingham: Open University Press, 1996.

Office of National Statistics. *Psychiatric Morbidity among Adults Living in Private Households 2000* London: ONS, 2001.

Office of National Statistics, Social Survey Division. *Living in Britain: results from the 1995 General Household Survey* London: ONS, 1997.

Öhlin B, Nilsson PM, Nilsson J-Å, *et al*. Chronic psychological stress predicts long-term cardiovascular morbidity and mortality in middle-aged men *European Heart Journal* 2004; 25: 867–73.

Ormel J, Von Korff M. Synchrony of change in depression and disability *Archives of General Psychiatry* 2000; 57: 381–2.

Oyebode J. Assessment of carers' psychological needs *Advances in Psychiatric Treatment* 2003; 9: 45–53.

Parikh RM, Robinson RG, Lipsey JR, *et al*. The impact of post-stroke depression on recovery in activities of daily living over a 2 year follow-up *Archives of Neurology* 1990; 47: 785–9.

Park H, Hong Y, Lee H, et al. Individuals with type 2 diabetes and depressive symptoms exhibited lower adherence with self-care *Journal of Clinical Epidemiology* 2004; 57(9): 978–84.

Paschalides C, Wearden AJ, Dunkerley R, *et al*. The associations of anxiety, depression and personal illness representations with glycaemic control and health-related quality of life in patients with type 2 diabetes mellitus *Journal of Psychosomatic Research* 2004; 57(6): 557–64.

Pettigrew M, Bell R, Hunter D. Influence of psychological coping on survival and recurrence in people with cancer: a systematic review *British Medical Journal* 2002; 325: 1066–75.

Portegijs PJ, van de Horst FG, Proot IM, *et al*. Somatisation in frequent attenders of general practice *Social Psychiatry & Psychiatric Epidemiology* 1996; 31(1): 29–37.

Raine R, Haines A, Sensky T, *et al*. Systematic review of mental health interventions for patients with common somatic symptoms: can research evidence from secondary care be extrapolated to primary care? *British Medical Journal* 2002; 325: 1082–92.

Rosengren A, Hawken S, Ounpuu S, *et al*. INTERHEART investigators. Association of psychosocial risk factors with risk of acute myocardial infarction in 11119 cases and 13648 controls from 52 countries (the INTERHEART study) *Lancet* 2004; 364(9438): 953–62.

Rozanski A, Blumenthal JA, Kaplan J. Impact of psychological factors on the pathogenesis of cardiovascular disease and implications for therapy *Circulation* 1999; 99: 2192–217.

The Sainsbury Centre for Mental Health. *Economic and Social Costs of Mental Illness in England*, Policy Paper 3, 2003.

Schleifer SJ, Macari-Hinson MM, Coyle DA, *et al*. The nature and course of depression following myocardial infarction *Archives of Internal Medicine* 1989; 149(8): 1–8.

Schulz R, O'Brien AT, Bookwala J, *et al*. Psychiatric and physical morbidity effects of dementia care giving: prevalence, correlates and causes *Gerontologist* 1995; 35: 771–91.

Stenager EN, Madsen C, Stenager E, *et al*. Suicide in patients with stroke: an epidemiological study *British Medical Journal* 1998; 316: 1206.

Strine TW, Beckles GL, Okoro CA, *et al*. Prevalence of CVD risk factors among adults with diabetes by mental distress status *American Journal of Health Behavior* 2004; 28(5): 464–70.

Timonen M, Laakso M, Jokelainen J, *et al*. Insulin resistance and depression: cross sectional study *British Medical Journal* 2005; 330: 17–18.

Wade DT, Legh-Smith J, Hewer RA. Depressed mood after stroke: a community study of its frequency *British Journal of Psychiatry* 1998; 151: 200–5.

Williams RB, Barefoot JC, Califf RM, *et al*. Prognostic importance of social and economic resources amohg medically treated patients with angiographically documented coronary artery disease *Journal of the American Medical Association* 1992; 267: 520–4.

3 | Mental illness prevention and mental health promotion

Hilary Guite

What this chapter contributes:

it introduces the concepts of risk and protective factors for mental health and wellbeing

based on these factors, it identifies practical tasks that the primary care team can undertake both with individuals at different life stages and with wider community structures.

Too vast and 'woolly' for primary care?

At face value preventing mental illness and promoting positive mental health in primary care may seem too vast, since it could span from prevention of birth injury to promotion of social cohesion. It may also seem woolly as the evidence base was barely developing when most of us left formal education. In the last 10 to 15 years all this has changed.

A document called *Making it Happen*[1] provided a framework for structuring an approach to mental health promotion within Primary Care Trusts that can work equally well within an individual practice. This framework consisted of three elements:

- strengthening individuals

- strengthening communities

- reducing structural barriers to good mental health.

This approach combined with an understanding of the risk and protective factors for mental health and wellbeing (see Tables 3.1 and 3.2) can help to identify some practical tasks that can be carried out by the primary care team operating with the individual patient and within wider community structures.

Table 3.1: Protective factors potentially influencing the development of mental health problems and mental disorders in individuals (particularly children)

Individual factors	Family factors	School context	Life events and situations	Community and cultural factors
Easy temperament	Supportive, caring parent	Sense of belonging	Involvement with significant other person (partner/mentor)	Sense of connectedness
Adequate nutrition	Family harmony	Positive school climate	Availability of opportunities at critical turning points or major life transitions	Attachment to and networks within the community
Attachment to family	Secure and stable family	Pro-social peer group	Economic security	Participation in church or other community groups
Above average intelligence	Small family size	Required responsibility and helpfulness	Good physical health	Strong cultural identity and ethnic pride
School achievement	More than two years between siblings	Opportunities for some success and recognition of achievement		Access to support services
Problem-solving skills	Responsibility within the family (for child or adult)	School norms against violence		Community/ cultural norms against violence
Internal locus of control	Supportive relationship with other adult (for a child or adult)			
Social competence	Strong family norms and morality			
Social skills				
Good coping style				
Optimism				
Moral beliefs				
Values				
Positive self-related cognitions				

Source: Mental Health and Special Programs Branch. *Promotion, Prevention and Early Intervention for Mental Health: a monograph* Canberra: Commonwealth Department of Health and Aged Care, 2000.[2] Copyright Commonwealth of Australia reproduced by permission.

Table 3.2: Risk factors potentially influencing the development of mental health problems and mental disorders in individuals (particularly children)

Individual factors	Family factors	School context	Life events and situations	Community and cultural factors
Prenatal brain damage	Having a teenage mother	Bullying	Physical, sexual and emotional abuse	Socioeconomic disadvantage
Prematurity	Having a single parent	Peer rejection	School transitions	Social or cultural discrimination
Birth injury	Absence of father in childhood	Poor attachment to school	Divorce and family break-up	Isolation
Low birth weight	Large family size	Inadequate behaviour management	Death of family member	Neighbourhood violence and crime
Birth complications	Antisocial role models (in childhood)	Deviant peer group	Physical illness/ impairment	Population density and housing conditions
Physical and intellectual disability	Family violence and disharmony	School failure	Unemployment, homelessness	Lack of support services including transport, shopping, recreational facilities
Poor health in infancy	Marital discord in parents		Incarceration	
Insecure attachment in infant/child	Poor supervision and monitoring of child		Poverty/economic insecurity	
Low intelligence	Low parental involvement in child's activities		Job insecurity	
Difficult temperament	Neglect in childhood		Unsatisfactory workplace relationships	
Chronic illness	Long-term parental unemployment		Workplace accident/injury	
Poor social skills	Criminality in parent		Caring for someone with an illness/disability	
Low self-esteem	Parental substance misuse		Living in nursing home or aged care hostel	
Alienation	Parental mental disorder		War or natural disasters	
Impulsivity	Harsh or inconsistent discipline style			
	Social isolation			
	Experiencing rejection			
	Lack of warmth and affection			

Source: Mental Health and Special Programs Branch. *Promotion, Prevention and Early Intervention for Mental Health: a monograph* Canberra: Commonwealth Department of Health and Aged Care, 2000.[2] Copyright Commonwealth of Australia reproduced by permission.

As for the evidence base for mental health promotion being woolly, the rapid expansion of trials in this area meant that Friedli identified over 20 systematic reviews or meta-analyses of mental health promotion interventions dating between 1994 and 2002.[3] The preface to the World Health Organization summary of the evidence base for the prevention of mental disorders in 2004 noted that, even though there had been a summary in 1998, just six years earlier, 'this scientific field has seen rapid development of ideas and research evidence, necessitating a fresh review'.[4,5]

This new evidence base has helped to clarify the meaning behind the statement 'there is no health without mental health'.[5] The links between physical and mental health are better understood, and many interventions now routinely provided in primary care, such as good antenatal care and promotion of physical exercise,[6] can also be understood as mental health promotion activities. The new evidence base also means that mental health promotion activities that complement existing interests and patterns of working for the primary care team can be given a new emphasis – such as the effective non-pharmaceutical management of insomnia or a greater involvement with local housing policy. The rest of this chapter will identify a range of interventions at individual, community and structural level that reduce risk factors and promote protective factors for good mental health that can be undertaken by members of the primary care team.

What is mental illness prevention and mental health promotion?

For the purposes of this chapter mental health promotion will encompass mental illness prevention and mental health promotion. This includes primary measures to promote positive mental health and to prevent mental illness, as well as screening for mental illness to provide treatment for early disorder or symptoms.

The effective approaches to preventing specific mental illnesses and to promoting positive mental health have been found to overlap considerably.[3,5] What is important in defining the promotion of mental health and mental wellbeing and preventing mental illness is that we concentrate on primary prevention, i.e. before significant disorder is established. Guite and Bywaters report that the current policy emphasis on widening access to psychological therapies and other aspects of social exclusion, whilst welcome, sometimes pushes primary mental health promotion off the agenda.[7]

It is of note that suicide prevention is often used as a proxy albeit narrow measure for mental health promotion. The England suicide prevention strategy identifies six goals, including secondary prevention measures such as the appropriate treatment of those with existing mental illness, and reduction of access to means.[8] Where suicide prevention overlaps with mental health promotion is in the goal to promote 'mental wellbeing to the wider population'. We therefore do not cover suicide prevention separately since the secondary prevention measures will be covered elsewhere. The social inclusion agenda for people with severe mental illness, including promoting their physical health, which is also often subsumed within mental health promotion, is dealt with in Chapter 18.

Individual level

The following section brings together action that can be taken by the primary care team to promote protective factors and reduce risk factors (see Tables 3.1 and 3.2, pp. 52 and 53) with the individual by life stage and by setting.

Pregnancy/child birth

Antenatal care

Several of the risk factors for mental health problems listed in Table 3.2 can be reduced by good antenatal care and encouraging family spacing of two years or more. The risk factors include prenatal brain damage, prematurity, birth injury, low birth weight, physical and intellectual disability.

Teenage pregnancies

Reducing the risk factor of having a teenage mother requires action within schools and the community, but also needs to be supported by good primary care including: family outreach, involving teenagers' parents in information and prevention campaigns; early pregnancy testing; quick referral to unbiased advice and counselling; speedy referral for abortion is this if what is chosen; and promoting uptake of antenatal and postnatal care.[9]

Early years and family life

Parenting support and parenting programmes

Home-based preschool support for parents and parenting programmes in classes improve mental health outcomes for children and mothers.[10,11] Parenting programmes have also been shown to reduce antisocial behaviour.[12] These programmes reduce key early risk factors for mental health problems, including family violence, disharmony and harsh discipline. Spencer found that exposure to ridicule at home was associated with antisocial behaviours, depression and post-traumatic stress disorders.[13] Exposure to corporal punishment at home was associated with 'aggression and internalizing disorders'. Early recognition of child abuse and neglect, and provision of parenting support and parenting programmes, are important elements of the work of the primary care team.

Postnatal support

The identification of women at high risk of postnatal depression and provision of intensive postnatal support has been found to reduce the onset of postnatal depression.[14] Interestingly, provision of antenatal support was not found to alter levels of postnatal depression.

Screening of mothers and their partners in the postnatal period for relationship problems can lead to a four-fold increase in identification and a six-fold increase in people being offered help.[15]

Physical health

Poor physical health in infancy can be improved by good, evidence-based, physical health care of children, especially the management of chronic conditions to reduce hospital stays for children with conditions such as asthma, diabetes or cerebral palsy.

Adults and older adults

Promoting positive mental health

There is a case for all adults and older adults to be advised to regularly check the extent to which they are following the 12 steps to positive mental health (see Box 3.1).[16] The 12 steps promote factors that protect against mental health problems and are well supported by the evidence base. A quiz is included in Appendix I for patients and practice staff to assess their current level of wellbeing.

Box 3.1: Positive steps to improve mental health and wellbeing

- Keeping physically active.
- Eating well.
- If you do drink, drinking in moderation.
- Valuing yourself and others.
- Talking about feelings.
- Keeping in touch with friends and loved ones.
- Caring for others.
- Getting involved and making a contribution.
- Learning new skills.
- Doing something creative.
- Taking a break.
- Asking for help.

Source: Care Services Improvement Partnership 2005[16] and Department of Health 2006.[17]

Seligman found that identifying three good things that went well each day and writing down their causes every night for one week resulted in higher levels of happiness and lower levels of depression at 1, 3 and 6 months.[18] Similarly, the group in this study allocated to identifying their 'signature strengths' online (www.authentichappiness.org) and working out a way to use one of these top strengths in a new and different way every day for one week also experienced increasing levels of happiness at 3 and 6 months, and lower levels of depression at 1, 3 and 6 months.

Relationships

The capacity for loving relationships was the only predictor of life satisfaction for middle-aged adults in a US study.[19] For older adults hope, citizenship and loving relationships all predicted life satisfaction.[19] The quality of interpersonal and couple relationships has been identified as a key element of happiness and satisfaction in life by others.[20,21] Provision of a Prevention and Relationship Enhancement Programme (PREP), which aimed to decrease risk factors for marital distress and increase protective factors for marital functioning (identification of danger signs, speaker–listener techniques, problem solving, identifying issues and planning events), increased positive behaviour and reduced negative behaviour at 1 year. This was particularly so for those receiving the intervention from religious organisations.[22] Even relationships that are relatively happy can be enhanced further, leading to increases in relationship satisfaction, autonomy, relatedness, closeness, acceptance of one another and reduction in relationship distress.[23]

For those with relationship problems and depression, both individual and couple therapy improves the depression, but only couple therapy improves the relationship.[24–26] There is some concern about referring couples with violence in their relationships for couple counselling, and the general advice is to refer each partner for individual counselling or to use multi-couple groups.[27]

Social prescribing

Friedli describes social prescribing as providing a framework to 'develop alternative responses to mental distress and a wider recognition of the influence of social and cultural factors on mental health outcomes across the whole spectrum of disorders'.[28] She includes specific schemes such as Exercise on Prescription, Prescription and Arts on Prescription, and a wider range of signposting and linking of patients to local resources. Positive outcomes include: reduced low mood; greater confidence; better self-esteem; increased sense of ability to achieve things; and transferable skills.[29]

Sleep

Poor sleep often develops at the time of stressful life events listed in Table 3.2 (see p. 53) and can become the primary problem. In one study only 28 per cent of people with severe insomnia described the quality of their lives as good compared with 68 per cent of those with no sleep problems.[29] Depression was found in 21–40 per cent of insomniacs compared with 0-1 per cent of those without sleep problems; anxiety disorders were present in 13–24 per cent of insomniacs compared with 3–10 per cent of non-insomniacs.[30] Simple insomnia is characterised as either difficulty falling asleep, difficulty maintaining sleep or waking too early where there are no other physical problems and snoring is not a major issue. Lasting improvement using non-drug-based treatments has been found in 70–80 per cent of people using a range of behavioural or cognitive (thought-based) techniques.[31] There is good evidence for the interventions listed in Box 3.2.[31–35]

Box 3.2. Effective interventions for simple insomnia
(see Appendix II for fuller descriptions)

Single interventions:

- stimulus control (reducing the amount of stimulus before sleep and in the bedroom (described in www.holistic-online.com)

- sleep restriction or compression

- paradoxical intention

- biofeedback.

Multi-modal interventions:

- stimulus control and sleep restriction with:
  – cognitive restructuring
  – progressive muscle relaxation
  – sleep hygiene education
  – exercise.

Isolation

There is some evidence that home visiting programmes for people at risk of isolation improve mental wellbeing.[36,37]

Physical exercise

There is good evidence that increases in physical exercise benefit mind and body.[6]

Community

Work

Primary care practitioners are well aware of the impact of community issues such as availability of employment and the practices of local employers on their population. There is good evidence that organisation-wide approaches improve wellbeing of workers.[38] Addressing work–life balance is just as important.[39] Awareness of local issues, advocacy for patients affected by their work and promotion of a work–life balance are all legitimate roles for the primary care team.

Housing

Other issues within the community, particularly to do with housing, are important for a sense of wellbeing. Halpern found that during a period when demolition of an estate was expected the ratio of consultations in affected residents compared with non-affected residents increased by 50 per cent. It fell back to pre-announcement levels after a reprieve and rose again by 50 per cent after re-confirmation of the decision to demolish the estate.[40] Guite *et al.* have identified 12 factors that predict people falling into the lowest quartile of a mental health score indicating significantly poor mental wellbeing.[41] Many of these factors will be known to the primary care team: damp; ugly buildings; neighbour noise; feeling overcrowded; poor access to green spaces, community amenities and social and entertainment facilities; being afraid to go out in the day- and night-time; needles and syringes lying around; lack of places to stop and chat, and few events to get people together. The primary care team can advocate on many of these issues on behalf of patients. The team will also be aware of new residents who may need help integrating into the local area.

Local events

The availability of local arts programmes can lead to improvements in mental wellbeing in participants.[42] Knowledge of local resources is important for all members of the primary care team.

Health-promoting schools

Health-promoting school initiatives are effective where there is a focus on mental health rather than mental illness, mental health is discussed as part of the curriculum and a problem-solving rather than a topic-based approach is taken, and the initiative is part of a change to the school ethos and is implemented over several years. Specific programmes using skills-based approaches include tackling negative body image amongst teenagers by taking a problem-solving approach to improving self-esteem[43] and reducing drug misuse based on a social competence model (self-management, problem solving, communication and resisting negative social influences).[44] Health-promoting school initiatives using a range of approaches have shown improvements in the protective factors for mental health and reduction in risk factors.[45] Members of the primary care team might be involved in delivery of some sessions within the school. They can influence the approach to ensure that they are involved in problem-solving approaches rather than topic-based approaches. If the team is aware of the messages and approaches provided by the school, for example approaches to negative body image, drug taking or bullying, these can be reinforced within the practice setting.

Policy/structural level

Some of the services and approaches mentioned here that are effective for promoting mental wellbeing are not available in many areas or are not available in sufficient numbers to be effective for the whole of the practice population. Practices could become wellbeing-promoting practices by ensuring a systematic approach to monitoring and promoting mental wellbeing by practitioners in the team, and by lobbying at a policy level on a range of issues.

Examples of action for a mental wellbeing-promoting practice

There may not be sufficient voluntary-sector provision for mental health in the local area. Organisations such as Relate (for relationship problems), Cruise (for people who are bereaved) and Mind (for people with mental health problems) provide access to support and counselling. These organisations need premises and funding. A large practice may have rooms available in the evening. There may be poor access to evidence-based counselling such as CBT, which needs to be highlighted. A wellbeing-promoting practice could comment on local planning applications to identify early issues such as noise and the need for events for new residents. Local Area Agreements are agreements between key local players to produce gains in health and wellbeing through joint working. It is important that mental wellbeing targets are identified here so that joint work to promote mental wellbeing between the local authority and NHS can be identified and supported.

Summary

Many of the examples we have given here for promoting positive mental health and preventing mental illness (summarised in Table 3.3 on p. 61) are already part of the work of primary care teams, which operate holistically. We have shown that there is evidence for the importance of activities that may be seen as peripheral to promoting good health but are in fact central to promoting wellness in individuals and their communities. With the advent of Practice-Based Commissioning it is important to emphasise the value of such activities and ensure that they continue to be provided and developed to meet the needs of the entire practice population. The adoption of a systematic approach to identifying ways to promote positive mental health at individual, community and policy levels will deliver benefits not just in improvements in mental health and wellbeing but also in overall social and physical health.

Table 3.3: Primary care mental health promotion interventions

Pregnancy and child- birth	Early years and family life	Adults and older adults	Community	Structural/ policy
Good antenatal care	Parent training and home visiting	Promote the 12 positive steps to mental health	Be an advocate for good working conditions	Become a wellbeing-promoting practice
Promote family spacing of more than two years	Recognise violence and abuse	Identify relationship enhancement skills programmes locally and promote them	Be an advocate for good local housing	Develop a systematic approach to promoting mental wellbeing by all practitioners
Support smaller family sizes	Identify women at risk of postnatal depression and provide high levels of postnatal support	Identify relationship problems and refer to couple therapy	Promote work–life balance	Adopt mental health-promoting working practices to benefit all staff groups
Practice strategy to reduce teenage pregnancy	Identify relationship problems postnatally	Use social prescribing schemes for mild depression	Identify new residents and support their integration into the local community	Lobby for resources via the primary care team and the local authority
		Identify simple insomnia and use behavioural and cognitive techniques	Be involved in local health-promoting schools initiatives	Comment on the wellbeing implications of local planning applications
			Reinforce problem-solving approaches	
		Arrange home visiting for groups at risk of isolation	Be aware of local arts and cultural programmes	Keep mental wellbeing in the Local Area Agreements and work with local counsellors

References

1. Department of Health. *Making it Happen: a guide to delivering mental health promotion.* Ref 24509. London: DH, 2001.

2. Mental Health and Special Programs Branch. *Promotion, Prevention and Early Intervention for Mental Health: a monograph* Canberra: Commonwealth Department of Health and Aged Care, 2000.

3. Friedli L. *Making it Effective: a guide to evidence based mental health promotion* London: Mentality, 2003.

4. World Health Organization. *Primary Prevention of Mental, Neurological and Psychosocial Disorders* Geneva: WHO, 1998.

5. World Health Organization. *Prevention of Mental Disorders: effective interventions and policy options.* Summary Report. A Report of the World Health Organization, Department of Mental Health and Substance Abuse in Collaboration with the Prevention Research Centre of the Universities of Nijmegen and Maastricht. Geneva: WHO, 2004.

6. Mutrie N. The relationship between physical activity and clinically defined depression. In: SJH Biddle S, Fox KR, Boucher SH (eds). *The Case for Exercise in the Promotion of Mental Health and Well-being,* pp. 46–62, London: Routledge, 2000.

7. Guite HF, Bywaters J. Mental health promotion. In: C Brooker, J Repper (eds). *Implementing the Mental Health Policy: principles, practice and research* Edinburgh: Elsevier, in press 2007.

8. Department of Health. *National Suicide Prevention Strategy for England* London: DH, 2002.

9. Health Development Agency. *Teenage Pregnancy and Parenthood: a review of reviews* (evidence briefing), 2003, www.nice.org.uk/page.aspx?o=502531 [accessed November 2007].

10. Olds DL, Eckenrode J, Henderson CR, *et al.* Long term effects of home visitation on maternal life course and child abuse and neglect: fifteen year follow up of a randomized trial *Journal of the American Medical Association* 1997; **278(8)**: 637–43.

11. Barlow J, Coren E, Stewart-Brown S. *Systematic Review of the Effectiveness of Parenting Programmes in Improving Maternal Psychosocial Health* Oxford: Oxford Health Services Research Unit, University of Oxford, 2001.

12. Scott S, Spender Q, Doolan M. Multi-centre controlled trial of parenting groups for childhood antisocial behaviour in clinical practice *British Medical Journal* 2001; **323**: 194–8.

13. Spencer MJ. Corporal punishment and ridicule: residual psychological effects in early adulthood. Implications for counsellors. *Dissertation Abstracts International Section A: Humanities and Social Sciences* 1999; **60(4-A)**: 1030.

14. Dennis C-L, Creedy D. Psychosocial and psychological interventions for preventing postpartum depression *British Medical Journal* 2005; **331(7507)**: 15, www.pubmedcentral.nih.gov/articlerender.fcgi?artid=558531 [accessed November 2007].

15. Simons J, Reynolds J, Morison L. Randomised controlled trial of training health visitors to identify and help couples with relationship problems following a birth *British Journal of General Practice* 2001; **51**: 793–9.

16. Care Services Improvement Partnership. *Making it Possible: improving mental health and well-being in England* Leeds: NIMHE, CSIP, 2005.

17. Department of Health. *Our Health, Our Care, Our Say: a new direction for community services* London: DH, 2006.

18. Seligman ME, Steen TA, Park N, *et al.* Positive psychology: empirical validation of interventions *American Psychologist* 2005; **60(5)**: 410–21.

19. Isaacowitz DM, Vaillant GE, Seligman MEP. Strengths and satisfaction across the life span *International Journal of Aging and Human Development* 2003; 57(2): 181–201.

20. Diener E, Seligman M. Beyond money: toward an economy of well-being *Psychological Science in the Public Interest* 2004; 5(1): 1–31.

21. Horwitz AV, Mclaughlin J, White HR. How the negative and positive aspects of partner relationships affect the mental health of young married people *Journal of Health and Social Behaviour* 1998; 39: 124–36.

22. Laurenceau J-P, Stanley SM, Olmos-Gallo A, *et al.* Community based prevention of marital dysfunction: multilevel modeling of a randomized effectiveness study *Journal of Consulting and Clinical Psychology* 2004; 72(6): 933–43.

23. Carson JW. Mindfulness-based relationship enhancement *Behavior Therapy* 2004; 35(3): 471–94.

24. Barbato A, D'Avanzo B. Marital therapy for depression *Cochrane Database of Systematic Reviews* 2006, Issue 2, Art. No. CD004188. DOI: 10.1002/14651858.CD004188.pub2.

25. Wood ND. What works for whom: a meta-analytical review of marital and couples therapy in reference to marital distress *American Journal of Family Therapy* 2005; 33(4): 273–87.

26. Denton WH. Depression, marital discord and couple therapy *Current Opinion in Psychiatry* 2003; 16(1): 29–34.

27. Stith SM, McCollum KH, Thomsen EE, *et al.* Treating intimate partner violence within intact couple relationships: outcomes of multi-couple versus individual couple therapy *Journal of Marital and Family Therapy* 2004; 30(3): 305–18.

28. Friedli L. Private minds in public bodies: the public mental health role of primary care *Primary Care Mental Health* 2005; 3: 41–6.

29. Hajak G. Epidemiology of severe insomnia and its consequences in Germany *European Archives of Psychiatry and Clinical Neuroscience* 2001; 251(1): 49–56.

30. Dealberto M-J. Epidemiology of sleep disorders and psychiatric diseases *Encephale* 1992; 18(4): 331–40.

31. Morin CM, Hauri PJ, Espie CA, *et al.* Nonpharmacologic treatment of chronic insomnia *Sleep* 1999; 22(8): 1134–56.

32. Chesson AL Jr, Anderson WM, Littner M, *et al.* Practice parameters for the nonpharmacological treatment of chronic insomnia *Sleep* 1999; 22(8): 1128–33.

33. Hajak G. Psychological, psychotherapeutical and other forms of nonpharmacological treatment of insomnia: statement by the expert group on insomnia of the German Society for Sleep Research and Sleep Medicine *Fortschritte der Neurologie Psychiatrie* 1997; 65(3): 133–44.

34. Shapiro CM, Bachmayer D. Epidemiological aspects of sleep in general public and hospital outpatient samples *Acta Physiologica Scandinavica* 1988; 134(suppl. 574): 41–3.

35. Vuori I, Urponene H, Hasan J, *et al.* Epidemiology of exercise effects on sleep *Acta Physiologica Scandinavica* 1988; 134(suppl. 574): 3–7.

36. Ciliska D, Hayward S, Thomas H, *et al.* A systematic overview of the effectiveness of home visiting as a delivery strategy for public health nursing interventions *Canadian Journal of Public Health* 1996; 87(3): 193–8.

37. Cattan M. *Supporting Older People to Overcome Social Isolation and Loneliness* London: Help the Aged, 2002.

38. Williams S, Michie S, Pattini S. *Improving the Health of the NHS Workforce: report of the partnership on the health of the NHS workforce* Leeds: The Nuffield Trust, 1998.

39. Donovan N, Halpern D with Richard Sargeant. *Life Satisfaction: the state of knowledge and implications for government* London: Prime Minister's Strategy Unit, 2002, www.cabinetoffice.gov.uk/strategy/downloads/seminars/ls/paper.pdf.

40. Halpern D. *More Bricks than Mortar? Mental health and the built environment* London: Taylor & Francis, 1995.

41. Guite HF, Clark C, Ackrill G. The impact of the physical and urban environment on mental well-being *Public Health* 2006; **120**: 1117–26

42. Matarasso F. *Use of Ornament? The social impact of participation in the arts* London: Commedia, 1997.

43. O'Dea J, Abraham S. Improving body image, eating attitudes and behaviours of young male and female adolescents: a new educational approach which focuses on self-esteem *Journal of Abnormal Psychology* 1999; **99**: 3–15.

44. Tobler NS, Stratton HH. Effectiveness of school-based drug prevention programs: a meta-analysis of the research *Journal of Primary Prevention* 1997; **18**(1): 71–128.

45. Wells J, Barlow J, Stewart-Brown S. *A Systematic Review of Universal Approaches to Mental Health Promotion in Schools* Oxford: Health Services Research Unit, Institute of Health Sciences, 2001.

Further reading

Department of Health. *Choosing Health* London: DH, 2004.

Diener E, Seligman M. Beyond money *Psychological Science in the Public Interest* 2004; **5**(1): 1–31.

Layard R. *Happiness: has social science a clue?* Lionel Robbins Memorial Lectures 2002/3, http://cep.lse.ac.uk/events/lectures/layard/RL030303.pdf [accessed November 2007].

4 | Identifying mental illness in primary care

Alan Cohen

What this chapter contributes:

the concept of 'caseness' – when is a mental illness a mental illness?

what influences the presentation and identification of mental illness?

the use of questionnaires to identify mental health problems.

The identification of a particular problem – making a diagnosis – is often difficult in primary care. We depend on what the patient tells us, or what we can elicit during a clinical examination, to make a clinical diagnosis. With physical disorders such as diabetes or asthma there are specific tests that can be performed to prove, one way or the other, if the patient is suffering from that condition.

The presentation, especially of mental health conditions, in general practice is chaotic and confused. Professor Paul Freeling, Emeritus Professor of General Practice at St George's Hospital Medical School, London, once said that the role of general practice was 'to organise the chaos of the first presentation'. In general practice, the consultation is much shorter than new patient assessments by psychiatrists and their teams. Frequently the patient may not present with a psychological problem. There are often external events or circumstances that influence the assessment of the problem, whether an exacerbation of an existing physical health condition, or problems at work or home that colour the way patients describe their problem. Finally, how patients perceive their own distress will influence the presentation. Is it 'acceptable' to have a mental health problem or is there a negative image, a sense of failure in some way, if the patient is to acknowledge that he or she is depressed, anxious or stressed?

All of these issues make the assessment of an individual difficult. Often, the difficulty lies in distinguishing between if the presenting problem is a normal reaction to an abnormal or distressing event, or an abnormal reaction to a normal event. It is not surprising therefore that extensive literature exists about how effective GPs are at 'identifying' people with mental health problems. For many years GPs were seen as 'poor' at identifying these problems, and that the solution was better training. More recently, with more research coming from primary care research specialists, the picture is becoming clearer. Identifying people with a mental health problem is difficult, and is often dependent on factors other than the clinical skills and acumen of the GP.

Nevertheless, it is not good enough to use these difficulties as an excuse for not making a diagnosis. Without a diagnosis, providing an effective intervention is not possible. There are effective interventions, ones that have been researched and studied, and if applied correctly these will significantly influence the patient's quality of life. Therefore as GPs we are duty bound, where possible, to make the best diagnosis, and to offer an effective, evidence-based intervention.

Levels of care

In 1980, Goldberg and Huxley[1] described five levels of care, and how individuals are filtered from one level to another (Figure 4.1).

Figure 4.1: The five levels of care

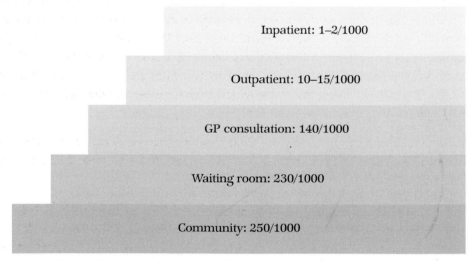

Inpatient: 1–2/1000

Outpatient: 10–15/1000

GP consultation: 140/1000

Waiting room: 230/1000

Community: 250/1000

Source: Goldberg D, Huxley P. *Mental Illness in the Community: the pathway to psychiatric care* London: Tavistock Publications, 1980. Reproduced by permission of Taylor & Francis Books.

Mental illness in the community

Mental illness in the community, that is the population before they choose to attend a GP surgery, has been assessed by a number of different screening questionnaires. The most elaborate questionnaire is the Index of Definition derived from a 140-item Present State Examination (PSE) by Wing.[2] This has become the gold standard of questionnaires, against which all others are compared. The other frequently used questionnaire is the General Health Questionnaire (GHQ)[2,3] initially a 120-item questionnaire, but has been shortened to a 30-item, 24-item and even a 12-item questionnaire, developed by Goldberg and colleagues. Both questionnaires were derived from UK populations.

The concept of a 'case' – when the mental health problem is sufficient to warrant being considered 'just clinically significant' – is inevitably an arbitrary decision. The results from any questionnaire screening for a mental health problem will return a distribution of patients without a clear division between normal and abnormal. Therefore, where that division is created will decide which individuals do, or do not, have a mental health problem. It is for that reason that the decision is arbitrary.

What is more interesting is who makes that decision. Is the 'cut-off' for becoming a case set by psychiatrists, GPs or even patients themselves? Certainly the PSE questionnaire was validated by psychiatrists, and although the classification is more complex (there is not a simple level above or below which is normal) the questionnaire is validated by testing against the opinion of psychiatrists. The gold standard test for identifying levels of morbidity of mental disorder in the community and attending primary care practices is thus dependent on the opinion of psychiatrists. In the UK, few patients access psychiatrists directly; most have been seen, and in some cases assessed and treated, by their GP prior to referral. Indeed this is the case that Goldberg and Huxley make, that access to the psychiatric services is dependent on the skills, knowledge and attitudes of the GP, as well as the needs of the patient. What is important is that psychiatrists rarely see people who may or may not have a mental health disorder. They only see people who have been screened/assessed, usually by their GP. It is something of a mystery therefore as to why they are expected to be the experts in deciding where the division should be between a case and not a case.

Nevertheless, there is enormous value in understanding the level of distress in the community, and what can be done to ensure that those that need/want treatment have the opportunity to receive it.

Throughout this section there are figures quoted that describe different levels of morbidity. In describing the presence of a disorder, it is necessary to distinguish between the number of people who have that disorder at a particular time, as compared with those who develop the disorder.

The *incidence rate* refers to the number of people who develop the disorder (those with a new episode) each year per 1000 of the population at risk. The decision as to what constitutes a 'new episode' is arbitrary, and in mental health seems dependent on the opinion of psychiatrists.

The *point prevalence rate* refers to the number of people who at a given point in time have a particular disorder. This is usually referred to as a proportion or rate per 1000 at risk population.

In the waiting room

It seems from Figure 4.1 that nearly everybody who has a mental health problem in the community attends the surgery. Why *do* people see their doctor? Do people with mental health problems behave differently when they see their doctor from people who do not have a mental health problem? Do people with a mental health problem who attend their doctor know that this is the reason why they are attending?

A sociological explanation

In 1960 Mechanic and Volkert[4] described 'illness behaviour' as a way to explain why patients attend their doctor. Illness behaviour was later described by Mechanic[5] as 'the ways in which given symptoms may be differentially perceived, evaluated and acted upon (or not acted upon) by different kinds of people'. The role of medicine was to 'effect the arrival of "ill" persons at medical setting so that treatment can be effectively administered'.

So how many people get 'symptoms', and does the presence of symptoms always end in a visit to the doctor? There have been many surveys of the general population seeking either for participants to record in a 'health diary' the number of symptoms that a person may experience, or to recall how many symptoms were experienced in the preceding short period of time. In both types of survey, the number of symptoms were high – Dunnell and Cartwright[6] identified that people could recall four symptoms in the last two weeks, and Banks *et al.*[7] noted that most people experienced at least one symptom per day. What is interesting is that, despite the fact that people experience this number of symptoms, something else must happen before people make the decision to do something about these 'abnormal' feelings, and consult a doctor.

Lots of people get symptoms, but only a few consult their doctor. Armstrong[8] suggests that there are a number of potential questions that are posed by people considering consulting their doctor:

- are my symptoms normal or abnormal?

- should I go to the doctor on this occasion?

- what else can I do?

- what are the costs and benefits of seeing the doctor?

Whether or not a symptom is felt by the patient as being 'normal' or 'abnormal' depends on his or her own experience. Some symptoms are so common, such as a headache, that they are generally felt to be a normal experience not requiring a doctor's opinion. So a consultation for a headache is relatively unusual, and represents for the patient a significant concern/worry. Some symptoms are normal for a specific group of people, such as aches and pains in older people.

Having decided that a symptom is sufficiently abnormal then a decision is made whether or not to attend the doctor this time. There have been a number of different ways of categorising this process, with descriptions of triggers, or 'tickets of entry'. Zola[9] suggests the following five triggers:

- perceived interference with vocational or physical activity

- perceived interference with social or personal relations

- the occurrence of an interpersonal crisis

- a kind of 'temporalising of symptomatology' – setting a deadline for a symptom to resolve

- sanctioning – permission to attend from family/friend or from somebody in authority (such as a school nurse etc.).

There are a number of things that patients can do themselves, instead of consulting the doctor: they can do nothing, they can consult their friends and family, who may then offer advice based on their own experience and knowledge; they can use self-medications or self-help; or they can consult other health professionals prior to the consultation with the GP. This latter option is one that has been much explored recently with the development of NHS Direct, and the increasing role of pharmacists in offering more detailed clinical advice as part of their new contract.

There are two specific benefits for the patient seeing the doctor. The first is therapeutic, in that the doctor will provide treatment for the symptoms that the patient presents. Some people do not consult because they believe that there is 'nothing that can be done' for their symptom. This is a particular issue for depression, where the media has an important role to educate the public that there are effective treatments available. The other benefit that the doctor provides for the patient is a legitimisation of being 'unwell'. This granting of the sick role allows the patient to both temporarily be excused from his or her normal role or occupation, and be allowed not to feel responsible for the illness.

Practical considerations

Whilst the above represents a sociological perspective on the reasons why people attend surgery, it does not represent the entire problem. There has been considerable discussion and debate as to the quality and quantity of the appointment systems that GPs use to organise their surgeries.

- Surgery hours, or more correctly consultation hours, have been a bone of contention between the General Practitioners Committee (GPC) of the BMA (British Medical Association) and the Department of Health (DH) during negotiations over the 2004 nGMS (new General Medical Services) contract. Over the last ten years or so there have been a number of incentives and targets to encourage different types of consulting hours. It was usual for general practice to provide a Saturday morning surgery, or to run early and late surgeries, to accommodate those who work and are thus unable to attend during normal office hours. The development of NHS Direct was intended to provide an advice service that had always previously been provided by general practice; in the view of politicians general practice had not delivered this role successfully. The development of out-of-hours services, GP-run cooperative arrangements, has allowed general practitioners to now run an 8.00 a.m. to 6.00 p.m. service, and in large cities and conurbations few if any practices now provide their own out-of-hours services.

- A further area of difficulty is whether or not people can register with a practice, and was addressed in theory in the nGMS contract of 2004. The contract described two types of practice lists, a list that was 'open' and a list that was 'closed'. An open list would accept all people living within a previously described geographical area who made a request to register. A closed list is a list that is closed to all new requests to register, irrespective of the address at which they live. A closed list is associated with certain financial sequelae, remains closed usually for at least six months, and needs to be agreed with the Primary Care Trusts (PCTs), so that a plan can be agreed to solve the issues that have resulted in the closure. Confusingly there is a third alternative, 'an open but full' list, which is temporarily closed to new patients, and reflects temporary staffing problems such as sickness.

- During the 2005 General Election, the Prime Minister was embarrassed by a member of the public complaining of the way that access targets were being implemented by GPs: that appointments were only available within 48 hours. This was implemented rigorously across England as it was a performance target for PCTs. The member of the public was complaining that she was unable to book an appointment, and that appointments were only available 'on the day'.

- In 2005, the Disability Rights Commission (DRC) undertook a formal investigation into the access of people with mental health and learning disability problems to primary care services. The basis for undertaking this investigation was the poor health outcomes of people with mental health and learning disabilities. The DRC has compiled a very extensive literature review of the health outcomes of these two groups.

The above indicates some of the difficulties that individuals have in accessing primary care, above and beyond the sociological reasons that individuals choose to consult their doctor. The sociological reasons explain why people behave as they do, but there are the practical difficulties (real and imagined) by patients in actually making an appointment at a time that is convenient to them, in a location that is appropriate. The DRC inquiry makes the point that people with mental health problems are frequently not in a frame of mind to be able to negotiate with receptionists a complex set of alternatives about appointment times. The DRC makes several suggestions as to how the practice can alter and make more 'user friendly' the appointment system, to allow people who are distressed to access the service more easily.

Despite all of the above, the sociological reasons for consulting, and the perceived practical barriers to consulting, the data suggests that 230/1000 at risk do attend the surgery, from a community in which 250/1000 at risk have mental health problems (see Figure 4.1). Clearly there are some barriers, but they may not be as significant as some have suggested.

The National Institute for Mental Health in England (NIMHE) has recently developed a training tool for primary healthcare teams that, for the first time, sets out what primary healthcare teams need to know about mental illness. This includes what receptionists and administrative staff need to know, so that people are not intimidated out of a consultation (as they were by the stereotypical 'dragon receptionist'). The training package includes managing people who are distressed or angry, and why these can be a presentation for people with mental illness.

In the GP consultation

A superficial and naïve look at the transition from the identification of mental disorder in the waiting room to identification during the GP consultation would seem to demonstrate that GPs are poor at identifying people with mental health problems. It would appear from the prevalence figures that GPs 'miss' nearly half of those with mental heath problems. Indeed this figure has oft been quoted[8,21] as a reason why better training is needed for GPs.[1,10]

If that is the case, there are some questions that need to be asked to understand the underlying clinical context for these individuals.

1. Is the interpretation of this data appropriate?

2. What sort of disorders are identified?

3. What sort of patients are more, or less, likely to be identified as suffering from a mental health disorder?

4. What sort of doctor is more, or less, likely to make a diagnosis of a mental health problem?

5. What happens to people whose mental health problem is not identified?

Is the interpretation of the data appropriate?

The prevalence data in Goldberg's and Huxley's 'Levels of Care' are the amount of mental health problems identified by the use of the GHQ at a specific time. What the GHQ does not do is to follow up patients who were not acknowledged as suffering from a mental health problem.

As described above, the GHQ is an extremely well-validated, population-based questionnaire. During its development it was compared with a number of other assessment tools, as well as the clinical skills of the psychiatrist, to assess how accurately the new questionnaire would identify people with mental health problems. Like any new questionnaire, the difficulty is always in finding something to compare it with, since even other assessment tools needed to be validated first, to ensure that they are an accurate measure themselves. Ultimately, therefore, all the questionnaires that assess mental health problems are validated on the clinical skills of the psychiatrist, which is not unreasonable; they are specially trained to provide this care and assessment. Generally, a first appointment with new patients to make an assessment is about an hour, and in some cases the accurate assessment of a complex problem may take several days.

Therefore, when it is claimed that GPs are 'bad at identifying people with mental health problems', or that they 'miss 50% of people with mental health problems', a comparison is being made between the diagnostic skills in a 10-minute consultation with a GP and a 60-minute consultation with a psychiatrist. Figure 4.2 demonstrates how over six 10-minute consultations, at a 50 per cent identification rate, the final 'success' rate is little different between general practitioners and psychiatrists.

Figure 4.2: Identification rates for GPs

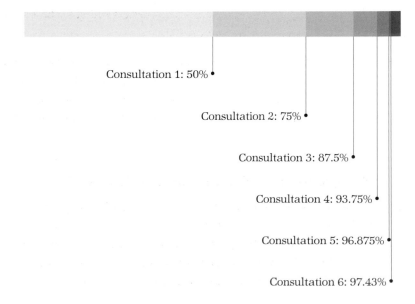

Consultation 1: 50%

Consultation 2: 75%

Consultation 3: 87.5%

Consultation 4: 93.75%

Consultation 5: 96.875%

Consultation 6: 97.43%

What sort of disorders?

Studies show that the most frequent disorders identified in primary care are the neuroses: disorders such as depression, anxiety and mixed anxiety and depression. Other disorders such as obsessive compulsive disorders, phobias and panic attacks are also seen but less frequently. The major psychoses are relatively uncommon, although they represent the majority of the work of the specialist mental health teams.

Further details of the types and numbers of disorders seen in primary care are included in Chapter 5.

What sort of patients?

Hesbacher et al. studied 1300 patients from seven family practices in Philadelphia, USA.[11] They found that social class is related to symptomatology of neuroses for males, and, more statistically significantly, for females. For both men and women, the higher social classes (I–III) were less symptomatic than the lower social classes (IV–V). Lower social class patients were 'sicker' than patients from the upper classes.

Cooper and Sylph found that new cases of neurotic illness were more likely than matched controls to have experienced life events in the three months preceding the onset of the illness.[12]

Gater et al. found that gender did not affect whether or not a mental health condition was recognised by the doctor.[13] However, other studies, such as by Marks et al., found that females were more likely to be recognised.[10]

Patients who are white, middle aged, bereaved or separated are more likely to be correctly identified as suffering from a psychological complaint.[10] Patients who have a co-morbid physical illness are more likely to be missed.[14]

Clearly the latter is important, as this reinforces the quote made by Professor Freeling – that the role of the general practitioner is 'to organise the chaos of the first presentation'. Disentangling the cause of a physical symptom, knowing that this is the most common way for a mental health problem to present, is one of the perennial challenges of modern practice.

What sort of doctors are more likely to make a diagnosis?

As with most clinical areas, GPs vary in their ability to identify people with mental health problems. Marks et al. showed that age and experience were not closely related to accurate identification,[10] but Goldberg et al., in a separate paper, showed that academically more competent GPs, with 'an appropriate concept of mental illness in primary care', were more likely to make accurate diagnoses.[15]

Howie *et al.* found that longer consultations improved recognition rates, and provided the patient with greater satisfaction with the consultation.[16] Goldberg *et al.* found that GPs who make more eye contact, interrupt less, don't appear rushed, use more open questions and are good listeners are more likely to recognise depression.[15]

What happens to those whose diagnosis was not acknowledged?

The case was made above that people with a mental health condition who continue to consult will be identified. It is likely that people whose condition is moderate or severe in character are more likely to consult. Hence those who need the intervention of a doctor are very likely to be correctly identified and treated. However, those with a mild disorder, who consult less frequently, are less likely to be identified.

What is not clear is what happens to those with mild depression or mild anxiety. There is evidence to show that some people with mild depression resolve spontaneously without the need for any specific intervention from the doctor.[17] The proportion of the total who do so is estimated at 52 per cent within the first three months.[17] Certainly the NICE guidelines for depression recommend that antidepressants are not used in cases of mild depression. It is clear that the presumption that all those with mild depression or mild anxiety naturally and completely go on to develop moderate or severe conditions is not true, but at present we are not able to identify which individuals are more or less likely to do so. It is for that reason that the phrase 'watchful waiting' was coined as part of the recognition of people with mental health problems.

Watchful waiting describes a pragmatic approach to people who have been identified as having a mild disorder, and who are then actively reviewed some four to eight weeks later to assess the progress (if any) of the disorder. If the condition has progressed or become more severe, then an evidence-based intervention should be offered as appropriate. If the condition has resolved completely, then, depending on clinical circumstances, it may be appropriate to follow up further.

Specialist mental health services

In the UK, specialist mental health services are required to prioritise those with a severe and enduring mental illness. This means that the majority of referrals to specialist mental health services from primary care should be for those with a severe and enduring mental illness. However, there is continuing anecdotal information that mental health services are overwhelmed by what they consider to be large numbers of 'inappropriate' referrals, i.e. conditions other than those with a severe and enduring mental illness.

The issue of what a 'severe and enduring mental illness' might mean, and the relationship between primary and secondary care, is dealt with in Chapter 7.

Questionnaires that can be used in primary care

The use of questionnaires in mental health research is well established. The use of such questionnaires to enable investigators to describe the presence and characteristics of specific disorders is clearly of value.

However, the questionnaires are also being used more and more frequently as both diagnostic and therapeutic tools. As diagnostic tools they can be used to assess the presence or absence of a specific disorder. As a therapeutic tool they can be used sequentially in the same individual to assess the progress of the disorder, or alternatively by sharing the results of the questionnaire with the patient. These can help the patient to gain insight into underlying psychological components of the presentation. Not all questionnaires are validated for use in primary care, and not all questionnaires can be used therapeutically as well as diagnostically. As the section on the nGMS contract describes in more detail, the use of specific questionnaires in the management of depression is included in the 2006 amendment to the Quality and Outcomes Framework.

The development of any questionnaire requires it to be validated or checked: that it really does measure what it purports to measure. Questionnaires now in development and in use are compared with previously developed questionnaires, and accepted by dint of careful validation as being both sensitive and specific. The original index questionnaire, which has been accepted by the World Health Organization, is the PSE – Index of Definition developed by Wing et al.[2] This questionnaire was checked for validity against the clinical acumen of psychiatrists. Subsequent questionnaires such as the Patient Health Questionnaire (PHQ) and Primary Care Evaluation of Mental Disorders (PRIME-MD), on which it was based, were validated against primary care physicians' opinion, and then patients were interviewed by psychiatrists for the 'definitive' diagnosis. So, although questionnaires may be validated for use in primary care, the standard of clinical diagnosis to which these questionnaires aspire is the diagnostic skills and acumen of psychiatrists, not experienced general practitioners. Certainly, in the UK, GPs see many more cases of mild and moderate mental disorder than psychiatrists, so that one could make the case that perhaps the validation technique for these questionnaires is not as appropriate to primary care as at first sight. Table 4.1 lists some questionnaires that see frequent use in primary care.

The newest questionnaire, the PMEQ (Patient Mental Health Experience Questionnaire), a scale developed by Dr Helen Lester at Birmingham Medical School, assesses the mental health character of a practice. 'Is the practice mental health friendly?' and 'Does it understand the special needs of people with mental health problems?' are the questions that the questionnaire addresses. It is therefore a very different type of questionnaire, which assesses the quality of care that is provided from a user/patient perspective, rather than a questionnaire that assists the GP to diagnose or manage a specific condition in a specific individual.

Table 4.1: Frequently used questionnaires in primary care:

Name	Disorder	Validated in primary care	Questionnaire completed by	Maps to ICD-10
PHQ-2	Depression	Yes	GP	No
PHQ-9	Depression	Yes	Patient	Yes
Beck Depression Inventory 2nd edition (BDI – II)	Depression	Yes	GP/patient	Yes
Hospital Anxiety and Depression Scale (HADS)	Anxiety scale and depression scale	Yes	GP	Yes
The CAGE	Alcohol misuse	Yes	GP	Yes
The SCOFF	Eating disorder	Yes	GP	Yes
PMEQ	Mental health character of practice	Yes	Patient	No
Edinburgh Postnatal Depression	Postnatal depression	Yes	Patient	Yes

The two-item and nine-item versions of the PHQ are derived from the PRIME-MD questionnaire developed by Spitzer *et al*. in the USA.[18] PRIME-MD is a questionnaire that diagnoses a number of common mental health conditions in a primary care setting, which map to specific ICD-10 categories (in the USA the equivalent is DSM-IV – *Diagnostic and Statistical Manual of Mental Disorders*, fourth edition). (Previous versions of DSM-IV and ICD-10 did not match completely, but the latest versions describe the same disorders.) PRIME-MD consists of a two-stage process: first, a 26-item self-completed questionnaire; and a second stage of algorithms and verification to be undertaken by the physician. It was noted during the validation stage that, although the questionnaire was of value in research, it took too long to be used in normal practice – this is a common feature of all questionnaires in normal clinical practice. To overcome this difficulty the authors developed a nine-item questionnaire that was completed by the patient. The strength of the questionnaire is that the nine items relate specifically to the nine items on the ICD-10 that describe the characteristics of depression in the ICD-10/DSM-IV classification. Thus the questionnaire not only is a diagnostic tool, but also allows a measure of the severity of the disorder to be made; this is of great value when implementing NICE guidelines for depression, as different interventions are recommended for different levels of severity. It is for this reason that the PHQ-9 (see Figure 4.3, p. 78) is recommended for UK general practice when participating in the Quality and Outcomes Framework of the nGMS contract, as it allows an accurate assessment of both diagnosis and severity to be made.

The PHQ-2 is, in contrast, a two-item questionnaire that is recommended for screening and case finding people who may be suffering from depression, or who are at greater risk of suffering from depression. The two questions are:

- During the last month, have you often been bothered by feeling down, depressed or hopeless?

- During the last month, have you often been bothered by having little interest or pleasure in doing things?

A positive response to either question would lead the clinician to administer the PHQ-9, to make a more formal assessment of the mental state of the patient.

There is a more recent three-question version of the PHQ-2 that adds the extra 'helping' question:

- Is this something with which you would like help?

As a result of this third question, the specificity (the chance of correctly identifying an individual with depression) rises to 87 per cent. If all three questions are replied to in the negative, the chance of the individual having depression is less than 1 per cent.

The PHQ-9 (see Figure 4.3, p. 78) is scored as follows:

1–4	minimal depression
5–9	mild depression
10–14	moderate depression
15–19	moderately severe depression
20–27	severe depression.

The Hospital Anxiety and Depression Scale (see Table 4.2, p. 79) is a second questionnaire approved for use in the Quality and Outcomes Framework, which unlike the PHQ-9 assesses both depression and anxiety. This questionnaire has been well validated for use in primary care and has been used for some years.

Figure 4.3: The PHQ-9

PATIENT HEALTH QUESTIONNAIRE (PHQ–9)

NAME: ______________________ **DATE:** ______________

Over the *last 2 weeks,* how often have you been bothered by any of the following problems? *(use "✓" to indicate your answer)*	Not at all	Several days	More than half the days	Nearly every day
1. Little interest or pleasure in doing things	0	1	2	3
2. Feeling down, depressed or hopeless	0	1	2	3
3. Trouble falling or staying asleep, or sleeping too much	0	1	2	3
4. Feeling tired or having little energy	0	1	2	3
5. Poor appetite or overeating	0	1	2	3
6. Feeling bad about yourself – or that you are a failure or have let yourself or your family down	0	1	2	3
7. Trouble concentrating on things, such as reading the newspaper or watching television	0	1	2	3
8. Moving or speaking so slowly that other people could have noticed. Or the opposite – being so fidgety or restless that you have been moving around a lot more than usual	0	1	2	3
9. Thoughts that you would be better off dead, or of hurting yourself in some way	0	1	2	3
	add columns:		+	+

(Healthcare professional: For interpretation of TOTAL please refer to accompanying scoring card) **TOTAL**

Source: reproduced by permission of Pfizer Inc.: www.phqscreeners.com. © Pfizer Inc.

Hospital Anxiety and Depression Scale (HADS)

Name: _____   Date: _____

Clinicians are aware that emotions play an important part in most illnesses. If your clinician knows about these feelings he or she will be able to help you more.

This questionnaire is designed to help your clinician to know how you feel. Read each item below and **underline the reply** which comes closest to how you have been feeling in the past week. Ignore the numbers printed at the edge of the questionnaire.

Don't take too long over your replies, your immediate reaction to each item will probably be more accurate than a long, thought-out response.

FOLD HERE

A D

I feel tense or 'wound up'
- Most of the time — 3
- A lot of the time — 2
- From time to time, occasionally — 1
- Not at all — 0

I still enjoy the things I used to enjoy
- Definitely as much — 0
- Not quite so much — 1
- Only a little — 2
- Hardly at all — 3

I get a sort of frightened feeling as if something awful is about to happen
- Very definitely and quite badly — 3
- Yes, but not too badly — 2
- A little, but it doesn't worry me — 1
- Not at all — 0

I can laugh and see the funny side of things
- As much as I always could — 0
- Not quite so much now — 1
- Definitely not so much now — 2
- Not at all — 3

Worrying thoughts go through my mind
- A great deal of the time — 3
- A lot of the time — 2
- Not too often — 1
- Very little — 0

I feel cheerful
- Never — 3
- Not often — 2
- Sometimes — 1
- Most of the time — 0

I can sit at ease and feel relaxed
- Definitely — 0
- Usually — 1
- Not often — 2
- Not at all — 3

I feel as if I am slowed down
- Nearly all the time — 3
- Very often — 2
- Sometimes — 1
- Not at all — 0

I get a sort of frightened feeling like 'butterflies' in the stomach
- Not at all — 0
- Occasionally — 1
- Quite often — 2
- Very often — 3

I have lost interest in my appearance
- Definitely — 3
- I don't take as much care as I should — 2
- I may not take quite as much care — 1
- I take just as much care as ever — 0

I feel restless as if I have to be on the move
- Very much indeed — 3
- Quite a lot — 2
- Not very much — 1
- Not at all — 0

I look forward with enjoyment to things
- As much as I ever did — 0
- Rather less than I used to — 1
- Definitely less than I used to — 2
- Hardly at all — 3

I get sudden feelings of panic
- Very often indeed — 3
- Quite often — 2
- Not very often — 1
- Not at all — 0

I can enjoy a good book or radio or television programme
- Often — 0
- Sometimes — 1
- Not often — 2
- Very seldom — 3

Now check that you have answered all the questions

A D   TOTAL [   ]

It is scored for depression as follows: 0–7 normal, 8–10 mild, 11–14 moderate, 15–21 severe

Source: reproduced by permission of GL Assessment.

The third questionnaire that has been approved for use in the Quality and Outcomes Framework is the Beck II questionnaire. It is available from Harcourt Assessment.[19]

Postnatal depression

According to Warner *et al.*, postpartum depression affects 10 per cent of new mothers, with the range being from eight to 15 per cent.[20] The Edinburgh Postnatal Depression Scale (EPDS) was developed in 1987 to act as a specific measurement tool to identify depression in new mothers. The scale has since been validated, and evidence from a number of research studies has confirmed the tool to be both reliable and sensitive in detecting depression.

The Edinburgh Postnatal Depression Scale[21]

Name .... EPDS Score ....

Assessment Date .... Assessor ....

As you have recently had a baby, we would like to know how you are feeling. Please underline the answer that comes closest to how you have felt in the past seven days – not just how you feel today.

Here is an example, already completed:
I have felt happy:
Yes, all the time
Yes, most of the time
No, not very often
No, not at all
This would mean 'I have felt happy most of the time during the past week'.
Please answer the following 10 questions by underlining the appropriate answer.
Thank you.

In the past 7 days:

1. I have been able to laugh and see the funny side of things:
As much as I always could
Not quite so much now
Definitely not so much now
Not at all

2. I have looked forward with enjoyment to things:
As much as I ever did
Rather less than I used to
Definitely less than I used to
Hardly at all

3. I have blamed myself unnecessarily when things went wrong:
Yes, most of the time
Yes, some of the time
Not very often
No, never

4. I have been anxious or worried for no good reason:
No, not at all
Hardly ever
Yes, sometimes
Yes, very often

5. I have felt scared or panicky for no good reason:
Yes, quite a lot
Yes, sometimes
No, not much
No, not at all

6. Things have been getting on top of me:
Yes, most of the time I haven't been able to cope at all
Yes, sometimes I haven't been coping as well as usual
No, most of the time I have coped quite well
No, I have been coping as well as ever

7. I have been so unhappy that I have had difficulty sleeping:
Yes, most of the time
Yes, sometimes
Not very often
No, not at all

8. I have felt sad or miserable:
Yes, most of the time
Yes, quite often
Not very often
No, not at all

9. I have been so unhappy that I have been crying:
Yes, most of the time
Yes, quite often
Only occasionally
No, never

10. The thought of harming myself has occurred to me:
Yes, quite often
Sometimes
Hardly ever
Never

Edinburgh Postnatal Depression Scale – guidelines for raters

Response categories are scored 0, 1, 2 and 3 according to increased severity of the symptom. Questions 3, 5, 6, 7, 8, 9 and 10 are reverse scored (i.e. 3, 2, 1, 0).

Individual items are totalled to give an overall score. A score of 12+ indicates the likelihood of depression, but not its severity. The EPDS score is designed to assist, not replace, clinical judgement.

Source: Cox JL, Holden JM, Sagovsky R. Detection of postnatal depression. Development of the 10-item Edinburgh Postnatal Depression Scale *British Journal of Psychiatry* 1987; 150: 782–6.[21]

Alcohol dependence

Using the CAGE questionnaire, alcohol dependence is likely if the patient gives two or more positive answers to the following questions:

- Have you ever felt you should Cut down on your drinking?

- Have people Annoyed you by criticising your drinking?

- Have you ever felt bad or Guilty about your drinking?

- Have you ever had a drink first thing in the morning to steady your nerves or get rid of a hangover (Eye-opener)?

The combination of the CAGE questionnaire and MCV and GGT activity will detect about 75 per cent of people with an alcohol problem.

Eating disorders

Using the SCOFF questionnaire,[22] patients receive one point for every yes; a score of 2 or more indicates a likely case of anorexia nervosa or bulimia nervosa with a sensitivity of 100 per cent and specificity of 87.5 per cent.

Sick: Do you make yourself *sick* because you feel uncomfortably full?

Control: Do you worry you have lost *control* over how much you eat?

One stone: Have you recently lost more than *one stone* (6.3 kg, or 14 lbs) in a 3-month period?

Fat: Do you believe yourself to be *fat* when other people say you are too thin?

Food: Would you say that *food* dominates your life?

References

1. Goldberg D, Huxley P. *Mental Illness in the Community: the pathway to psychiatric care* London: Tavistock Publications, 1980.

2. Wing JK, Nixon JM, Mann SA, *et al*. Reliability of the PSE (9th edition) used in a population study *Psychological Medicine* 1977; **7**: 505–16.

3. Vieweg BW, Hedlund JL. The General Health Questionnaire (GHQ): a comprehensive review *Journal of Operational Psychiatry* 1983; **14(2)**: 74–81.

4. Mechanic D, Volkert EH. Illness behaviour and medical diagnosis *Journal of Health and Human Behaviour* 1960; **1**: 86–94.

5. Mechanic D. The concept of illness behaviour *Journal of Chronic Disease* 1962; **15**: 189–94.

6. Dunnell K, Cartwright A. *Medicine Takers, Prescribers and Hoarders* London: Routledge and Kegan Paul, 1972.

7. Banks M, Beresford SA, Morrell DC, *et al*. Factors influencing demand for primary medical care in women aged 20–44 *International Journal of Epidemiology* 1975; **4**: 189–95.

8. Armstrong D. *An Outline of Sociology as Applied to Medicine* Oxford: Butterworth Heinemann, 1994.

9. Zola IK. Pathways to the doctor: from person to patient *Social Science and Medicine* 1973; **7**: 677–89.

10. Marks JN, Goldberg D, Hillier VF. Determinants of the ability of general practitioners to detect psychiatric illness *Psychological Medicine* 1979; **9**: 337–53.

11. Hesbacher PT, Rickels K, Goldberg D. Social factors and neurotic illness symptoms in family practice *American Journal of Family Practice* 1975; **65**: 148–55.

12. Cooper B, Sylph J. Life events and the onset of neurotic illness: an investigation in general practice *Psychological Medicine* 1973; **3**: 421–35.

13. Gater R, Tansella M, Korten A, *et al*. Sex differences in the prevalence and detection of depressive and anxiety disorders in general health care settings: report from the World Health Organization Collaborative Study on Psychological Problems in General Health Care *Archives of General Psychiatry* 1998; **55**: 405–13.

14. Tylee AT, Freeling P, Kerry S. Why do general practitioners recognise major depression in one woman patient yet miss it in another? *British Journal of General Practice* 1993; **43**: 327–30.

15. Goldberg DP, Jenkins L, Millar T, *et al*. The ability of trainee general practitioners to identify psychological distress among their patients *Psychological Medicine* 1993; **23**: 185–93.

16. Howie JGR, Porter AMD, Heaney DJ, *et al*. Long to short consultation ratio: a proxy measure of quality in general practice *British Journal of General Practice* 1991; **41**: 48–52.

17. Posternak MA, Solomon DA, Leon AC, *et al*. The naturalistic course of unipolar major depression in the absence of somatic therapy *Journal of Nervous and Mental Disease* 2006; **194**: 324–9.

18. Spitzer R, Kroenke K, Williams JB. Validation and utilization of a self report version of PRIME-MD *Journal of the American Medical Association* 1999; **282**: 1737–44.

19. Harcourt Assessment, http://harcourtassessment.com [accessed November 2007].

20. Warner R, Appleby L, Whitton A, *et al*. Demographic and obstetric risk factors for postnatal psychiatric morbidity *British Journal of Psychiatry* 1996; **168**: 607–11.

21. Cox JL, Holden JM, Sagovsky R. Detection of postnatal depression. Development of the 10-item Edinburgh Postnatal Depression Scale *British Journal of Psychiatry* 1987; **150**: 782–6.

22. Morgan JF, Reid A, Lacey JH. The SCOFF questionnaire: a new screening tool for eating disorders *British Medical Journal* 1999; **319**: 1467–8.

Further reading

British Medical Association. *New GMS Contract* London: BMA, 2003.

Hedlung JL, Vieweg BW. The Hamilton rating scale for depression *Journal of Operational Psychiatry* 1979; **10(2)**: 149–65.

WHO Guide to Mental Health in Primary Care London: WHO Collaborating Center for Mental Health Research & Training, Institute of Psychiatry, 2000.

5 | The range of disorders

Alan Cohen

What this chapter contributes:

mental health problems are common

mental health problems are frequently divided into two categories, 'severe and enduring mental illness' and 'common mental illness'

The term 'severe and enduring mental illness' is a 'password' to access specialist mental health services.

The previous chapter described some of the processes by which people attend their general practitioner, and the issues that affect how and when they make the choice to attend. Within the UK, the role of general practice was described thus:

> the essential unit of medical practice is the occasion when, in the intimacy of the consulting room or sick room, a person who is ill or believes himself to be ill, seeks the advice of a doctor whom he trusts. This is a consultation and all else in the practice of medicine derives from it. The purpose of the consultation is that the doctor, having gathered his evidence, shall give explanation and advice.[1]

This means – amongst other things – that people present with unorganised complaints. Professor Paul Freeling made the observation that the role of general practitioners was 'to organise the chaos of the first presentation' (see Chapter 4).

The consequence of this complex set of sociological and medical interrelationships is that most people attend their general practitioner for most of their perceived medical needs. In other countries of the world, there are opportunities to consult specialists directly, bypassing the general practitioner; in the UK general practitioners are the gatekeepers to secondary care services.

General practitioners are therefore likely to be involved in the care of everybody who has any form of mental health condition to some extent or another. That mental health condition could vary from a mild adjustment disorder, to the consequences of a severe psychosis. The International Classification of Diseases (ICD) developed by the World

Health Organization (WHO) provides a useful way of describing the different sorts of disorder that general practitioners can expect to see in their practice.[2]

The tenth version of this classification, ICD-10, is outlined below. It describes the broad range of disorders that are encountered in primary care.

Details of the clinical features of the more common disorders found in primary care are provided in the next chapters.

Table 5.1: ICD-10

Organic, including symptomatic, mental disorders

F10–F19	Mental and behavioural disorders due to psychoactive substance use
F20–F29	Schizophrenia, schizotypal and delusional disorders
F30–F39	Mood [affective] disorders
F40–F48	Neurotic, stress-related and somatoform disorders
F50–F59	Behavioural syndromes associated with physiological disturbances and physical factors
F60–F69	Disorders of adult personality and behaviour
F70–F79	Mental retardation
F80–F89	Disorders of psychological development
F90–F98	Behavioural and emotional disorders with onset usually occurring in childhood and adolescence
F99	Unspecified mental disorder

Source: World Health Organization. *International Classification of Diseases*, www.who.int/classifications /icd/en. Reproduced by permission of the World Health Organization.

The Office of National Statistics (ONS) undertakes a survey of the number of people with mental health problems in the general population on a regular basis.[3] The survey is based on the use of epidemiological questionnaires and survey tools, not those that are appropriate for identifying and managing individuals in the primary care setting. Nevertheless the results are helpful as they give an indication of the expected number of people with a specific problem, and therefore provide information on planning healthcare services. The results of the survey are subdivided into neurotic disorders, personality disorders, psychotic disorders, and substance and alcohol misuse.

What the survey demonstrates is that mental health problems are common. The WHO believes that by 2020 depression will be the second most common chronic disorder in the world. One hundred and sixty-four per 1000 cases of neurotic disorder (equivalent to one in six adults) make this a very common disorder. It is very much the responsibility of general practitioners.

Neurotic disorders

The ONS survey looked at both the presence of neurotic symptoms, and the presence of specific neurotic conditions. The presence of neurotic symptoms was assessed by the use of the revised Clinical Interview Schedule (CIS-R),[4,5] and the presence of specific neurotic conditions was calculated by applying algorithms to the responses to the CIS-R, to deliver diagnoses that conformed to the ICD-10 classification.

Figure 5.1 shows the proportion of people with neurotic symptoms in the community.

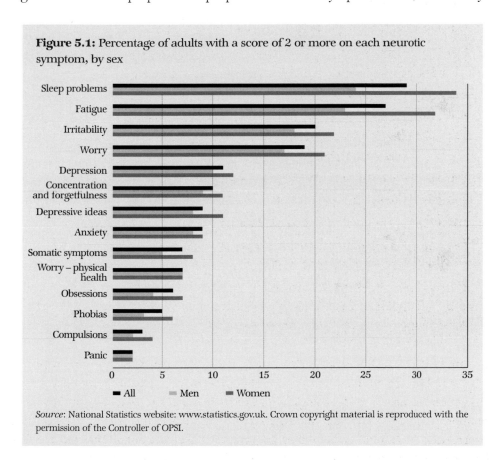

Figure 5.1: Percentage of adults with a score of 2 or more on each neurotic symptom, by sex

Source: National Statistics website: www.statistics.gov.uk. Crown copyright material is reproduced with the permission of the Controller of OPSI.

Twenty-nine per cent of the respondents to the survey reported problems with sleeping, with smaller proportions complaining of problems with fatigue, irritability and worry. Adding the scores across the 14 domains above provides an overall score that is a measure of the severity of the symptoms; the range is 0 to 57. Scores above 12 indicate a significant level of symptom, and scores of 18 or above indicate symptoms that are likely to need treatment. Figure 5.2, (p. 88) shows the distribution of these scores; 15 per cent of the sample were above the cut-off level of 12, and 7 per cent had symptoms significant enough to warrant treatment.

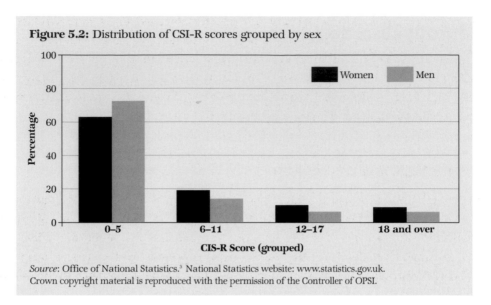

Figure 5.2: Distribution of CSI-R scores grouped by sex

Source: Office of National Statistics.[3] National Statistics website: www.statistics.gov.uk.
Crown copyright material is reproduced with the permission of the Controller of OPSI.

The types of neurotic disorders that the survey identified were mixed anxiety and depression, generalised anxiety disorder, depressive disorder, phobias, obsessive compulsive disorder, and panic disorder (see Figure 5.3). Overall, in the week preceding the survey, there were 164 cases per 1000 of neurosis, which is around 1 in 6 of all adults.

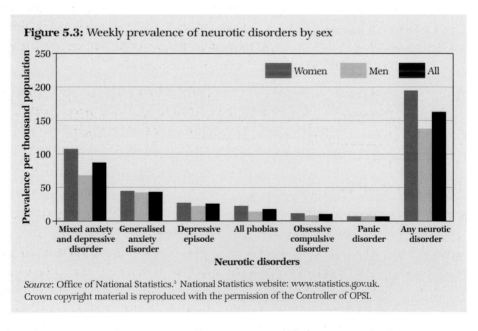

Figure 5.3: Weekly prevalence of neurotic disorders by sex

Source: Office of National Statistics.[3] National Statistics website: www.statistics.gov.uk.
Crown copyright material is reproduced with the permission of the Controller of OPSI.

There were 88 cases per 1000 of mixed anxiety and depression, a further 44 cases per 1000 had generalised anxiety disorder, 26 per 1000 had a depressive disorder, 18 per 1000 had all forms of phobia, 11 per 1000 had obsessive compulsive disorder, and 7 per 1000 had panic disorder.

The highest prevalence rates appeared amongst females aged 40–54, although men in this age range also had relatively high levels of prevalence. The study undertaken prior to the publication date of 2000 estimated variation by ethnicity, and observed that South Asian people had higher rates of neuroses, and black people lower, although in both circumstances the rates were not statistically significant. How these figures might change with differing classification of ethnicity remains unclear.

Personality disorder

The sample was relatively small, 626 individuals, but the results indicate that there were some 54 per 1000 men and 34 per 1000 women who had a personality disorder. The most common type of personality disorder was obsessive compulsive, while the least common were the dependent and schizotypal personality disorders, at a rate of only 1 per 1000. No cases of histrionic or narcissistic personality disorder were identified in the sample.

Psychoses and severe affective disorders

The sample was relatively small, and there were methodological problems with being able to identify exactly the numbers of individuals. Hence the authors of the ONS survey talked about 'probable' cases of psychoses. Nevertheless, they are able to estimate that there were likely to be 5 per 1000 women, and 6 per 1000 men, who in the year preceding the survey suffered from a probable psychotic disorder.

They were able to identify that black people had rates of psychosis that appeared to be three times greater than for white people (18 per 1000 compared with 6 per 1000), but because of the small sample size the data was not statistically significant.

Alcohol misuse

The ONS survey distinguishes between alcohol dependence and hazardous drinking. The latter was assessed using a WHO tool called the Alcohol Use Disorder Identification Test (AUDIT), and defines hazardous drinking as an established pattern of drinking that brings the risk of physical and psychological harm now or in the future. A score of 8 or above (from a range of 0 to 40) indicates that alcohol consumption is likely to be hazardous. Using this cut-off score, it was found that 38 per cent of men and 15 per cent of women were experiencing hazardous drinking. Alcohol dependence was assessed using the Severity of Alcohol Dependence Questionnaire (SAD-Q), which categorises the disorder into mild, moderate and severe dependency. Sixty-nine per 1000 were found to have mild alcohol dependence, 7 per 1000 had moderate dependence and 1 per 1000 had severe dependence. In all categories there was a statistically significant proportion of men to women, and younger age groups compared with older age groups. Young men were more likely to experience hazardous drinking and to be alcohol dependent than any other group.

Substance misuse

Any survey of private households that attempts to assess use of illegal substances is likely to be an underestimate of the prevalence. This is not only because the respondents are not likely to reply truthfully, but also because users are more likely to be living in institutions or to be homeless. Given those caveats, 27 per cent of all respondents replied that they had used illicit drugs at some time in the past; of which, a third of all men and a fifth of all women admitted use. Thirteen per cent of men and 8 per cent of women said that they had used illicit drugs in the last year.

The management of mental illness

The management of mental illness, as subsequent chapters will show, can vary from supportive talking therapy for relatively minor disturbances to the involvement of a multiprofessional team providing around-the-clock community support for those few people with very severe and complex disorders. Management can involve medication, a range of talking therapies, social care to ensure appropriate housing, access to benefits, employment, and activities of daily living. Social prescribing such as the use of exercise to manage depression is also of value. There is a multitude of different types of interventions, which will be described in more detail in later chapters, but it is important to note that the accessibility of some of these services is dependent on a referral to a specialist mental health trust. Thus access to cognitive behavioural therapy, or a multiprofessional community mental health team, is only through the individual being accepted for treatment by that mental health trust. Therefore the process of referral is of interest to both clinicians and more importantly to the patient. Which patients can be referred to a specialist mental health team? What problems are appropriate to be referred? What happens if the referral is deemed appropriate by the referring GP, or the patient, and the mental health team does not feel that it can offer any support?

To try and answer some of these questions, the appropriateness of referrals to specialist mental health services has been studied and a referral tool developed by psychiatrists working at the Institute of Psychiatry, London. This tool, the Threshold Assessment Grid (TAG), which was developed by Slade and colleagues,[6,7] provides a simple way of assessing the appropriateness of referrals to a mental health team, based on an assessment of seven domains:

1. Intentional self-harm

2. Unintentional self-harm

3. Risk from others

4. Risk to others

5. Survival needs/disabilities

6. Psychological needs/disabilities

7. Social needs/disabilities.

Domains 2, 3, 6 and 7 are scored 0–3 for increasing severity of disorder, and the remaining three domains, 1, 4 and 5, have an extra level of severity, 4, for very severe disorder, which may require immediate attention. The tool has been validated against two definitions of severe mental illness, one generated by Kendrick and colleagues (see below),[8] which is a primary care definition, and the second definition based on Department of Health (DH) guidance.[9]

Slade *et al.*'s second paper in 2002,[7] as part of the introduction to the study on validity of the TAG, makes some interesting points, which are reproduced here:

> Specialist mental health services are a scarce resource, and need to be effectively targeted towards people with more severe and enduring mental health problems. This apparently simple goal has proved difficult to achieve, yet the need to match referrals with available services is becoming more pressing: referral rates from primary to secondary care for mental health problems have increased by a factor of 4.5 from 1971 to 1997....[[10]] The difficulty in getting the right patients referred to specialist mental health services is highlighted by the mismatch between this increasing rate of referral and the patient preference for primary-care level talking therapy over medication or referral to a mental health professional....[[11]] Maximizing the proportion of appropriate referrals requires at least two developments: shared agreement about who the severely mentally ill are, and a currency for communication between primary care services (such as health and social services) and specialist mental health services.

This short paragraph makes several telling points that underline some of the difficulties experienced by professionals and more importantly the users of the service at the interface between primary and specialist care services.

- '[N]eed to be effectively targeted towards people with more severe and enduring mental health problems.'

  This is DH policy, but as the subsequent section below demonstrates there is no consistent agreement as to what constitutes 'severe mental illness'.

- '[T]he need to match referrals with available services is becoming more pressing.' The implication is that the eligibility criteria of suffering from a severe mental illness is based on managing demand, rather than delivering a service that meets the needs of the population. Since the definition is described and implemented by specialist mental health services, it serves its purpose extremely well.

- '[S]hared agreement about who the severely mentally ill are, and a currency for communication between primary care services (such as health and social services) and specialist mental health services.'

  These two developments are now much closer than the authors of the paper supposed in 2002, as there is an effective definition of severe and enduring mental illness, developed by Kendrick. There is also a currency for communication that has recently been introduced, called Practice-Based Commissioning (PBC). Although at present there is no national tariff for mental health conditions, it is clear that this is being developed and that mental health services are amongst those that should be commissioned by practices or localities through the PBC route. No doubt this opportunity will offer the chance to both primary and secondary care professionals to discuss afresh the appropriateness of referrals.

McEvoy described some of the pressures as a consequence of gate-keeping access to specialist mental health services.[12] He recognised that there were a number of factors that made it difficult to establish consistent priorities, including the uneven distribution of specialist services, the lack of a consensus on the definition of 'severe mental illness', and the difficulty in weighing the potential benefits of care for the individual against the need to ensure that resources are distributed fairly.

Severe mental illness

The term 'severe mental illness' (SMI) or 'severe and enduring mental illness' (SEMI) are used extensively by mental health professionals, and in writing about mental health, to describe those who are the most vulnerable, the most needy, the most socially excluded group of people for whom prioritisation of services is appropriate. It seems entirely reasonable that services should be directed at those who are the neediest, providing of course that this group of people can be described clearly by the term 'SMI'. Indeed there is guidance from the DH that makes this prioritisation explicit.[13–15]

Therefore there is value in being clear about the definition of the term 'severe mental illness' as it provides access to specialist mental health services, an opportunity for assessing the number of patients within the community, and as a consequence it will inform the planning of services.

The evolution of the definition

In 1987 the National Institute of Mental Health – the US department not the National Institute for Mental Health in England (NIMHE) – described how individuals could be categorised as suffering from a severe mental illness if they fulfilled three criteria:[16]

- *diagnosis* – a diagnosis of non-organic psychosis or personality disorder

- *duration* – prolonged illness and long-term treatment, and operationalised as a two-year or longer history of mental illness or treatment

- *disability* – which was described as at least three of the eight specified criteria.

In 1990 Schinnar *et al*. reviewed 18 definitions of severe mental illness by using the definitions provided by 13 authors, as applied to 222 patients receiving care in an inner-city mental health service in Philadelphia, USA.[17] They found that the range of severe mental illness varied from 4 per cent to 88 per cent, but that if the NIMH criteria were used the incidence was between 45 per cent and 55 per cent, and that this range was covered by eight of the 13 authors.

In 2000 Ruggeri and colleagues undertook a similar study but investigated patients from Verona, Italy, and Southeast London, originally part of a larger study in the early 1990s.[18] They acknowledged that ten years on from Schinnar *et al*.'s paper there was still no internationally accepted definition of severe and enduring mental illness. They refined the definition to a three-dimensional definition of:

- *diagnosis* – non-organic psychosis

- *duration* – more than two years

- *dysfunction* – as measured by the Global Assessment of Functioning, an American Psychiatric Association scale.

The legislative definition

There are a number of descriptions and definitions of mental disorder in relation to the Mental Health Act (1983) and the amended act (2007). These serve a different purpose from the definition of severe mental illness, which is used as a way of prioritising access to specialist mental health services.

The 1995 DH publication *Building Bridges: a guide to arrangements for inter-agency working for the care and protection of severely mentally ill people* defined severe mental illness as:[13]

- *diagnosis* – suffering from some sort of mental illness (typically people suffering from schizophrenia or a severe affective disorder, but including dementia)

- *disability* – suffering substantial disability as a result of their illness, such as an inability to care for themselves independently, to sustain relationships or to work

- *duration* – suffering from a chronic, enduring condition

- *informal/formal care* – having suffered recurring crises leading to frequent admissions/interventions

- *safety* – occasioning significant risk to their own safety or that of others.

It can be seen that the major change in the 1995 publication was the addition of two extra criteria, the need for care, and the aspect of safety.

The most recent definition

The most recent definition of severe mental illness can be found in the National Service Framework (NSF) for Mental Health in the following terms:[15]

- there must be a mental disorder as designated by a mental health professional (psychiatrist, mental health nurse, clinical psychologist, occupational psychologist, occupational therapist or mental health social worker) *and either*

- there must have been a score of 5 (very severe problem) on at least one, or a score of 4 (moderately severe problem) on at least two, of the Health of the Nation Outcome Scale (HoNOS) items 1–10 (excluding item 5 'physical illness or disability problems') during the previous six months *or*

- there must have been a significant level of service usage over the past five years as shown by:
  – a total of six months in a psychiatric ward or day hospital *or*
  – three admissions to hospital or day hospital *or*
  – six months of psychiatric community care involving more than one worker or the perceived need for such care if unavailable or refused.

HoNOS is an outcome measure commissioned by the DH in 1993 to measure the health and social functioning of the severely mentally ill.[19] The HoNOS has been recommended by the NSF for Mental Health, and provides scales for working-age adults, children and adolescents (HoNOSCA), the older population (HoNOS65+), the secure population (HoNOSsecure), people with learning disability (HoNOS-LD), and those with acquired brain injury (HoNOS-ABI).

HoNOS for working-age adults has 12 scales:

1. Overactive, aggressive, disruptive or agitated behaviour

2. Non-accidental self-injury

3. Problem drinking or drug-taking

4. Cognitive problems

5. Physical illness or disability problems

6. Problems associated with hallucinations and delusions

7. Problems with depressed mood

8. Other mental and behavioural problems

9. Problems with relationships

10. Problems with activities of daily living

11. Problems with living conditions

12. Problems with occupation and activities.

Each scale is rated as follows:

1. No problem

2. Minor problem requiring no action

3. Mild problem but definitely present

4. Moderately severe problem

5. Severe to very severe problem.

The definition of severe mental illness is interesting in that general practitioners are not one of the professional groups able to make the 'designation', not a diagnosis, of mental disorder, and that without this designation an individual cannot have prioritised access to specialist mental health services. The practical implication of this is that, to access specialist mental health services, a person has to have a severe mental illness, but such a designation cannot be made until the person has accessed mental health services.

The definition requires that the person has a very severe problem on one scale, or a moderately severe problem on at least two scales. This is excluding physical illness or disability. So an individual whose physical health is exacerbated by the presence of a mental disorder, sufficient to be moderately severe, would still not be 'severely mentally ill' and unlikely to have access to specialist mental health services. A person, for example, with depression and diabetes, whose diabetes was deteriorating because of his or her depression, would be unable to access specialist mental health services, even though it is there that the complex care that this person needs, in the form of psychological care, might be found.

Finally the definition depends on the subjective analysis of a mental health professional that the person might need community care, even if that care was refused or wanted by the patient him or herself.

Clearly the definition of such a complex condition is difficult, and the interpretation tends to vary from mental health trust to mental health trust, and from one mental health professional to another. In practice what seems to happen is that a referral letter is considered either by an individual in the community mental health team or by the assessment team, to decide if the conditions are met to allow access and a complete assessment by that team. It is not surprising therefore that many referrals are apparently 'bounced back' to general practitioners, saying that specialist mental health services are not appropriate. Practically, it appears that this definition is applied by most mental health trusts to mean people with psychosis and those who are suicidal. In some areas of the country where there is extreme demand for services that access is only permitted if a person is likely to be compulsorily detained under the Mental Health Act.

The primary care definition

The foregoing demonstrates that the definition of severe mental illness lies with the psychiatrists and mental health teams providing the care, not the GPs referring patients for the care that they or their patients may perceive as being appropriate. In 1995 Kendrick *et al.* published a study that included a primary care-orientated definition of severe mental illness, which, whilst retaining the characteristic 'three Ds' basis, had been amended to reflect the primary care origins of the definition:[8]

- *diagnosis* – the diagnosis may be one of the psychoses; a severe and chronic, non-psychotic disorder, including depression, anxiety and phobic disorders; obsessional neurosis; severe personality disorder; eating disorder; alcohol or drug misuse; or a mental illness that has not been given a specific label

- *duration* – one, who for two years or more, has been disabled by impaired social behaviour as a consequence of a mental illness

- *disability* – disability is the defining criterion; the patient is unable to fulfil any one of four roles:
  – holding down a job
  – self-care and personal hygiene
  – performing necessary domestic chores
  – participating in recreational activities.

The disability must be due to any one of four types of impairment of social behaviour:
– withdrawal and inactivity
– responses to hallucinations or delusions
– bizarre or embarrassing behaviour
– violence towards others or self.

This definition has much to recommend it, being both simple and also more inclusive of people who are severely affected by a mental illness. It does not require the medical label of a psychosis (designated by a mental health professional), and puts the emphasis on the explanation of what 'disability' means for the sufferer. That current policy in mental health care is to ensure social inclusion and reduce stigma is reflected by this definition, which preceded the change in emphasis of policy by nearly ten years.

Whilst the Kendrick *et al.* definition may be more acceptable, useful to primary care clinicians, and more closely reflect the needs of people who are severely affected by a mental illness, it remains an academic exercise unless there can be some way of using the definition in clinical care. One of the major roles of the definition was to provide criteria for treatment by specialist mental health services. Specialist mental health services are a provider service commissioned by the Primary Care Trust, or more recently by Practice-Based Commissioning. If commissioning is to be effective in developing services that meet the needs of the user of the service, then perhaps varying the definition of 'severe mental illness' to more closely fit Kendrick *et al.*'s diagnosis would be a useful step change in improving access to specialist mental health services.

Disability

One of the features of the definitions of 'severe mental illness' is the concept of disability. Whilst the explanation of what disability meant in the 1987 definition from the USA was clear then, there has been considerable development in the way that the term is used, as Kendrick *et al.* demonstrated in the primary care definition of SMI. The Disability Discrimination Act (DDA) (2005) further defined disability in quite specific terms.[20]

Definition of disability under the Disability Discrimination Act

The DDA defines a disabled person as someone who has a physical or mental impairment that has a substantial and long-term adverse effect on his or her ability to carry out normal day-to-day activities.

The definition

For the purposes of the act:

- substantial means neither minor nor trivial

- long term means that the effect of the impairment has lasted or is likely to last for at least 12 months (there are special rules covering recurring or fluctuating conditions)

- normal day-to-day activities include everyday things like eating, washing, walking and going shopping

- a normal day-to-day activity must affect one of the 'capacities' listed in the act, which include mobility, manual dexterity, speech, hearing, seeing and memory.

Some conditions, such as a tendency to set fires and hay fever, are specifically excluded. Provisions allow for people with a past disability to be covered by the scope of the act. There are also additional provisions relating to people with progressive conditions. The DDA amends the definition of disability, removing the requirement that a mental illness should be 'clinically well-recognised'.

People with HIV, cancer and multiple sclerosis will be deemed to be covered by the DDA effectively from the point of diagnosis, rather than from the point when the condition has some adverse effect on their ability to carry out normal day-to-day activities.

The guidance, from which the above is quoted, also makes particular reference to people with a mental impairment:

Mental illness

A9. The Act previously required that where any impairment arose from, or consisted of, a mental illness, that illness had to be clinically well-recognised in order for it to be regarded as a mental impairment for the purposes of the Act. The Disability Discrimination Act 2005 amended the original Act to remove this requirement with effect from December 2005. However, anyone who has a mental illness will still need to meet the requirements of the definition as set out in paragraph A1, in order to demonstrate that they have a disability under the Act.

This means that somebody is disabled under the DDA who has a mental health impairment (including a mental illness) that has a significant and long-term adverse effect on their ability to carry out normal day-to-day activities. This feels very like the original spirit of the 'three Ds' definition of severe mental illness: 'diagnosis, duration and disability'.

The particular areas of distinction between the 1987 US definition and the 2005 UK definition of disability lies predominantly in the fact that the diagnosis has to be a psychotic illness, or a personality disorder, rather than any mental illness.

The 1999 definition in the NSF does not specify that the diagnosis has to be a psychotic illness; it can be any mental illness, but it has to be designated by a mental health professional – not a general practitioner.[15] Further, the definition of severe mental illness, the category prioritised by the specialist mental health services, excludes from the definition the impact of the mental illness on physical health (scale 5), employment (scale 11) and accommodation (scale 12). It is these scales that have the greatest impact on an individual, on their social functioning, their inclusion into society, their opportunity to participate in a meaningful fashion, and it is these areas that are specifically excluded from the definition of severe mental illness, so that they are not taken into account when considering if a person can access specialist mental health services.

It seems perverse that the access to specialist mental health services is based on a definition of severe mental illness that excludes those aspects of disability that are most important to the people who suffer. It also seems perverse that the definition is dependent on those who provide the care, since the accuracy of the definition and its use becomes self-fulfilling. Far more effective would be a definition used by the commissioners of the service that is perhaps based on the Kendrick *et al.* definition. It would certainly make much clearer the appropriateness of the referral process, improve relationships between primary and secondary care, and more importantly provide access to specialist mental health services for a larger number of people, who currently do not benefit from some of the more specialised talking therapies.

References

1. Royal College of General Practitioners. The consultation. In: *The Future General Practitioner: learning and teaching*, p. 13, London: RCGP, 1972.

2. World Health Organization. *International Classification of Diseases*, www.who.int/classifications/icd/en/ [accessed November 2007].

3. Office of National Statistics, www.statistics.gov.uk/CCI/nscl.asp?ID=6437 [accessed November 2007].

4. Lewis G, Pelosi AJ. *Manual of the Revised Clinical Interview Schedule (CIS-R)* London: Institute of Psychiatry, 1990.

5. Lewis G, Pelosi AJ, Araya RC, *et al*. Measuring psychiatric disorder in the community: a standardised instrument for use by lay interviewers *Psychological Medicine* 1992; 22: 465–86.

6. Slade M, Powell R, Strathdee G, *et al*. Threshold Assessment Grid (TAG). The development of a valid and brief scale to assess the severity of mental illness *Social Psychiatry and Psychiatric Epidemiology* 2000; 35: 78–85.

7. Slade M, Cahill S, Kelsey W, *et al*. Threshold 2: the reliability, validity, and sensitivity to change of the Threshold Assessment Grid (TAG) *Acta Psychiatrica Scandinavica* 2002; 106: 453–60.

8. Kendrick T, Burns T, Freeling P. Randomised controlled trial of teaching general practitioners to carry out structured assessments of their long term mentally ill patients *British Medical Journal* 1995; 311: 93–7.

9. Department of Health. *National Service Framework for Mental Health* London: DH, 1999.

10. Verhaak PF, Van de Lisdonk EH, Bor JH, *et al*. GPs' referrals to mental health care during the past 25 years. *British Journal of General Practice* 2000; **50**: 307–8.

11. Brody DS, Khaliq AA, Thompson TL. Patients' perspectives on the management of emotional distress in primary care settings *Journal of General Internal Medicine* 1997; **12** 403–6.

12. McEvoy P. Gatekeeping access to services at the primary/secondary interface *Journal of Psychiatric Nursing and Mental Health* 2000; **7**: 241–7.

13. Department of Health. *Building Bridges: a guide to arrangements for inter-agency working for the care and protection of severely mentally ill people* London: DH, 1996.

14. Department of Health. *A First Class Service: quality in the new NHS* London: DH, 1998.

15. Department of Health. *A National Service Framework for Mental Health* London: DH, 1999.

16. National Institute of Mental Health. *Towards a Model for a Comprehensive Community-Based Mental Health System* Washington DC: NIMH, 1987.

17. Schinnar A, Rothbard AB, Kanter R, *et al*. An empirical literature review of definitions of severe and persistent mental illness *American Journal of Psychiatry* 1990; **147**: 1602–8.

18. Ruggeri M, Leese M, Thornicroft G, *et al*. Definition and prevalence of severe and persistent mental illness *British Journal of Psychiatry* 2000; **177**: 149–55.

19. Royal College of Psychiatrists. *Health of the Nation Outcome Scale (HoNOS)*, www.rcpsych.ac.uk/crtu/healthofthenation/whatishonos.aspx [accessed November 2007].

20. *Disability Discrimination Act. Consultation document: guidance on matters to be taken into account in determining questions relating to the definition of disability* London: Department of Work and Pensions, 2005.

6 | Common mental health problems

Paul Walters and Andre Tyleé

> **What this chapter contributes:**
>
> epidemiology of common mental health problems
>
> diagnosis and prognosis of common mental health problems
>
> managing specific common mental health problems.

Mental health problems are common in primary care. Over 90 per cent of patients with mental health problems are treated in primary care alone, and nearly 15 per cent of patients registered with a general practitioner (GP) will consult for mental health problems in any one year.[1,2] This means that common mental health problems make up a considerable part of primary care's work. Common mental health problems, or common mental disorders, are umbrella terms for the mental health problems that commonly present to primary care. These are, broadly, depression, anxiety, stress-related disorders and the somatoform disorders. This chapter will discuss the diagnosis and management of these common mental disorders.

Epidemiology of common mental health problems in primary care

Between a quarter and a half of GP attendees have at least one psychiatric disorder as defined by the ICD-10 Classification of Mental and Behavioural Disorders criteria.[3–6] Overall the prevalence of current ICD-10 disorders in the World Health Organization's (WHO) Collaborative Study of Psychological Problems in General Health Care was: depression 10.4 per cent, generalised anxiety disorder 7.9 per cent, harmful use of alcohol 3.3 per cent, alcohol dependence 2.7 per cent, somatisation disorder 2.7 per cent, panic disorder 1 per cent, agoraphobia 1.5 per cent and hypochondriasis 0.8 per cent.[7] Women were almost twice as likely as men to suffer from depression, but men were more likely to suffer from alcohol problems. In the UK general population, one in six adults suffer from a common mental disorder, the commonest being mixed anxiety and depression (7 per cent of men and 11 per cent of women), anxiety (4 per cent of men and 5 per cent of women) and depression (2 per cent of men and 3 per cent of women).[8]

Diagnosing common mental health problems in primary care

Diagnosing common mental health problems in primary care can be complex. Patients usually present with a mixture of physical and psychological symptoms such that it may be difficult to disentangle which symptoms are due to physical illness and which are due to a psychiatric illness.

Diagnosis is also complicated in primary care because of the numerous classification systems available. This can lead to confusion, especially when classifications differ from those used in guidelines. A number of different approaches have been taken to classify mental health problems in primary care. Examples of different classification systems include the International Classification of Health Problems in Primary Care (ICHPPC-2), the Read code system, specialist classification systems (e.g. ICD-10 and DSM-IV) and the ICD-10 PHC (ICD-10 Primary Health Care Version). All have limitations, but in the UK 97 per cent of practices use the Read code system, which has the advantage of allowing classification by diagnoses, symptoms and problems.[9] The main disadvantage of this is that it may be at the expense of reliability and validity.[10] In this chapter we will use the ICD-10 and ICD-10 PHC diagnostic criteria.

Prognosis of common mental health problems in primary care

Patients with mental health problems in primary care tend to have a poor prognosis and only about 25 per cent are fully recovered after 12 months. About 50 per cent have intermittent symptoms and another 25 per cent have persistent symptoms over the same period.[11] In the longer term, over 50 per cent of patients are still unwell 11 years later, with nearly 40 per cent having a relapsing or chronic course over this time.[12] In another study, 45 per cent of severely depressed patients recognised by their GP remained depressed after 12 months, and of these nearly 30 per cent remained severely depressed.[13]

Depression

By 2020 depression will be the second commonest cause of disability worldwide after ischaemic heart disease.[14] Depression, therefore, will be an ever-increasing part of the GP's and other primary care professional's workload.

Classification

The ICD-10 classifies depression as a *depressive episode* for a single episode of depression, and a *recurrent depressive disorder* for patients who have suffered repeated episodes. The ICD-10 also classifies two persistent mood disorders in which symptoms are chronic but not of the severity necessary to diagnose a depressive episode. These are *dysthymia* and *cyclothymia*. The ICD-10 classification system makes no aetiological assumptions about depression (see Box 6.1).

Box 6.1: ICD-10 classification of depression[3]

F32 Depressive episode

    F32.0 Mild depressive episode

    F32.1 Moderate depressive episode

    F32.2 Severe depressive episode without psychotic symptoms

    F32.3 Severe depressive episode with psychotic symptoms

F33 Recurrent depressive disorder

    F33.0 Recurrent depressive disorder, current episode mild

    F33.1 Recurrent depressive disorder, current episode moderate

    F33.2 Recurrent depressive disorder, current episode severe without psychotic symptoms

    F33.3 Recurrent depressive disorder, current episode severe with psychotic symptoms

    F33.4 Recurrent depressive disorder, currently in remission

F34 Persistent mood disorders

    F34.0 Cyclothymia

    F34.1 Dysthymia

Depressive episodes can be further classified according to severity as mild, moderate or severe. In the case of recurrent depressive disorders, the current episode is classified as mild, moderate or severe, e.g. recurrent depressive disorder, current episode moderate. Whether a depressive episode or recurrent depressive disorder is classified as mild, moderate or severe depends upon the number and intensity of symptoms. However, in each case symptoms must have been present for at least two weeks (see Box 6.2, p. 104).

In addition to severity, a depressive episode can be defined as having a somatic syndrome depending on the presence of somatic symptoms frequently associated with depression (see Box 6.3, p. 104). Severe depressive episodes are further classified as with or without psychotic symptoms.

Box 6.2: ICD-10 guidelines for a depressive episode or recurrent depressive disorder

At least two-week history of:

- depressed mood
- loss of interest/enjoyment
- poor energy and fatigue.

Other symptoms:

1. Reduced concentration
2. Reduced self-esteem
3. Ideas of guilt/worthlessness
4. Pessimistic views of the future
5. Ideas of self-harm/suicide
6. Disturbed sleep
7. Diminished appetite.

Mild depression: two core symptoms plus two others.

Moderate depression: two core symptoms plus three others. Depression interferes with social, work or domestic activities.

Severe depression: three core symptoms plus at least four others. Person unable to continue with social, work or domestic activities.

Source: adapted from World Health Organization. *The ICD-10 Classification of Mental and Behavioural Disorders*.[3]

Box 6.3: Somatic symptoms of depression

- Loss of interest and enjoyment.
- Loss of emotional reactivity to normally pleasurable experiences.
- Early morning waking (at least two hours earlier than usual).
- Diurnal variation in mood (often feeling worse in the mornings).
- Psychomotor retardation or agitation.
- Loss of appetite.
- Weight loss.
- Loss of libido.

At least four of these symptoms should be present to diagnose a somatic syndrome.

Diagnosis

The key diagnostic features of depression are low mood, loss of interest and enjoyment, and a reduction in energy levels. The change in mood is pervasive, though may show a diurnal variation, typically patients complaining of feeling worse in the mornings. Other typical symptoms are shown in Box 6.2. In primary care, patients often present with physical symptoms rather than with the classical symptoms of depression.[15,16] Common presenting symptoms in primary care are non-specific aches and pains, fatigue and lethargy. Often, if psychosocial problems are mentioned by patients it is towards the end of the consultation. Therefore a high index of suspicion of depression is needed in patients presenting with medically unexplained symptoms and general non-specific somatic symptoms. Patients often fail to attribute the many, often seemingly disparate, symptoms to a depressive illness, and often think they are due to a physical illness (see the section on somatisation, p. 121).

Measurement of severity

Severity of depressive episodes can be measured using a number of instruments. Using a standardised instrument has advantages over a clinical impression of severity as symptom severity, and allows comparisons to be made in subsequent consultations. In the UK, GPs are now remunerated through the Quality and Outcomes Framework (QOF) for measuring the severity of a depressive episode at baseline. The instruments recommended by the QOF for measuring severity are the Hospital Anxiety and Depression Scale (HADS),[17] the Beck Depression Inventory (BDI),[18] and the Patient Health Questionnaire-9 (PHQ-9), a short nine-question instrument.[19]

Differential diagnosis

There are many disorders that can present with depressive symptoms. Physical illnesses in which depressive symptoms are common need to be excluded, e.g. thyroid dysfunction. Medications too can cause depressive symptoms and these should be reviewed. Psychiatric disorders that can present with depression include a depressive phase of bipolar affective disorder, schizophrenia, alcohol and substance misuse, stress-related disorders such as post-traumatic stress disorder, somatoform disorders, and anxiety disorders.

Screening for depression in primary care

As of 1 April 2006, the QOF in the UK remunerates GPs for depression screening (or more correctly case-finding) in patients with ischaemic heart disease and patients with diabetes mellitus. The use of a two-question screening instrument has been recommended by the QOF. The two questions are:

1. Over the past two weeks, have you felt down, depressed or hopeless?

2. Over the past two weeks have you felt little interest or pleasure in doing things?

These questions have a sensitivity of 96 per cent and a specificity of 57 per cent.[20] Anyone screening positive needs to be clinically assessed to rule out a false positive diagnosis.

Management

The National Institute for Health and Clinical Excellence (NICE) has recommended a stepped-care approach to the management of depression:[21]

Step 1: The recognition and assessment of depression in primary care and general hospital setting. In primary care this is the responsibility of the GP and practice nurse, and should include a full risk assessment.

Step 2: The treatment of mild depression in primary care. This is the responsibility of the primary care team.

Step 3: The treatment of moderate or severe depression by the primary care team.

Step 4: Referral to, and treatment by, mental health specialists for patients with treatment-resistant, recurrent, atypical, psychotic depression or those at significant risk.

Step 5: Inpatient care or crisis team treatment for depressed patients at risk of dying through suicide or severe self-neglect.

Mild depression

For mild depressive episodes NICE has recommended watchful waiting, guided self-help, computerised cognitive behavioural therapy (cCBT), exercise or brief psychological interventions. Antidepressant medications are not recommended.

Moderate or severe depression

NICE has recommended treatment with antidepressant medication, psychological interventions such as cognitive behavioural therapy (CBT) and social support. In terms of medication, the selective serotonin reuptake inhibitors (SSRIs) are recommended as the first-line antidepressant.

Referral

Referral to specialist mental health services should be considered as an emergency for patients at serious risk to themselves or others, and for patients with psychotic depression. Referral should also be considered for patients who fail to respond to a trial of at least two antidepressants from different classes at an adequate dose for an adequate length of time (at least four weeks), and if a patient fails to respond to a combination of psychological therapy and antidepressant treatment. Because of the complexities of management, patients with co-morbid alcohol and drug misuse problems should also be considered for referral.

Anxiety disorders

Anxiety disorders are common, often chronic, and are associated with significant distress and disability. They frequently go undiagnosed and untreated in primary care.

Prevalence

Anxiety disorders are amongst the commonest mental health problems encountered in primary care. The WHO's Study of Mental Illness in General Health Care found the prevalence in consecutive primary care attenders of generalised anxiety disorder (GAD) was 7.1 per cent, agoraphobia 3.8 per cent, and panic disorder 3.5 per cent.[1] Amongst the general population, the Office for National Statistics survey found that the most common neurotic disorder was mixed anxiety and depression (8.8 per cent), followed by GAD (4.4 per cent), phobic disorders (1.8 per cent) and panic disorder (0.7 per cent).[8]

Factors associated with GAD are being divorced, living alone or being a lone parent. GAD is commonest between the ages of 35 and 54 years, and is about twice as common in women as in men.[7,8] Agoraphobia, too, is about twice as prevalent in women. There does not appear to be a sex difference in the prevalence of panic disorder.

Classification

In the ICD-10 classification, anxiety disorders are classified under 'Neurotic, stress-related and somatoform disorders' (see Box 6.4, p. 108).[3]

Essentially, the anxiety disorders can be divided into three main disorders: phobic disorders, panic disorder and GAD (with or without panic disorder). Though, as with most classification systems, divisions between these disorders appear quite distinct, in practice and especially in primary care these distinctions are frequently blurred. Symptoms of anxiety, depression and panic attacks often all co-exist and it can be difficult to determine which disorder if any is predominant. A detailed history of the chronology of symptoms may help primary care professionals come to a firm diagnosis. This may require a number of consultations. Complicating diagnosis further, anxiety is an important symptom of most other mental disorders. In depressed patients attending their GP, over half (57 per cent) had significant symptoms of anxiety.[22]

Box 6.4: ICD-10 classification of neurotic, stress-related and somatoform disorders (abbreviated)[3]

F40 Phobic anxiety disorders

    F40.0 Agoraphobia

        F40.00 without panic disorder

        F40.01 with panic disorder

    F40.1 Social phobia

    F40.2 Specific phobia

    F40.8 Other phobic anxiety disorders

    F40.9 Phobic anxiety disorder, unspecified

F41 Other anxiety disorders

    F41.0 Panic disorder

    F41.1 Generalised anxiety disorder

F41.2 Mixed anxiety and depressive disorder

F41.3 Other mixed anxiety disorders

F41.8 Other specified anxiety disorders

F41.9 Anxiety disorder, unspecified

F42 Obsessive-compulsive disorder

F43 Reaction to severe stress, and adjustment disorders

    F43.0 Acute stress reaction

    F43.1 Post-traumatic stress disorder

    F43.2 Adjustment disorders

    F43.8 Other reactions to severe stress

    F43.9 Reaction to severe stress, unspecified

F44 Dissociative (conversion) disorders

F45 Somatoform disorders

    F45.0 Somatisation disorder

    F45.1 Undifferentiated somatoform disorder

    F45.2 Hypochondriacal disorder

    F45.3 Somatoform autonomic dysfunction

    F45.4 Persistent somatoform pain disorder

    F45.8 Other somatoform disorders

    F45.9 Somatoform disorder, unspecified

F48 Other neurotic disorders

Generalised anxiety disorder

Diagnosis

As in depressed patients, patients with GAD often present with somatic symptoms associated with anxiety (e.g. headaches, muscle aches due to muscle tension, palpitations). The key feature of GAD however is 'free-floating' anxiety: anxiety that is persistent and not directly related to a particular stressor (though is often associated with chronic environmental stresses). Anxiety can be split into three components: apprehension (e.g. worries about the future, poor concentration, irritability, excessive worrying over minor problems, disturbed sleep); muscle tension (e.g. tension headaches, other aches and pains such as backache, restlessness, trembling, feeling shaky); autonomic hyperactivity (e.g. palpitations, nausea, feelings of suffocation or choking, attacks of shortness of breath, sweating, lightheadedness, dry mouth).

Patients should have been symptomatic for at least a number of weeks, though usually will have been present for months and typically 5–10 years before diagnosis. GAD frequently runs a fluctuating course, exacerbated by times of stress.

Differential diagnosis

Anxiety may be a presenting symptom of many physical illnesses (e.g. thyrotoxicosis) and is also common in alcohol and substance misuse disorders. Other common differential diagnoses include depression, panic disorder, phobic disorders and post-traumatic stress disorder.

As anxiety is a common symptom of depression it is important that this is excluded, and if low mood accompanied by other symptoms consistent with a depressive disorder are the central features of the presentation then these should take priority. Likewise if intermittent panic attacks, or anxiety provoked by particular stimuli, are the main symptoms then panic disorder or a phobic disorder should be considered.

Management

General management

Information about GAD should be provided to help the patient make an informed choice about treatment options. Patients should be encouraged to limit caffeine intake and stop alcohol and substances of misuse. Anxiety management and relaxation training may be helpful, and physical exercise should be encouraged. Problem solving may also be useful. If sleep disturbance is a problem patients should be educated in good sleep hygiene habits. Patients should be encouraged to use self-help materials to cope with anxiety. There is evidence that psychological interventions have the longest duration of effect, followed by pharmacological therapy and then self-help.[23]

Psychological treatments

CBT has the largest evidence base for clinical effectiveness and has better long-term outcomes than medication alone.

Medication

Benzodiazepines should not normally be prescribed for anxiety disorders unless immediate relief from anxiety is necessary. If they are used, they should not be prescribed for longer than 2–4 weeks.

SSRIs are the first-line pharmacological treatment for GAD. However, patients with GAD may initially suffer an exacerbation in symptoms when first started and they should be warned of this. Starting at a low dose may minimise any exacerbation (though this should then be gradually increased to the treatment dose).

Self-help

Bibliotherapy, self-help groups and exercise may be of benefit.[22]

Referral

If a patient fails to respond to at least two interventions then referral to specialist mental health services should be considered.

Panic disorder

Panic disorder is characterised by episodic panic attacks. A panic attack is a subjective feeling of terror and anxiety accompanied by somatic symptoms that reach a crescendo before dying away. An unexpected panic attack is defined as one that isn't immediately associated with a situational trigger, either external or internal.[23] Panic disorder can be extremely disabling with up to 50 per cent of sufferers no longer able to drive and 75 per cent having to give up their employment.[24]

Diagnosis

Symptoms of panic include palpitations, chest pain, feelings of choking or suffocation, dizziness often accompanied by an intense fear of impending death, loss of control or of going mad. The symptoms start rapidly reaching a crescendo. They can last from minutes to an hour and frequently the sufferer will be left exhausted after the attack. The person is left with an extreme fear of having another.

To diagnose panic disorder the patient must have suffered several attacks over a period of a month or longer, and be relatively free from anxiety between attacks. Panic attacks should not be triggered by predictable situations.[2]

Differential diagnosis

The symptoms associated with panic attacks can be caused by many medical conditions. These include cardiovascular disease, asthma, exacerbations of chronic obstructive pulmonary disease, cerebrovascular disease and endocrine disorders such as thyrotoxicosis. Panic attacks may also accompany alcohol and substance misuse, and as part of a withdrawal syndrome. To further complicate diagnosis, panic attacks may be symptomatic of depression, phobic disorders and post-traumatic stress disorder. Careful history taking, examination and relevant investigations to exclude physical illness are usually necessary to confirm the diagnosis, though repeated investigations should be avoided. If a patient meets criteria for a depressive episode, then this should be diagnosed rather than panic disorder. However, depression is also a relatively common sequelae of panic disorder and nearly 50 per cent of patients with panic disorder go on to develop co-morbid depression. Again, attention to the chronology of symptoms should enable the correct diagnosis to be made.

Management
General management
The general management strategies are the same as for GAD. Patients should be educated about the 'panic cycle' and given information on panic disorder. They should be taught self-help techniques such as breathing and relaxation exercises that they can perform if they feel a panic attack starting. They should be advised to avoid caffeine, alcohol and drugs of misuse, and should be reviewed regularly. A stepped-care approach, as for GAD, should be taken.

Psychological treatment
As for GAD, CBT is the psychological treatment of choice for panic disorder.

Medication
An SSRI licensed for panic disorder is the first choice. If a patient fails to respond to an SSRI then imipramine or clomipramine may be considered.

Self-help
Bibliotherapy based on the principles of CBT, self-help groups and computerised CBT, where available, may be of benefit.

Referral
If a patient fails to respond to at least two interventions then referral to specialist mental health services should be considered.

Phobic anxiety disorders

Phobic disorders are a group of disorders characterised by anxiety in response to a specific external stimulus. The degree of anxiety is beyond that which would normally be expected. There are three symptom components to phobic anxiety disorders; *anxiety* in response to a specific stimulus that results in *avoidance* and *anticipatory anxiety* of the stimulus.

Phobias are often co-morbid with depression, and may be a symptom of depression. Phobic disorders affect about 2 per cent of women and 1 per cent of men.[25]

Agoraphobia

Agoraphobia is not restricted to the fear of open spaces, but includes the fear of crowds and public places, travelling on buses, trains, cars or planes, and leaving or being alone at home. Patients suffering from agoraphobia often fear a lack of an immediate exit from the anxiety-provoking situation.

Diagnosis

The main clinical feature of agoraphobia, as with other phobias, is the avoidance of the feared situation and anticipatory anxiety associated with that situation. This can be very disabling with patients avoiding leaving their houses. This in itself can interfere with their ability to get appropriate help.

Social phobia

Social phobia is the only phobic disorder equally common in men and women. Its onset is usually earlier than agoraphobia, often starting in adolescence.

Diagnosis

Anxiety only occurs in social situations, such as being in small groups, eating in public, public speaking or social encounters with members of the opposite sex.[3] Patients become anxious that they are being scrutinised by others and often feel the symptoms of their anxiety are visible to others (shaking, blushing, sweating, etc.). This results in a 'vicious circle' leading to avoidance of the particular social situations.

Differential diagnosis of phobic anxiety disorders

Depression often coexists with phobias, and may be a symptom of depression if they develop within the context of a depressive episode. Panic attacks may be a feature of agoraphobia and social phobias. As with any anxiety disorder alcohol and substance misuse should be ruled out before making a diagnosis.

Management of phobic anxiety disorders

Self-help measures for dealing with anxiety may be useful. Patients should be informed of the link between avoiding the feared situation and its role as a maintaining factor. Management should include a systematic programme of gradual exposure together with relaxation techniques to help deal with the accompanying anxiety. Patients should be encouraged to gradually increase their exposure to the feared situation. It is useful if specific goals are set out in the programme, starting with small goals and gradually increasing as they learn to tolerate and overcome their anxiety associated with each goal. Patients may need frequent review to support them in attaining each goal. Social skills training may be helpful for patients with social phobia.[26]

As with other anxiety disorders CBT-based bibliotherapy may be helpful. If panic attacks are a significant feature of the phobia then management strategies, as for panic disorder, should be followed.

Medications should rarely be required. If they are, benzodiazepines should be avoided and treatment with an SSRI or tricyclic antidepressant may be helpful. Beta blockers can help treat the autonomic responses to anxiety but do little for the psychological experience of anxiety. Medications may also be helpful if there is a significant mood component to their presentation.

Referral

Patients should be referred if they fail to respond to treatment in primary care, or when symptoms are so severe that the patient is housebound, making treatment in primary care unrealistic.[26]

Mixed anxiety and depressive disorder

In the ICD-10 classification, mixed anxiety and depressive disorder is a category reserved for patients who suffer from both anxiety and depressive symptoms with neither predominating. This is the commonest mental health problem in the community with a population prevalence of 8.8 per cent.[25]

Diagnosis

Mixed anxiety and depressive disorder should be diagnosed when there are significant symptoms of both depression and anxiety, but *neither* are severe enough to constitute a depressive disorder or an anxiety disorder in their own right.

Differential diagnosis

If symptoms meet criteria for a depressive episode or anxiety disorder then this should be diagnosed rather than mixed anxiety and depressive disorder. Alcohol and substance misuse disorders should be excluded. If the symptoms are a response to a particular stressor then an adjustment disorder may be the more appropriate diagnosis.

Management

NICE recommends following its stepped-care depression guidelines for patients with mixed anxiety and depressive disorder as above.[21]

Obsessive-compulsive disorder

Obsessive-compulsive disorder (OCD) has a community prevalence of about 1 per cent and is more common in women (61 per cent).[25] It often runs a chronic fluctuating course.

Obsessions are recurrent, unwanted, intrusive ideas, images or impulses. The thoughts are distressing because of their nature, and patients will frequently try unsuccessfully to resist them. The commonest obsessions in OCD are a fear of contamination (38 per cent), fear of harm (24 per cent), a need for order and symmetry (10 per cent), obsessions about physical symptoms (7 per cent), obsessions of a religious or blasphemous nature (6 per cent), sexual thoughts (6 per cent), urges to hoard (5 per cent) and violent or aggressive thoughts (4 per cent).[27]

Compulsions can be thought of as the motor equivalent to obsessions, and are repetitive acts or rituals that the patient feels compelled to perform. They are recognised by patients as being pointless and, initially at least, they will attempt to resist the compulsion, often with mounting anxiety until the act is completed. Compulsions are purposeless apart from minimising anxiety and are not in themselves pleasurable. The most common compulsions are checking (e.g. doors locked, cooker switched off) (30 per cent), cleaning and washing (27 per cent), mental compulsions, such as repeating special words (11 per cent), ordering objects (6 per cent), hoarding and/or collecting (4 per cent), and counting (2 per cent). Patients often have a combination of compulsions and obsessions.

Diagnosis

Obsession and/or compulsions must have been present on most days over a two-week period for a diagnosis to be made. The distressing symptoms should be severe enough to disable the patient in some way. Patients with OCD should have insight into their obsessions and compulsions as being unreasonable.

Differential diagnosis

Obsessions and compulsions are also common symptoms of depression. Complicating diagnosis, depression and OCD are often co-morbid. In determining whether symptoms are secondary to depression or co-morbid with depression, the chronology of symptom development can help. Other anxiety disorders and psychotic disorders should also be considered.

Management
Psychological Treatments

For patients with mild impairment NICE recommends brief, low-intensity CBT. This may be with structured self-help materials, or with therapy by phone or in a group. For those patients with moderate impairment more intensive CBT with exposure and response prevention (ERP) is recommended, and for patients with severe impairment CBT with ERP may be combined with medication.[27]

Medication

For patients with moderate impairment an SSRI may be used, either alone or in combination with a course of CBT. In patients with severe impairment a combination of an SSRI with CBT should be used.

Referral

Referral to specialist mental health services should be considered for patients with severe OCD, patients with co-morbidity and those that fail to respond to initial treatment strategies.

Reactions to stress

These include acute stress reactions, adjustment disorders and post-traumatic stress disorder. The prevalence of these disorders in primary care is unclear.

Acute stress reactions

Acute stress reactions are defined in ICD-10 as transient reactions in response to 'exceptional physical and/or mental stress'. Symptoms usually last for hours or sometimes days.[3]

Diagnosis

For an acute stress reaction to be diagnosed there must be a clear temporal connection between the stressor and the onset of symptoms. This is usually within a few minutes of the stressor. Initially there is a state of 'daze', which may be accompanied by confusion. This can be followed by depression symptoms, anxiety, anger, despair, withdrawal and/or hyperactivity. The symptoms are usually time-limited and resolve rapidly within hours, or if the stressor continues by 2–3 days.[3]

Management

Acute stress reactions are by definition time-limited and so no specific intervention is usually necessary. Patients should be reassured on the time-limited nature of the symptoms and, where appropriate, may benefit from advice about managing the practical implications of the stressor and on managing the stressor itself.[26]

If the symptoms are so severe that the patient is unable to tolerate them then a short course (three days or less) of a low-dose benzodiazepine may be considered. There is no evidence that critical-incident debriefing has any beneficial effect.[26]

Adjustment disorders

Adjustment disorders are 'states of subjective distress and emotional disturbance, usually interfering with social functioning and performance, and arising in the period of adaptation to a significant life change or the consequences of a stressful life-event'.[3]

Diagnosis

The onset of symptoms should be within a month of the stressful experience or life change and symptoms should not last longer than six months. The clinical presentation can vary with symptoms of depression, anxiety, worry, anger and difficulty coping, resulting in social or occupational disability. The symptoms should not be severe enough to justify a diagnosis of a depressive or anxiety disorder.

Management

The management of adjustment disorders is similar to that for acute stress reactions. Counselling may be helpful to assist the patient 'work through' the effects of the stressor. The patient should be encouraged to return to life as normal as soon as possible. Problem-solving strategies may also help the patient tackle the aftermath of the stressful experience.[26]

Post-traumatic stress disorder

PTSD is a disorder that arises as a result of exposure to a 'stressful event or situation of an exceptionally threatening or catastrophic nature, which is likely to cause pervasive distress in almost anyone'.[3] Up to 30 per cent of people will develop PTSD following exposure to a severely traumatic experience. There is little data available on the incidence or prevalence of PTSD in the UK, but in the USA and Australia the 12-month prevalence is 3.6 per cent and 1.3 per cent respectively.[28] The onset of symptoms following the traumatic experience can be months later, though onset is rarely longer than six months after the trauma. PTSD frequently runs a fluctuating course, though prognosis is usually good.

Diagnosis

For a diagnosis of PTSD to be made the patient must have been exposed to a severely traumatic event within the previous six months. Typical symptoms of PTSD include persistent, repetitive and intrusive 'reliving' of the trauma through memories, 'flashbacks' and/or dreams. Patients can feel emotionally detached and often complain of feeling 'numb'. This is accompanied by anhedonia and an avoidance of circumstances associated with the trauma. Autonomic hyperarousal, hypervigilance and insomnia are common. Symptoms of depression and anxiety are also common, and PTSD may be complicated by alcohol or drug misuse.[3]

In primary care, patients often present with symptoms of depression, anxiety, somatic complaints, irritability or sleep problems.[28] The diagnosis of PTSD may be missed unless the occurrence of a traumatic event is specifically asked about. The NICE PTSD guidelines recommend that a traumatic experience be asked about in any patient repeatedly presenting with unexplained somatic symptoms.[28]

Differential diagnosis

Other disorders that may be caused by exposure to a traumatic event include depression, anxiety disorders (especially phobic anxiety disorder and GAD) and adjustment disorders. Psychosis may also present with symptoms similar to those found in PTSD.

Management

For patients with mild symptoms of less than four weeks' duration, watchful waiting should be considered with a follow-up appointment arranged within a month. For patients with more severe and disabling symptoms, or with symptoms that do not resolve within four weeks, psychological treatments and medication can be used.[28]

Psychological treatments

Trauma-focused CBT or eye movement desensitisation and reprocessing (EMDR) are the psychological treatments for which there is the largest evidence base.

Medication

Medication should be used in patients who express this as a preference over psychological treatments, or in those who fail to engage in psychological treatments. NICE recommends paroxetine or mirtazapine for general use, and amitriptyline or phenelzine for use by mental health specialists. It may take up to eight weeks for patients to improve.

Referral

Referral should be considered for patients with severe or complicated PTSD and those who fail to respond to initial treatment strategies.

Eating disorders

The two main eating disorders are anorexia nervosa (AN) and bulimia nervosa (BN). The community prevalence of AN in the UK is unclear but a community prevalence of AN in Sweden was found to be 0.7 per cent in females and 0.1 per cent in men.[29] In the UK the community prevalence of BN has been estimated at between 0.5 per cent and 1 per cent, with 90 per cent being female.[30] A GP with a list of 2000 patients could expect to have two patients with AN and seven with BN.[31]

Diagnosis

AN is characterised by deliberate weight loss. It most commonly affects adolescent girls and young women. AN presents as:

- a body mass index (kg/[height(m)^2]) of 17.5 or less

- the weight loss is self-induced through dieting. Patients may also induce vomiting, purge, use excessive exercise and/or appetite suppressants and diuretics

- patients have a morbid fear of being fat and a distorted body image, and aim for a low body weight

- women may have amenorrhoea due to endocrine dysfunction. They may also have elevated levels of growth hormone, changes in thyroid hormone and abnormalities in insulin secretion.[3]

BN is characterised by recurrent food binges followed by compensatory vomiting, purging, fasting, exercise, or the misuse of laxatives or stimulants to prevent weight gain. The body mass index should not drop below 17.5 kg/m^2, in which case a diagnosis of AN should be made in precedence. For BN to be diagnosed the following should be present:

- a persistent preoccupation with eating together with a craving for food. Patients are unable to resist the cravings, resulting in large quantities of food being consumed over short periods of time

- patients then purge by inducing vomiting, using purgatives or appetite suppressants, diuretics or thyroxine

- as in AN there is a preoccupation with weight and a morbid fear of being fat.[3]

Differential diagnosis

Physical illnesses that cause weight loss should be considered (e.g. malabsorption syndromes, inflammatory bowel disease, diabetes mellitus and other chronic debilitating diseases). Depressive disorders, personality disorders, anxiety disorders, OCD, and substance misuse disorders may be co-morbid with eating disorders.

Management

Anorexia nervosa

The majority of patients with AN are referred on to specialist mental health services. Patients with AN can be difficult to treat as they are frequently ambivalent about treatment and often deny they have a problem. Patients should be educated about food and weight, and weighed regularly. Rate of weight loss should be recorded together with any physical signs of malnutrition. Routine blood tests should be conducted in case of metabolic disturbances secondary to malnutrition. The family may play an important supportive role.

NICE recommends cognitive analytic therapy, CBT, interpersonal psychotherapy, focal psychodynamic therapy or family interventions focused on eating disorders. These should be of at least six months' duration.[32]

Bulimia nervosa

Initially patients should be encouraged to use cognitive behaviour-based self-help books written specifically for BN. Patients should be seen regularly whilst working through these to monitor progress and provide support and encouragement. If unsuccessful then formal CBT for BN should be considered. This should be of 16 to 20 sessions over the course of four to five months.

Antidepressant medications can reduce the frequency of binge eating and purging, and fluoxetine can be used as an alternative first step or in addition to self-help bibliotherapy. Doses are higher than for depression, e.g. fluoxetine 60 mg. Patients should improve in 2–4 weeks if there is going to be a beneficial effect. If patients with BN are vomiting frequently or using laxatives, urea and electrolytes should be monitored.[32]

Referral

Referral should be considered for patients who fail to respond to initial treatment strategies, and urgent referral for those physically unwell as a result of an eating disorder.

Personality disorders

Personality disorders are deeply ingrained, pervasive, maladaptive personality traits that have a detrimental effect on the patient and/or others. They tend to manifest in adolescence and continue into adulthood. Personality disorders appear relatively common in primary care, with 24 per cent of consecutive attenders diagnosed as having a personality disorder.[33] Patients with personality disorders tend to be high healthcare utilisers, and personality disorder is associated with other common mental disorders.

Diagnosis

For a personality disorder to be diagnosed the patient has to display problematic attitudes and behaviour in several areas of functioning such as emotions, arousal, impulse control and ways of relating to others. Personality traits are enduring, and not limited to episodes of mental illness. They result in considerable personal, social and/or occupational disability.

Personality disorders can be broadly divided into three groups because of similarities and overlap of personality traits that the disorders within each group demonstrate:

group A: paranoid and schizoid personality disorder

group B: dissocial (antisocial), emotionally unstable (impulsive type and borderline type) and histrionic personality disorders

group C: anankastic (obsessive), anxious (avoidant) and dependent personality disorders.

In primary care, groups B and C most commonly come to attention. Group B often does so because of impulsive self-harm attempts, or with co-morbid alcohol or substance misuse and/or dependence. Group C does so because of excessive anxiety or the drive to have dependency needs met by others including primary care professionals.[3]

Differential diagnosis

Many mental health problems are accompanied by changes in personality (e.g. depression, anxiety, substance misuse). However, the history should reveal whether changes in personality are enduring and longstanding, or more recent and in the context of another mental health problem. If they are in the context of another mental health problem then personality disorder should not be diagnosed and the mental health problem takes precedence.

Management

Management is often difficult as the problematic characteristics are usually longstanding and deeply engrained. Clear boundaries between health professional and patient are vital. For patients with emotionally unstable personality disorder it is often useful to have an agreed crisis management plan that all members of the team should be aware of. Particular management plans are dependent upon individual patients, their type of personality disorder and their particular personal, social and occupational problems.[26]

Psychological treatments

These are usually the mainstay of treatment for patients with severe personality problems. Therapies include psychodynamic (insight-orientated) therapy, dialectical behaviour therapy, and cognitive analytic therapy.

Medication

For patients with emotionally unstable personality disorder SSRIs have been used to decrease impulsive behaviour. Low-dose antipsychotics have also been used to decrease levels of arousal and occasionally mood stabilisers in patients with marked affective lability.

Referral

Referral should be considered for any patient at ongoing risk of self-harm or harm to others, or for patients with co-morbid mental illnesses or substance misuse disorders.

Somatisation and the somatoform disorders

Somatisation can be defined as the expression of psychological distress through physical symptoms. It is common in primary care, and patients with mental health problems more often present physical symptoms at the onset of a psychiatric illness.[15] Therefore a high index of suspicion of mental health problems should be maintained for all patients presenting with unexplained somatic symptoms.

Somatoform disorders proper (as opposed to somatisation [see p. 123]) also appear to be common in primary care. One study of Dutch general practice found a prevalence of somatoform disorders of 16 per cent with significant co-morbidity with anxiety and depression.[34] The Manchester arm of the WHO Collaborative Study of Mental Illness in General Health Care found a prevalence in consecutive GP attenders of 0.4 per cent for somatisation disorder, 0.5 per cent for hypochondriasis and 9.7 per cent for neurasthenia.[7] Somatoform disorders are about three times more common in women.

Classification

The classification of somatoform disorders is complicated because people with mental disorders (especially depressive and anxiety disorders) commonly present with physical symptoms, especially in primary care. The classification of somatoform disorders has been criticised and there has been debate about the face validity and practical utility of these diagnoses. It has been argued that, given the frequency with which mental disorders present with somatic complaints, the somatoform disorder diagnoses could be subsumed under symptoms of other mental disorders.[35] Though ICD-10 attempts to remove aetiological assumptions from the classification of mental disorders (with the exception of the stress-related disorders), there is an underlying assumption within the somatoform disorders that symptoms are secondary to a mental health problem. This in effect reinforces the Cartesian mind–body dichotomy rather than accepting that physical symptoms are a 'normal' feature of many mental disorders and vice versa. This dichotomy is also of dubious clinical use since patients often find it difficult to accept that physical symptoms may be the result of a mental health problem. With this in mind, ICD-10 classifies the somatoform disorders as shown in Box 6.5.

Box 6.5: ICD-10 classification of somatoform disorders[3]

F45 Somatisation disorder

    F45.1 Undifferentiated somatoform disorder

    F45.2 Hypochondriacal disorder

    F45.3 Somatoform autonomic dysfunction

        F45.30 Heart and cardiovascular system

        F45.31 Upper gastrointestinal tract

        F45.32 Lower gastrointestinal tract

        F45.33 Respiratory system

        F45.34 Genitourinary system

        F45.38 Other organ system

F45.4 Persistent somatoform pain disorder

F45.8 Other somatoform disorders

F45.9 Somatoform disorder, unspecified

Diagnosis

Somatoform disorders are characterised by frequent consultations for physical symptoms for which no physical cause can be found. Patients often request further investigations despite adequate investigations being completed with negative findings.[3] In primary care, the GP is faced with the difficult task of determining whether unexplained somatic symptoms are due to a physical illness, are symptoms of another mental disorder such as an anxiety or depressive disorder, or are core symptoms of a somatoform disorder. The task is further complicated by significant co-morbidity between the somatoform, depressive and anxiety disorders.

Somatisation disorder

Patients must have had at least two years of multiple, changing physical symptoms with no identifiable physical cause. Patients cannot be reassured and their symptoms result in significant impairment.

Undifferentiated somatoform disorder

This diagnosis is reserved for patients who have multiple unexplainable physical symptoms but not of the severity required for somatisation disorder either in number of symptoms, requests for further investigations and/or impairment as a result of the symptoms.

Hypochondriacal disorder

Patients with hypochondriacal disorder have a conviction that they have a serious physical illness. They present with persistent physical symptoms that may be due to a misevaluation of normal bodily sensations. Patients cannot be reassured that there is no underlying pathology and seek repeated investigations and examinations, often from a number of doctors.

The emphasis on having a serious underlying illness distinguishes patients with hypochondriacal disorder from those with somatisation disorder. There is also an emphasis on finding the nature of the underlying illness rather than on symptom relief, whereas in somatisation disorder the patient emphasises symptom relief rather than a search for the underlying cause.

Body dysmorphic disorder also falls under this category. In body dysmorphic disorder patients hold a strong belief that there is something wrong with their physical appearance. Patients cannot be reassured and may attempt to rectify the perceived problem, sometimes through plastic surgery.

Somatoform autonomic dysfunction

The physical symptoms in this disorder are associated with one organ system under the control of the autonomic nervous system (see Box 6.4, p. 108). In addition, ICD-10 guidelines require autonomic arousal (e.g. flushing, sweating, tremor, palpitations), and a preoccupation with the possibility of having a serious disorder that is not amenable to reassurance despite adequate examinations and investigations, all of which are negative.

Disorders that fall under this diagnosis include 'cardiac neurosis' and irritable bowel syndrome.

Persistent somatoform pain disorder

In this disorder patients complain of persistent and severe pain for which no underlying physical cause can be found. There is often an element of secondary gain associated with the painful symptoms and the patient's history often reveals evidence of psychosocial problems.

Differential diagnosis

The main differential diagnosis is of an underlying physical problem causing the symptoms. Clinical judgement is necessary to decide which investigations are necessary to exclude a physical cause, though multiple referrals to medical specialists and multiple investigations should be avoided. The patient's physical condition should be kept under review so that any emerging physical illness is not missed.

Other differential diagnoses include a depressive disorder, anxiety disorder, substance misuse disorder and a psychotic disorder.

Management

The most important, and difficult, part of managing somatoform disorders is making the diagnosis. Once a diagnosis has been made the management of all somatoform disorders is similar. Though relief from symptoms should be a goal, this is not always attainable, and it is therefore important to limit iatrogenic harm caused by unnecessary investigations and treatments. Primary care is well placed to manage patients with somatoform disorders as it can coordinate the patient's care. A strong therapeutic alliance with the patient is vital in order to do this.

Reduction of disability and rehabilitation should be the aim of treatment rather than a search for a 'cure'. A search for a 'cure' can result in the doctor becoming frustrated as successive attempts at symptom relief fail, or work initially only for another set of symptoms to manifest. Patients should be offered appointments at regular intervals so that their care is not dependent on them presenting with symptoms.

One model of treatment for somatisation is the reattribution model.[36] This has three stages:

Stage 1

The first stage is to help the patient feel understood. This can be accomplished by taking a detailed history and examination, exploring a typical pain day, asking about associated symptoms, looking at his or her health beliefs and at any family or social issues.

Stage 2

In the second stage the doctor broadens the agenda by acknowledging the reality of the pain, feeding back the results of the examination and any investigations (which are usually negative or non-specific), and summarises any mood symptoms and life events.

Stage 3

The third stage involves the doctor helping the patient to make the link between his or her physical symptoms, social stresses, life events and/or symptoms of depression or anxiety. This can be done in a number of ways. A practical demonstration of how depressive or anxious symptoms can cause physical symptoms may be given, or the pain can be related to the 'here and now', life events or stresses in the family.

Once the patient has made the link then problems in the patient's life that act to reinforce and perpetuate symptoms can be tackled. At this stage it may be useful to obtain the help of a practice counsellor or psychologist, though this should not be at the expense of regular contact with the GP.

Referral

Referral to a mental health specialist (a liaison psychiatrist may be most appropriate) should be considered for any patients whose symptoms cause significant disability in terms of social or occupational functioning, and have not responded to treatment in primary care. Sometimes a joint appointment with GP and psychiatrist can be helpful. Patients with a persistent somatoform pain disorder may benefit from referral to a multidisciplinary pain clinic if available.

Chronic fatigue syndrome

Chronic fatigue syndrome (a.k.a. myalgic encephalomyelitis (ME), post-viral fatigue syndrome and neurasthenia) is a disorder characterised by severe persistent fatigue. Though symptoms of feeling tired all the time are relatively common, the prevalence of chronic fatigue syndrome in community and primary care populations is about 0.2 per cent, and is up to twice as common in women.[37] Prognosis can be poor. Up to 50 per cent of patients show some improvement, but only 6 per cent return to a pre-morbid level of functioning.

Diagnosis

To make a diagnosis patients should have:

- severe, disabling fatigue of at least six months' duration that affects both physical and mental functioning, and is present for more than 50 per cent of the time

- other symptoms such as myalgia, sleep and mood disturbance may be present.[35]

Differential diagnosis

Chronic fatigue syndrome should not be diagnosed if there is an underlying cause of the fatigue, such as a physical illness, anorexia or bulimia nervosa, or psychotic disorder. Other disorders that can present with severe fatigue include depression, the anxiety disorders and somatoform disorders. Depression is frequently co-morbid with chronic fatigue syndrome.

Management

The main evidence-based treatment strategies for managing chronic fatigue syndrome are graded exercise programmes and CBT. There is little evidence for the efficacy of steroids, antidepressants, dietary supplements or immunotherapy; prolonged rest should be discouraged. A detailed daily record of activities over a period of weeks should be kept by the patient. This will often show an 'all or nothing' pattern of activities with the patient doing as much as possible when feeling less tired, followed by periods of complete incapacitation due to fatigue. It is important that patients avoid this by scheduling activities *regularly* that are not over-strenuous. These can then be slowly built up using the activity records.

Referral

Services for patients with chronic fatigue syndrome vary. In some areas specialist clinics are run by physicians, in others by psychiatrists. Patients should be referred if symptoms are disabling and fail to respond to such measures as a graded exercise programme.

Conclusion

Mental health problems are common in primary care and make up a considerable part of primary care professionals' workload. Though common, they cause significant suffering and disability. There is an increasing evidence base for the effect management of these disorders in primary care. Paradoxically, despite the growing evidence for effective treatments, access to many of these treatments in primary care, especially psychological therapies, remains limited. Though guidelines emphasise the importance of the patient's preferences in deciding which treatment options to pursue, the realities of treatment availability mean, in practice, choices are limited. Layard has recently documented the difficulties in accessing psychological therapies and estimated the expansion in services necessary to provide treatment in line with national guidelines.[38] He has estimated that an extra 10,000 therapists would be needed, and has recommended the establishment of 250 'psychological treatment centres' across England. The challenge then is not only pursuing more effective treatments, but also, perhaps more importantly, being able to provide the treatments already proven effective to patients in primary care.

References

1. Shepherd M, Cooper B, Brown AC, *et al*. *Psychiatric Illness in General Practice* London: Oxford University Press, 1966.

2. Goldberg D, Huxley P. *Common Mental Disorders: a biosocial model* London: Routledge, 1992.

3. World Health Organization. *The ICD-10 Classification of Mental and Behavioural Disorders: clinical descriptions and diagnostic guidelines* Geneva: WHO, 1992.

4. Freeling P, Rao BM, Paykel ES, *et al*. Unrecognised depression in general practice *British Medical Journal (Clinical Research Ed.)* 1985; **290(6485)**: 1880–3.

5. Blacker CV, Clare AW. Depressive disorder in primary care *British Journal of Psychiatry* 1987; **150**: 737–51.

6. Tiemens BG, Ormel J, Simon GE. Occurrence, recognition, and outcome of psychological disorders in primary care *American Journal of Psychiatry* 1996; **153(5)**: 636–44.

7. Ustun TB, Sartorius N (eds). *Mental Illness in General Health Care: an international study* Chichester: John Wiley & Sons, 1995.

8. Office for National Statistics. *Surveys of Psychiatric Morbidity among Adults in Great Britain* Newport: ONS, 2000.

9. Saint-Yves IF. The Read clinical classification *Health Bulletin* (Edinburgh) 1992; **50**: 422–7.

10. Jenkins R, Smeeton N, Shepherd M. Classification of mental disorders in primary care *Psychological Medicine Supplement* 1988; **12**.

11. Mann AH, Jenkins R, Belsey E. The twelve-month outcome of patients with neurotic illness in general practice *Psychological Medicine* 1981; **11(3)**: 535–50.

12. Lloyd KR, Jenkins R, Mann A. Long-term outcome of patients with neurotic illness in general practice *British Medical Journal* 1996; **313(7048)**: 26–8.

13. Goldberg D, Privett M, Ustun B, *et al*. The effects of detection and treatment on the outcome of major depression in primary care: a naturalistic study in 15 cities *British Journal of General Practice* 1998; **48(437)**: 1840–4.

14. Murray CJ, Lopez AD. Alternative projections of mortality and disability by cause 1990–2020: Global Burden of Disease Study *Lancet* 1997; **349(9064)**: 1498–504.

15. Bridges K, Goldberg D. Somatic presentation of DSM-III psychiatric disorders in primary care *Journal of Psychosomatic Research* 1985; **29**: 563–9.

16. Kirmayer LJ, Robbins JM, Dworkind M, *et al*. Somatization and the recognition of depression and anxiety in primary care *American Journal of Psychiatry* 1993; **150(5)**: 734–41.

17. Zigmond AS, Snaith RP. The Hospital Anxiety and Depression Rating Scale *Acta Psychiatrica Scandinavica* 1983; **67**: 361–70.

18. Beck AT, Ward CR, Mendelson M. An inventory for measuring depression *Archives of General Psychiatry* 1961; **4**: 561–71.

19. Kroenke K, Spitzer RL, Williams JB. The PHQ-9: validity of a brief depression severity measure *Journal of General Internal Medicine* 2001; **16(9)**: 606–13.

20. Kroenke K, Spitzer RL, Williams JB. The Patient Health Questionnaire-2: validity of a two-item depression screener *Medical Care* 2003; **41(11)**: 1284–92.

21. National Institute for Health and Clinical Excellence. *Clinical Guideline 23, Depression: management of depression in primary and secondary care* London, NICE, 2004 www.nice.org.uk/CGO23NICEguideline [accessed November 2007].

22. Tylee A, Gastpar M, Lepine JP, *et al*. DEPRES II (Depression Research in European Society II): a patient survey of the symptoms, disability and current management of depression in the community. DEPRES Steering Committee *International Clinical Psychopharmacology* 1999; **14(3)**: 139–51.

23. National Institute for Health and Clinical Guidance. *Clinical Guideline 22, Anxiety: management of anxiety (panic disorder, with or without agoraphobia, and generalised anxiety disorder) in adults in primary, secondary and community care* London: NICE, 2004, www.nice.org.uk/nicemedia/pdf/ CG022NICEguidelineamended.pdf [accessed November 2007].

24. Sheehan DV. Current concepts in the treatment of panic disorder *Journal of Clinical Psychiatry* 1999; **60(suppl. 18)**: 16–21.

25. Singleton N, Bumpstead R, O'Brien M, *et al*. *Psychiatric Morbidity among Adults Living in Private Households, 2000* Norwich, HMSO, 2001.

26. Jenkins R (ed.). *WHO Guide to Mental and Neurological Health in Primary Care* (second edn) London: Royal Society of Medicine Press, 2004.

27. National Institute for Health and Clinical Guidance. *Clinical Guideline 31, Obsessive-Compulsive Disorder: core interventions in the treatment of obsessive-compulsive disorder and body dysmorphic disorder* London: NICE, 2006, www.nice.org.uk/nicemedia/pdf/cg031niceguideline.pdf [accessed November 2007].

28. National Institute for Health and Clinical Guidance. *Clinical Guideline 26, Post-Traumatic Stress Disorder (PTSD): the management of PTSD in adults and children in primary and secondary care* London: NICE, 2005, www.nice.org.uk/nicemedia/pdf/cg026niceguideline.pdf [accessed November 2007].

29. Rastam M, Gillberg C, Garton M. Anorexia nervosa in a Swedish urban region: a population-based study *British Journal of Psychiatry* 1989; **155**: 642–6.

30. Bacaltchuk J, Hay P, Trefiglio R. Antidepressants versus psychological treatments and their combination for bulimia nervosa *Cochrane Database of Systematic Reviews* 2001, Issue 4, Art No: CD003385.

31. Hoek HW. The incidence and prevalence of anorexia nervosa and bulimia nervosa in primary care *Psychological Medicine* 1991; **21(2)**: 455–60.

32. National Institute for Health and Clinical Guidance. *Clinical Guideline 9, Eating Disorders: core interventions in the treatment and management of anorexia nervosa, bulimia nervosa and related eating disorders* London: National Institute for Clinical Excellence, 2004, www.nice.org.uk/nicemedia/pdf/cg009niceguidance.pdf [accessed November 2007].

33. Moran P, Jenkins R, Tylee A, *et al*. The prevalence of personality disorder among UK primary care attenders *Acta Psychiatrica Scandinavica* 2000; **102(1)**: 52–7.

34. de Waal MW, Arnold IA, Spinhoven P, *et al*. The reporting of specific physical symptoms for mental distress in general practice *Journal of Psychosomatic Research* 2005; **59(2)**: 89–95.

35. Sharpe M, Mayou R, Walker J. Bodily symptoms: new approaches to classification *Journal of Psychosomatic Research* 2006; **60(4)**: 353–6.

36. Gask L, Goldberg D, Porter R, *et al*. The treatment of somatization: evaluation of a teaching package with general practice trainees *Journal of Psychosomatic Research* 1989; **33(6)**: 697–703.

37. Reid S, Chalder T, Cleare A, *et al*. Chronic fatigue syndrome *Clinical Evidence* 2005; **14**: 1366–78.

38. Layard R. The case for psychological treatment centres *British Medical Journal* 2006; **332**: 1030–2.

Further reading

Jenkins R (ed.). *WHO Guide to Mental and Neurological Health in Primary Care* (second edn) London: Royal Society of Medicine Press, 2004.

National Institute for Health and Clinical Guidance. *Clinical Guideline 22, Anxiety: management of anxiety (panic disorder, with or without agoraphobia, and generalised anxiety disorder) in adults in primary, secondary and community care* London: NICE, 2004, www.nice.org.uk/nicemedia/pdf/CG022NICEguideline amended.pdf [accessed November 2007].

National Institute for Health and Clinical Excellence. *Clinical Guideline 23, Depression: management of depression in primary and secondary care* London: NICE, 2004, www.nice.org.uk/CG023NICEguideline [accessed November 2007].

National Institute for Health and Clinical Guidance. *Clinical Guideline 9, Eating Disorders: core interventions in the treatment and management of anorexia nervosa, bulimia nervosa and related eating disorders* London: National Institute for Clinical Excellence, 2004, www.nicc.org.uk/nicemedia/pdf/cg009niceguidance.pdf [accessed November 2007].

National Institute for Health and Clinical Guidance. *Clinical Guideline 31, Obsessive-Compulsive Disorder: core interventions in the treatment of obsessive-compulsive disorder and body dysmorphic disorder* London: NICE, 2006, www.nice.org.uk/nicemedia/pdf/cg031niceguideline.pdf [accessed November 2007].

World Health Organization. *The ICD-10 Classification of Mental and Behavioural Disorders: clinical descriptions and diagnostic guidelines* Geneva: WHO, 1992.

7 | Severe mental illness
The primary care response

David Shiers and Helen Lester

What this chapter contributes:

this chapter will examine two parts of the care pathway of psychosis, the early
   phase and the later established phase. We will argue that:

- primary care is an important partner in providing good-quality holistic
  care for this group of patients and their families
- the relationship between primary and specialist care lies at the heart of
  what needs to change if we are to achieve integrated care that makes
  sense to practitioners, patients and families.

Introduction

The last decade has witnessed an extraordinary shift in how we understand, treat and
organise care for people with severe mental illnesses, heralding new hope for patients
and their families. Significant advances in understanding the nature of psychosis have
created a range of new treatment options including psychological interventions, family
work and an overt emphasis on recovery.[1] These treatment advances have been accompanied by major investment and redesign of community-based specialist mental health
provision with the creation of new functionalised mental health teams for people with
severe mental illness.[2] However, although this focus on specialist services is welcome,
there is a risk that it may perpetuate the myth that primary care has only a minor role
to play in the treatment of patients with psychosis. In this chapter we will argue that
primary care is an important partner in providing good-quality holistic care for this
group of patients. Indeed we believe there is now an overwhelming case for changing
the nature of the ongoing relationship between primary and specialist care to ensure
that both are working together in an integrated manner to provide care that makes
sense to practitioners, patients and families.

Terminology in this area can be fraught with difficulty. The Primary Care Version of the International Classification of Diseases (ICD-10)[3] offers a condensed ICD-10 with 23 diagnostic categories for use by generalists in primary care settings. We have selected two main categories that we feel are of most relevence to this chapter:

F23 Acute psychotic disorder

F20 Chronic psychotic disorder.

Much of ths chapter, however, also applies to patients with an ICD-10 diagnostic category of:

F31 Bipolar affective disorder.

We add just two caveats. Since psychoses have, historically, been regarded as disorders of adulthood, the ICD-10 has yet to classify adolescent psychosis. However, psychosis may start in adolescence (though rarely before puberty) and indeed early onset predicts a more persistent and difficult course. We have therefore used the term psychosis to indicate a disorder that can commence in young people. We are also excluding people with a psychosis caused by an 'organic' brain illness.

The chapter is divided into three sections. In the first section, we will give an overview of current practice in the UK, suggest a different way of thinking about serious mental illness in terms of a 'stress/vulnerability' model, describe traditional service structures and processes, and propose new ways of organising care for people with serious mental illness. In the second section, we will describe the potential for primary care to respond differently in the care of young people experiencing their first episode of psychosis. In the third section, we will discuss general practitioner (GP) and patient views of good-quality primary care for people with psychosis, the importance of providing good-quality physical health care, new ways of working and the advent and potential of the Quality and Outcomes Framework (QOF).

An overview of current practice

Severe mental illness can be difficult to define. If you include people with schizophrenia, bipolar disorder or chronic psychosis, it affects 3 per cent of the population in the UK.[4] The impact of the diagnosis is, however, out of proportion to the raw prevalence figures, magnified by the fact that 80 per cent of first-episode psychoses (FEP) occur in people aged between 16 and 30 years, at a point when they have their whole life ahead of them. Social exclusion (see Box 7.1), poor physical health (see Box 7.2) and family burden (see Box 7.3) add to the impact and the diagnosis. Indeed the World Health Organization (WHO) has calculated that, at a family level, the burden and human suffering caused by psychosis is exceeded only by quadriplegia and dementia.[5]

Box 7.1: Social exclusion and serious mental illness

- In 1997, a Department of Health survey found strong support for community care services but only 13 per cent of people would be happy if their son or daughter were in a relationship with somebody with schizophrenia.[6]

- In 2003, whilst 83 per cent of people agreed that we need to adopt a far more tolerant attitude towards people with mental illness in our society, this still means that nearly 1 in 5 believe there is no need to do so.[7]

- It has been estimated that someone with a serious mental illness is four times more likely than an 'average' person to have no close friends.[8]

- In England, only 24 per cent of people with mental health problems are currently in work, the lowest employment rate of any group of people.[9]

Box 7.2: Physical health issues for people with serious mental illness

- People with serious mental illness often have poorer physical health and a lower life expectancy than the general population.

- Patients with psychosis (compared with those without) are less likely to be offered blood pressure, cholesterol, urine or weight checks, or to receive advice on smoking cessation, alcohol, exercise or diet from primary care.[10]

- A person with schizophrenia can expect to live for ten years less than someone without a mental health problem, mainly because of physical health problems.[11]

- Deaths from infectious diseases, endocrine, circulatory, respiratory, digestive and genitourinary system disorders are all significantly more likely for adults with serious mental health problems.[12]

Box 7.3: Family burden and serious mental illness[13]

- 95 per cent of carers are members of service users' families.

- 29 per cent provide support and care in excess of 50 hours per week.

- 90 per cent of carers are adversely affected by the caring role in terms of leisure activities, career progress, financial circumstances and family relationships.

- 60 per cent of carers have a significantly or moderately impacted reduced social life.

- 33 per cent of carers' family relationships are seriously affected.

- 41 per cent of carers' mental and physical health has been significantly or moderately reduced.

These health and social impacts create spirals of decline and a loss of autonomy that can quickly become entrenched and difficult to address. This situation, we suggest, would be unacceptable in almost any other area of health care. It is time, therefore, to re-examine not only how practitioners think about people with serious mental illness, but also how we can better organise health services in the UK to provide 21st-century care for our patients.

The stress/vulnerability model

Kraepelin's original description (1896) of 'dementia praecox' (literally *dementia of young mind*) as a single disease entity, schizophrenia, with a universally poor outcome has dominated a whole century of treatment approaches. This concept of a relentless, downward, deteriorating course survived, virtually unchallenged, until Manfred Bleuler's classic observations published in 1977[14] of the course of schizophrenia over 20 years in 208 patients and families. Bleuler discovered that even the most severely affected person could achieve a partial or even complete recovery. Subsequent long-term follow-up studies have suggested that approximately half the people diagnosed with a psychotic illness have a favourable outcome.[15]

During the last 30 years, a growing evidence base has demonstrated the impact of environmental factors such as family behaviour,[16] social networks, psychosocial treatments, sociocultural factors[17] and life events on the origins and outcomes of psychosis. These, in turn, have led to schizophrenia and affective psychoses being conceptualised as two ends of a single continuum, each influenced by different aspects of stress and vulnerability.

In this model, psychoses in people with an 'endogenous' vulnerability manifest at a younger age, tend to be more insidious and are associated with poorer outcomes (the schizophrenias). Vulnerability may be conferred by:

- a family history (first-degree relatives have a ten-fold increased risk)
- cannabis use under the age of 15, which creates a causal link for certain genotypes
- pre-morbid factors such as obstetric complications, structural brain changes, cognitive dysfunction in the form of delayed milestones, reading and motor impairment
- being male.

Psychoses linked to 'exogenous' stressors tend to start when people are a little older, are 'affective' in nature and have a better prognosis. Stressors may include:

- adverse life events
- drug misuse
- urbanisation
- social deprivation.

The 'stress/vulnerability model' has opened up a whole range of new treatment options including psychoeducation for patients and families, and social interventions to support access to education, employment and housing. It has also helped to create a feeling of therapeutic optimism in early intervention and has deposed the old Kraepelinian model of inexorable decline.

Traditional organisation of services

From a historical perspective, modern psychiatric care has evolved largely out of the context of the 'water tower' psychiatric hospitals built in the nineteenth century.[18] However, from the 1950s onwards, the development of neuroleptic medication, the cost inflation of mental hospitals[19] and new ways of thinking about health care, including the growing importance of social networks,[20] led to an increasing move away from hospital-based care towards community care.[21]

However, the policy-led shift from asylum-based to community-based provision of care for patients with psychosis resulted, in many cases, in overstretched community specialist services using limited resources to case-manage patients with long histories. In 1954 there were, for example, 154,000 residents in UK mental hospitals. By 1982, this figure had fallen to 100,000 and by 1998 to 40,000. But this was not always matched by a sufficient infrastructure of community-based services to support the people who had been discharged into the community, prompting notions of a 'careless community.'[22] Society was, in effect, allowing people to drift quietly into community ghettos of disability in which the Kraepelinian mindset maintained a stronghold. Although subsequent research has highlighted the possibility of positive outcomes of discharging people from hospitals into the community, this has not been the case for everyone.[23]

With little support from specialist teams, these patients often relied, by default, on primary care and social care until they reached a crisis point. The effect on primary care was to feel both unsupported in providing care for people with chronic psychosis in the community and unable to access specialist services whose referral thresholds prioritised only the most severely ill. This helped to create a legacy in the 1980s and 1990s where many primary care and specialised services communicated poorly,[24] worked in quite distinct ways, rarely implemented referral protocols, or agreed the roles and responsibilities of either sector.[25]

Creating new ways of working

The 1990s saw 'care in the community' become severely criticised for, one might argue, all the wrong reasons. In the late 1980s and early 1990s there was significant media coverage of a small number of untoward incidents involving people with severe mental illness, for example the killing of Jonathan Zito by Christopher Clunis. Although much of this was alarmist, a net result was a growing public concern about safety and a change in policy towards control as well as care in the community. This included the introduction of supervision registers to identify and provide information on service users 'who are liable to be at risk of committing serious violence or suicide or serious self neglect'.[26] At a macro-level, therefore, decisions were being taken to prioritise people with serious mental illness rather than focusing policy on those with common mental health problems.

However, the services available, particularly for young people with a first episode of psychosis, were far from ideal. The quality of treatment and care traditionally provided was often poor.[27] Pharmacological approaches sometimes used outmoded regimens for this age and phase of illness, whilst often neglecting psychosocial treatments and family therapy. Treatment issues dominated at the expense of practical help and education about psychosis to promote personal adaptation, functional recovery, relapse prevention and meeting carer needs. Little wonder the majority of these patients became lost to follow-up within six months and that the majority (55 per cent) relapsed within five years[28] (see Figure 7.1).

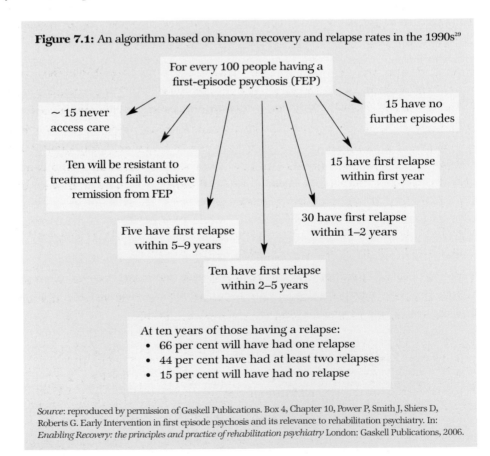

Figure 7.1: An algorithm based on known recovery and relapse rates in the 1990s[29]

For every 100 people having a first-episode psychosis (FEP)

~ 15 never access care

15 have no further episodes

Ten will be resistant to treatment and fail to achieve remission from FEP

15 have first relapse within first year

30 have first relapse within 1–2 years

Five have first relapse within 5–9 years

Ten have first relapse within 2–5 years

At ten years of those having a relapse:
- 66 per cent will have had one relapse
- 44 per cent have had at least two relapses
- 15 per cent will have had no relapse

Source: reproduced by permission of Gaskell Publications. Box 4, Chapter 10, Power P, Smith J, Shiers D, Roberts G. Early Intervention in first episode psychosis and its relevance to rehabilitation psychiatry. In: *Enabling Recovery: the principles and practice of rehabilitation psychiatry* London: Gaskell Publications, 2006.

In the 1990s, user and carer organisations such as the National Schizophrenia Fellowship (NSF) (now Rethink) and the Initiative to Reduce the Impact of Schizophrenia (IRIS) were key to raising awareness of poor services, particularly for young people, and acted both as pressure groups and think tanks for redesigning services.

At the same time, during the 1990s, evidence began to reveal typically long treatment delays for FEP and the benefits of intervening early in terms of recovery. Studies across the world measured delays of one to two years between the onset of psychotic symptoms and the start of treatment.[30] This so-named Duration of Untreated Psychosis (DUP) was longer in those with poor pre-morbid functioning, poor psychosocial support,[31] insidious presentations with predominantly negative symptoms[32,33] and if male. Factors generating such delay include stigma and fear,[34] a lack of knowledge about mental illness and mental health services in the general community, methods of healthcare delivery and the educational system.[35] Studies showed that, despite the reduction of symptoms once treatment began,[36] those with longer DUP could expect poorer functional and symptomatic outcomes at 12 months, increasing behavioural disturbance and family difficulty (often involving multiple failed attempts to access care), and life-threatening behaviour.[37] Added to which, with each relapse the speed and quality of remission becomes progressively impaired, further relapse becomes more likely and persisting symptoms[38] and service costs increase.[39]

Coinciding with the understanding about the adverse impact of long DUP, the key concept of a 'critical period' was being developed by Birchwood *et al*.[40] The notion that the first few years form a 'critical period' when therapeutic, illness and life experiences can have important long-term consequences was supported by evidence that clinical progress in the first two years strongly predicts outcome at 15 years.[15] Importantly this encourages the potential identification from an early stage of individuals who can be predicted to develop long-term 'treatment resistant' symptoms, and who may experience a 'revolving door' pattern of repeated relapse.

Each of these discoveries, acting synergistically, meant that the stage was set for a radical change in the mental health care of people with psychosis.

In 1998, the government announced in *Modernising Mental Health Services* that Early Intervention Services (EIS) for young people in the early phase of psychosis would form part of the new structure of services for the severely mentally ill:

> Early intervention matters to prevent relapse, reduce the risk of suicide and ensure public safety … professionals in primary care and in specialist services need the proper education and training to recognise early symptoms and risk and to take appropriate action.
>
> (*Modernising Mental Health Services*, p. 35)[41]

The National Service Framework for Mental Health in 1999[2] and *The National Plan for the NHS*[42] the following year heralded the replacement of the traditional single-community specialist team approach with the development of a range of new functionalised teams with discrete roles and responsibilities to deliver more intensive and directed support at key points. Such intensive case management at specified key phases of the care pathway should reduce the need for hospitalisation and coercion. These different 'functionalised' teams would provide:

- *early intervention*: intensive case management in the early phase of psychosis

- *assertive community treatment*: where the patient resides, e.g. to patients prone to a pattern of disengagement and relapse in crisis

- *home treatment/crisis response*: at the point of crisis to avoid hospital admission.

The success of these new specialist services within a whole system will, however, ultimately hinge on their ability to integrate with primary care. In the following sections, we will go on to consider how primary care can respond in more detail.

The role of primary care in acute psychosis

Treatment as usual – the case for change

> Our overwhelming feeling was of an opportunity missed for someone so young and at such an important stage of her life – to what extent she was needlessly disabled by those first four years of care we'll never know.
>
> (Mother commenting on her daughter's prospects, 1998)

In considering the role and responsibilities of primary care, we want to focus on the typical situation of an acute mental health crisis – the issues apply both to an emerging first episode of psychosis or a relapse. We are using material gained from a series of audits that were particularly influential in shaping Early Intervention (EI) policy development. For many people, the care pathways they experienced could be more accurately characterised as providing *late intervention*, reflecting the difficulties in negotiating the traditional interface between primary and specialist care, as well as interfaces within specialist services such as that between children/adolescents and adult mental health services. The net effect for a 16-year-old with emerging psychosis and the family may be a first-service experience of 'children's services that don't do psychosis, to be followed by adult services that don't do young people'. Box 7.4 illustrates some of the consequences.

Box 7.4: Pathways to care in the West Midlands Audit*

- Duration of untreated psychosis was 21 months on average.

- 80 per cent were hospitalised.

- 52 per cent required use of the Mental Health Act (1983).

- 45 per cent of these involved the police or criminal justice system.

- Only one person achieved effective engagement via a psychiatric outpatient clinic appointment (n = 45).

*An audit of Pathways to Care for 45 people with FEP in the West Midlands 1998/9.[43]

Pathway audits also highlight the complexity of patient and family journeys involving many other community agencies (see Table 7.1).

Table 7.1: Pathway players in the West Midlands Audit

General psychiatrist	45	General physician	1
Health visitor	3	Teacher/tutor	4
Family member	37	Learning difficulties psychiatrist	1
Work colleagues	3	Neighbour	4
GP	36	Forensic psychiatrist	1
Private landlord	2	Police surgeon	4
Police	22	Substance misuse service	1
Church	2	Hostel staff	4
Community psychiatric nurse	18	Homeless service	1
Occupational health	2	Probation office	3
A&E	13	Solicitor	1
Friends	2	Prison staff	3
Social worker	11	Ambulance service	1
Occupational health	1	Resource centre	3
Psychologist	5	Public health	1

The GP's role in this pathway is often crucial, and yet for any individual GP diagnosing FEP is uncommon (usually no more than once per 1–2 years). Nevertheless GPs are frequently consulted along the developing illness pathway,[44] and are the most common final referring agency. Their involvement also reduces the use of the Mental Health Act.[45]

The development of new EIS, however, heralded a new way of working across the interface to provide better services for people with acute psychosis (both first episode and relapse). Indeed, primary care and EIS share a number of philosophical and clinical concerns. Both have a low threshold for referral, work with diagnostic uncertainty and are used to seeing and trying to help distressed families. These shared issues provide fertile ground for primary care and EI services to work closely together with a common objective of ensuring that a young person and his or her family access appropriate quality services in a timely fashion.

How can primary care be more involved in people with acute psychosis?

Primary care must address some critical issues if it is to play a more active role in the care pathways of young people with acute psychosis:

Greater awareness about key 'alert' indicators for FEP

Psychosis usually emerges when people are young; 80 per cent of FEP emerges between the ages of 16 and 30 years; the average age is about 22, slightly younger in males.[46] A Primary Care pathways audit in North Staffordshire (n = 45)[43] showed that:

- 75 per cent live with either parent(s) or spouse
- 29 per cent have parenting roles
- 41 per cent are employed or in full-time education.

Psychosis rarely presents 'out of the blue'. Warning symptoms of possible psychological vulnerability include:

- irritability
- loss of concentration
- depression
- anxiety
- feelings of unease
- constant tiredness
- suspiciousness
- rudeness
- withdrawal from friends.

> Steve came from a close-knit family, enjoyed a happy childhood and was academically bright. Aged 16 he lost interest in school and became defiant. He consulted his GP and was referred to psychology. The records describe treatment for anxiety with over-valued ideas. He stopped after three attendances.

A prodromal phase heralds the onset of psychosis. This can last several months during which there may be varying psychological and social disturbances without clear-cut psychotic symptoms.

Steve left home for a bed-sit. He withdrew from his friends and at intervals appeared agitated and depressed. He muttered to himself and began to be suspicious of his father. His mother worried increasingly about his failure to use heating, eat adequately or generally self-care. She convinced him to return home.

Psychosis rarely presents with a neat symptom parcel. It is important to look for evidence of poor personal hygiene, delusional or bewildered mood, abstract or vague speech and outbursts of anger or irritation. Positive and negative symptoms are rarely volunteered spontaneously and may need to be actively sought. If you suspect the person may be developing a psychosis, ask about changes in:

- social functioning, e.g. problems in relationships with friends and family

- cognition, e.g. poor concentration and memory

- mood, e.g. feeling depressed, anxious or irritable

- thought content, e.g. preoccupation with strange thoughts or ideas (ideas of reference, delusions of harm, persecution or grandeur, auditory hallucinations)

- drug misuse

- suicidal ideas.

With some difficulty his mother took Steve to the family GP and assertively requested he should see a psychiatrist. But Steve failed to keep an urgent outpatient appointment made for the following week. A few days later a GP was summoned urgently because Steve was very agitated, with delusions of grandeur. Steve required urgent admission under the Mental Health Act (1983).

Perhaps, above all, where there are concerns, it is important to keep an 'active watching brief'– to ensure that a line of communication and offer of care is maintained wherever possible through follow-up appointments, home visit or a telephone call. See Lester *et al.*[47] for a description of the impact of training materials on GP recognition of young people with FEP.

Low threshold for access to specialist advice and assessment for suspected FEP cases

Steve's case, typical of other cases in the audits, demonstrates important issues about access and help-seeking. In the prospective audit, only one of 45 successful pathway engagements came through a traditional outpatient route, highlighting the need for both primary care and specialist services to provide more flexible and accessible pathways for this young client group. GPs need both a lower threshold for seeking help and advice, and a more responsive specialist service. Although the development of new services now means that GPs in many part of England have access to EIS, coverage is not universal and does not extend to the other devolved nations in the UK. There are, however, a range of measures that could be usefully agreed at a local level in areas both with and without access to EIS. For instance:

- GP concerns could be discussed at an early stage with a nominated local mental health team

- outpatients could be avoided as a setting for specialist assessment by encouraging the use of primary care settings or the patient's home

- shared primary care/specialist educational meetings, which discuss care pathways and cases of mutual concern, could be set up.

Acting on family concerns

In the West Midlands audits, between 59–80 per cent of family members initiated help-seeking on an individual's behalf. In the vast majority of cases, this was done through primary care and highlights the importance of GPs being sensitive to and acting on the concerns of the family. Indeed primary care can play a pivotal role in supporting families through this time of emerging psychosis by providing information, practical assistance and emotional support.

Early Intervention Services development – the current state of play

In March 2005, an audit by the National Institute for Mental Health in England (NIMHE)/Rethink National Early Intervention programme found that 86 new 'functionalised' EI teams had been implemented and were able to deliver services to approximately one-third of the population in England.[48] For primary care, this still means that the most common route of access is to the existing community mental health teams. However, when even good-quality 'standard' mental health services are compared with EIS, the latter report shorter DUP, lower use of legal detention, reduced hospital admissions,[49] lower relapse rates,[50] better recovery,[51] better service engagement and client/carer satisfaction and lower suicide rates.[38] A number of cost-effectiveness studies are underway, but we know that EIS reduces hospitalisation and can therefore reduce NHS Costs.[52]

Achieving EI at the moment hinges on changing the care pathway of this young client group and their families by more integrated working between primary, specialist and community agencies. We have now included two case studies that demonstrate how some of these new services can make a difference in practice.

Case study 1: Gloucestershire Recovery in Psychosis service, Gloucestershire Partnership NHS Trust and Cheltenham Community Projects

The Gloucestershire Recovery in Psychosis (GRIP) approach emphasises the development of coherent links between a number of interagency organisations, both statutory and non-statutory. GRIP provides its service from a low-stigma community-based setting, shared with a youth agency, Cheltenham Community Projects (CCP). A service specification was drawn up by the steering group with the key strategic aim to reduce DUP, which led to a series of operational service deliverables that include:

- allowing direct access for potential users and concerned family members

- offering a lower threshold for GPs to refer on suspicion rather than certainty, supplemented by communicating rapid feedback of assessments and treatment proposals

- offering a programme of awareness raising, conducted across the community

- including formal presentations to GPs, statutory and secondary teams, and also to the non-statutory sector; supporting information and leaflets were distributed and a number of helpful suggested initial assessment questions

- distributing a screening tool, developed by GRIP, to potential referrers.

The majority of service users are seen and assessed at home, whilst having the choice of being seen in GRIP offices. For those requiring continuing GRIP services, the community-based nature encourages an emphasis on recovery. This supports not just clinical improvement but also helps the service user reintegrate with social networks and explore the opportunity to access meaningful functional activity either in terms of vocation or unpaid or paid employment.

A number of clear operational targets have been defined within the *Mental Health Service Response to First Episode Psychosis in Gloucestershire Research* document (see www.gripinitiative.org.uk).

To date, GRIP has measured an impressive reduction in DUP, use of the Mental Health Act (1983) and suicide rates, together with increased user and carer satisfaction levels, and employment/occupation rates for service users. In order to sustain the improvement, an audit cycle has been set in place to continually listen to and learn from GPs, carers and users of the service.

Case study 2: Northumberland Early Interventions Team, Northumberland Care Trust

Northumberland Early Interventions Team (NEIT) focuses on improving engagement of service users with FEP. NEIT particularly works with families and service users to promote hope and prevent social exclusion, by encouraging service users to reintegrate with their social and occupational networks.

Research suggests that by reducing DUP people will have less traumatic entry into services, and an admission at presentation can be avoided. The NEIT developed two practical local measures:

1. Care coordinators from the NEIT offer education to GPs on the importance of early detection and referral of possible cases of psychosis to the service

2. Enhanced Family Work (Family Interventions) have been developed that work proactively with families to acknowledge and help them deal with their own needs, and to help them be more effective in their caring role.

The following vignette displays how care pathways were used to decide who to target and what information to give them. This illustrates what can be achieved if people are referred earlier and the service is prepared and able to work with families as co-therapists.

Following an educational session a GP approached a care coordinator to ask for advice. A mother had asked them to see her son, who was behaving oddly; however, he had refused to see the GP. The care coordinator's subsequent attempts to see the young man were met with refusal but, through the policy of encouraging family work, an alternative approach could be offered. The use of legal detention was discussed, but the family felt this should be a last resort. Thus having defined some clear boundaries around risk, it was agreed that the young man be offered a formulation-based psychosocial intervention approach, conducted by the mother and supervised by the care coordinator. Improvement slowly followed and over many months he was able to re-engage with some old friends, eventually returning to work.

Future possibilities

As the markers for those at highest risk become more refined, there is hope that very early detection and intervention could reduce the progression to psychosis. Several studies are currently testing whether Cognitive Behavioural Therapy (CBT) and/or low-dose antipsychotic medication offered to individuals at ultrahigh risk of psychosis can reduce the risk of subsequent psychosis as well as ameliorate prodromal symptoms. Two such trials have already reported promising results. The PACE study in Melbourne[53] has shown a reduction in the risk of FEP from 35 per cent to 10 per cent whilst in treatment with low-dose atypical antipsychotics and CBT, but the benefits disappeared when the treatment was withdrawn. Morrison *et al.* (2004)[54] demonstrated almost the same lowered conversion rate to psychosis (i.e. 12 per cent) with CBT alone in a similar group of patients. So far, however, these studies have been conducted in relatively small, selected samples of people at high risk of psychosis, willing to seek help and in a research setting. It remains to be seen if they can be translated into a practical intervention that is widely available to individuals with at-risk mental states. Nevertheless, for primary care, the implications of these studies are considerable. They could, for example, shift the focus towards GP recognition and flagging up of those with key 'alert' indicators and a different access route to a youth-orientated specialist assessment and psychological treatment service.

The role of primary care for people with chronic psychosis

In the final section of the chapter, we are going to explore some of the challenges that face primary care in providing quality care for people with chronic psychosis. In particular, we are going to look at GPs' and patients' views of the value, roles and responsibilities of primary care, the importance of providing good-quality physical health care, new ways of working and the advent and potential of the QOF.

People with chronic psychosis can present to primary care in a number of different ways. Although many may have an established history of psychosis, others may have a more insidious presentation or may have disengaged from services for some time. It is interesting to note that approximately 50 per cent of homeless people have serious mental illness and have often fallen through the health and social care safety net.[55]

Patients may present with the following issues:[56]

- difficulties with thinking or concentrating (e.g. they think that the television is talking to them, or that their thoughts are being read)
- reports of hearing voices or seeing visions
- strange beliefs (e.g. having supernatural powers or being persecuted)
- extraordinary physical complaints (e.g. strange sensations or having unusual objects inside their body)
- problems or questions related to antipsychotic medication
- problems in managing work, studies or relationships
- physical healthcare problems (e.g. weight, respiratory or cardiac problems)
- lack of energy or motivation and an inability to feel emotion
- depression or suicidal thinking.

Families may also seek help because of apathy, withdrawal, poor hygiene or strange behaviour.

One of the most important shifts in thinking that EI offers is to challenge the traditional approach that suggests people with psychosis require exclusive mental health specialist care for the rest of their life. Most people in the UK who have such an illness live in the community and are registered with a GP. Indeed a GP with a list of 2000 patients will care at any one time for 10–20 patients with chronic psychosis. People with chronic psychosis consult primary care practitioners three to four times more frequently[57] and are in contact with primary care services for a longer cumulative time than patients without mental health problems.[58,59] Indeed, 30–50 per cent of people with severe mental illness (SMI) are seen only in the primary care setting.[60] Recent national policy guidance[61] also suggests that primary care is now seen as the key locus for care for improving mental health services for all patients.

However, in spite of the prevalence and the considerable use people with chronic psychosis make of primary care services, many GPs still feel that, in contrast with patients with complex diabetes or heart failure, holistic care of such patients is beyond their remit. The majority see their role as limited to physical illness and prescribing, with only a minority regarding themselves as involved in the monitoring and treatment of mental illness.[62] There is also some evidence that people with SMI are perceived as 'difficult' and as creating work, with the attitudes of inner-city GPs particularly negative.[63] This of course simply reflects the negative stereotypes held by many in wider society. From the patients' perspectives, previous work has concentrated on the content of the consultation and has highlighted a perceived lack of information and explanation for patients about diagnosis and treatment,[64] overuse of medication and delay in obtaining a diagnosis,[65] and barriers created by stigmatised attitudes.[66] More recently, focus groups with patients who had a chronic psychosis, GPs and practice nurses, and then a mixed group of all participants, provided further insights into this area of care (see Box 7.5).[67]

An important 'bottom line' here is that, although GPs may feel that lack of knowledge inhibits greater involvement in care, patients with chronic psychosis value continuity of care, listening skills, advocacy and willingness to learn more than specific knowledge about mental health. A GP who knows his or her patient, listens and can access help for mental health problems when required would be viewed by almost all patients as 'good enough'.

The importance of good-quality physical health care

Patients with a chronic psychosis require, if anything, a better standard of primary care than the general population. People with schizophrenia, in particular, have a higher risk of medical illness than does the general population and have an increased (two- to four-fold) relative risk of premature death, dying at least ten years earlier that age-matched contemporaries.[68,69] The Office of National Statistics survey, *Psychiatric*

Box 7.5: Providing 'good enough' primary care

- Most patients in the study viewed primary care as the *'cornerstone'* of their physical and mental health care.

- Patients and health professionals agreed that the latter had a responsibility to continue prescribing drugs started in secondary care, monitor side effects, and tackle physical health issues. Both groups recognised, however, that it was sometimes difficult to present with or diagnose physical complaints once a mental health disorder has been diagnosed. Some GPs suggested this was related to difficulties in communicating effectively with people with serious mental illness.

- Most health professionals perceived the mental health care of people with serious mental illness as too specialised for routine primary care and felt they lacked sufficient skills and knowledge.

- All participants felt that interpersonal and longitudinal continuity was vital for good-quality care. However, most health professionals felt continuity was threatened by other national primary care policies.

- Patients felt that continuity helped to ensure accurate diagnosis, particularly at times of mental health crisis, prevented the retelling of painful stories, enabled trust to develop that in turn facilitated discussions of treatment options, and, above all, allowed patients and health professionals to understand each other as people.

- Most patients favoured seeing the same GP for their physical and mental health needs, preferring a continuous doctor–patient relationship and a positive attitude and willingness to learn, rather than the opportunity to consult a different GP with special expertise in mental health.

- Most patients knew that their GP had little formal training in mental health and did not expect expert advice from primary care professionals.

Morbidity among Adults Living in Private Households,[70] found that 62 per cent of people with psychosis reported a physical condition, compared with 42 per cent of those without a psychosis. Diabetes, for example, is up to five times as frequent in patients with schizophrenia and bipolar affective disorder than in the general population.[71]

There are a number of possible reasons for these statistics, including lifestyle, diet, physical activity, smoking, obesity, drug side effects and a relative lack of healthcare promotion and prevention. Brown *et al*. prospectively surveyed the lifestyles of 140 people with schizophrenia, and found that their diet was unhealthy (higher in fat and lower in fibre than the reference population), they took less exercise than the reference population, and also had significantly higher levels of cigarette smoking (90 per cent of people with schizophrenia smoke and about 30 per cent of people with bipolar disorder smoke).[72] A number of psychotropic drugs have a high risk of cardiotoxicity.[73] Phenothiazines, and the newer atypical antipsychotics, have also been shown to increase both central obesity and to be associated with diabetes.[74]

There is also evidence that health prevention and promotion activities in primary care are different for people with and without a diagnosis of chronic psychosis. Burns and Cohen[75] found that, although the annual general practice consultation rate was significantly higher than normal for people with chronic psychosis (13–14 consultations a year compared with approximately three for the general population), the amount of data recorded for a range of health promotion areas was significantly less than in consultations with the general population. Cardiovascular risk factors, in particular, are less likely to be recorded in primary care records or acted upon.[76] It is perhaps not surprising, therefore, that the standardised mortality rate (SMR) for all causes of death for people with schizophrenia is high and that deaths from infectious diseases, endocrine, circulatory, respiratory, digestive and genitourinary system disorders are all significantly more likely for adults with a chronic psychosis.[77] We are therefore left with a situation where people with SMI require particularly good primary care, yet appear, for a variety of reasons, to not always receive it.

New models of care

There has been a variety of policy initiatives during the last decade that have aimed to increase the role of primary care in the delivery of health care to people with chronic psychosis. Primary care, for example, has specific responsibility for delivering standards two and three of *The National Service Framework for Mental Health*[2] and is also integrally involved in the delivery of the other five standards. Since 1997 and the election of a new Labour government, there has also been an emphasis on partnership working, with a firm commitment to developing 'joined-up solutions' to 'joined-up problems'. Mental health is complex, with a range of different agencies involved (including health care, social care, housing, welfare advice and the employment services). Many patients with a diagnosis of chronic psychosis are vulnerable and have limited capacity to negotiate complex bureaucracies. They therefore need services that are well integrated at the point of contact, are easy to negotiate and are focused on their needs. Partnership working can also help to minimise bureaucracy and duplication. Above all, partnership working is seen to be beneficial for patients and their carers, who can often experience fragmented services, a lack of continuity and conflicting information in situations where local agencies fail to collaborate effectively.[78] This has been described by Preston *et al.* in terms of being 'left in limbo', with users and carers feeling that they are failing to make progress through the healthcare system:

> Separate clinics don't talk to each other or ring each other. I find the whole thing incredible the length of time it takes; it's just been horrendous, waiting weeks to see a consultant to be told 'I don't know why you've been referred to me.'
> … It can make you feel very insignificant.
>
> (patient, quoted in Preston *et al.*, p. 19)[79]

The expansion of 'shared care' schemes between primary care and secondary care (community- and hospital-based services) similarly reflects the importance of partnership working. One model of shared care is 'shifted-out patient clinics', where psychiatrists hold outpatient clinics in primary care surgeries, attaching mental health workers such as CPNs to a primary care surgery rather than basing them in the community. Another is 'consultation liaison' where primary care teams meet up regularly with the local lead psychiatrist to discuss issues and be supported in managing more challenging patients in a primary care setting. Each of these models of course has its own set of strengths and weaknesses,[80] with no 'ideal' model.

The advent and impact of the Quality and Outcomes Framework

Perhaps the biggest sea change in the delivery of primary care for people with chronic psychosis was precipitated by the introduction of a type of performance-related pay into the UK primary healthcare system in April 2004.[81] The Quality and Outcomes Framework (QOF) (see Chapter 1 on the nGMS) is a voluntary mechanism that pays practices for achieving health-related targets across specified disease areas (and a variety of organisational, patient experience and additional services). There are 1050 points attached to over 170 evidence-based indicators, with each point equating to £120.00 that can be earned by the practice on an annual basis. There are currently six indicators related to the care of people with psychoses in the QOF, representing 39 points (see Table 7.2, p. 150). The indicators encourage the development of a register of patients with a diagnosis of schizophrenia, bipolar disorder and other psychoses, monitoring of patients on lithium therapy and an annual review of physical health, medication and coordination arrangements with secondary care including offering appropriate health promotion and prevention advice.

Two new indicators introduced in 2006 encourage GPs to document a 'comprehensive care plan' in the primary care record that should include a list of the patient's early warning signs (their illness signature)[82] and discussion of financial benefits and employment opportunities. Discussion of benefits and work may be relatively challenging for some practices, but should also raise awareness within primary care of the social exclusion faced by the majority of people with psychosis. Unemployment rates for this popu-

Table 7.2: Mental health indicators in the QOF

Indicator	Points	Payment stages
Records		
MH8: The practice can produce a register of people with schizophrenia, bipolar disorder and other psychoses	4	
Ongoing management		
MH9: The percentage of patients with schizophrenia, bipolar affective disorder and other psychoses with a review recorded in the preceding 15 months. In the reviews there should be evidence that the patients have been offered routine health promotion and prevention advice appropriate to their age, gender and health status	23	40–90%
MH4: The percentage of patients on lithium therapy with a record of serum creatinine and thyroid-stimulating hormone (TSH) in the preceding 15 months	1	40–90%
MH5: The percentage of patients on lithium therapy with a record of lithium levels in the therapeutic range within the previous six months	2	40–90%
MH6: The percentage of patients on the register who have a comprehensive care plan documented in the records agreed between individuals, their family and/or carers as appropriate	6	25–90%
MH7: The percentage of patients with schizophrenia, bipolar affective disorder and other psychoses who do not attend the practice for their annual review who are identified and followed up by the practice team within 14 days of non-attendance	3	40–90%

lation range from 8 per cent to 20 per cent with particularly low rates (4 per cent to 12 per cent) for people with schizophrenia.[83] The second new indicator requires the practice to actively follow up any patient who has not attended his or her annual health check since there is evidence that people who fail to attend may do so because of worsening symptoms rather than a desire to waste a primary care appointment.[67]

It is still far too soon to see if these largely process measures have had an effect on patient health outcomes, but it is encouraging to see that practices across England achieved an average of 89 per cent of the points in the mental health domain in 2004/5. Since the indicators are evidence based, there is every reason to expect positive changes in the morbidity and mortality of people with a chronic psychosis over the next decade.

Conclusion

Primary care is a valued and valuable part of the care system of these patients. There are huge opportunities for primary care to impact on the health improvement of this neglected and marginalised group of patients and families. We have described some of the transformations in understanding, the new treatment options available and the different systems of care. The QOF currently offers an important opportunity for systemised improvements along that care pathway. Within this longer-term context, primary care can shift its focus from *disease maintenance* to *health improvement*. Such a system will, however, amount to little if delivered in a mechanised way that excludes individualised care.

We believe that the biggest hurdle primary care has to overcome is neither the acquisition of some new specialist skill nor some new specialist service configuration that might *sort out* all the problems. It is the self-realisation that the contribution of generalism and family practice is essential and a valued aspect of effective health care. Indeed, we would argue that the key clinical tool required is an ethical, respectful and trustworthy therapeutic doctor–patient relationship. Primary care is uniquely placed by the nature of its long-term view of the care pathway, allowing it to make the connections between early detection of emerging illness and relapse, health promotion, physical illness and support for patients and families with longer-term difficulties. A primary care response to psychosis feels timely and long overdue.

References

1. National Institute for Clinical Excellence. *Schizophrenia: full national clinic guidelines on core interventions in primary and secondary care* London: Royal College of Psychiatrists and the British Psychological Society, 2003.

2. Department of Health. *The National Service Framework for Mental Health* London: DH, 1999.

3. World Health Organization. *Guide to Mental and Neurological Health in Primary Care* London: Royal Society of Medicine Press, 2004.

4. Bird L. *The Fundamental Facts about Mental Illness* London: Mental Health Foundation, 1999.

5. World Health Organization. *Mental Health: new understanding, new hope* Geneva: WHO, 2001.

6. Department of Health. *Omnibus Survey of Public Attitudes to Mental Illness* London: DH, 1997.

7. Department of Health. *National Statistics on Adults' Attitudes to Mental Illness in Great Britain* London: DH, 2003.

8. Huxley P, Thornicroft G. Social inclusion, social quality and mental illness *British Journal of Psychiatry* 2003; **182**: 298–90.

9. Office for National Statistics. *Labour Force Survey, Autumn 2003* London: ONS, 2003.

10. *Not All in the Mind – the physical health of mental health service users – briefing paper 2* London: mentality, 2003.

11. Allebeck P. Schizophrenia: a life-shortening disease *Psychiatric Bulletin* 1989; **15**(1): 81–9.

12. Harris EC, Barraclough B. Excess mortality of mental disorder *British Journal of Psychiatry* 1998; **173**: 11–53.

13. Rethink. *Under Pressure* London: Rethink, 2003.

14. Bleuler M. *The Schizophrenic Disorders*, trans. Siegfried M Clemens, New Haven and London: Yale University Press, 1977.

15. Harrison G, Hopper K, Craig T, *et al*. Recovery from psychotic illness: a 15 and 25-year international follow-up study *British Journal of Psychiatry* 2001; **178**: 506–17.

16. Vaughan CE, Leff JP. The influence of family factors on the course of psychiatric illness *British Journal of Psychiatry* 1976; **129**: 125–37.

17. Warner R. *Recovery from Schizophrenia: psychiatry and political economy* (third edn) London: Brunner-Routledge, 2003.

18. Weller MPI, Muijen M. *Dimensions of Community Mental Health Care* Kent: Saunders, 1993.

19. Scull A. *Decarceration: community treatment and the deviant – a radical view* Englewood Cliffs, NJ: Prentice-Hall, 1977.

20. Prior L. Mind, body and behaviour theorizations of madness and the organisation of therapy *Sociology* 1991; **25**: 403–22.

21. Rogers A, Pilgrim D. *Mental Health Policy in Britain* Basingstoke: Palgrave, 2001.

22. Harrison P. Careless community *New Society*, 1973, 28 June.

23. Leff J. *Care in the Community: illusion or reality?* Chichester: John Wiley & Sons, 1997.

24. Goldberg D, Jackson G. Interface between primary care and specialist mental health care *British Journal of General Practice* 1992; **42**(360): 267–9.

25. Kendrick T, Sibbald B, Burns T, *et al*. Role of general practitioners in the care of long term mentally ill patients *British Medical Journal* 1991; **302**: 508–10.

26. NHS Executive. *Introduction of Supervision Registers for Mentally Ill People from 1 April 1994* HSG (84)5, 1994.

27. Garety P, Rigg A. Early psychosis in the inner city: a survey to inform service planning *Social Psychiatry and Psychiatric Epidemiology* 2001; **36**: 537–44.

28. Robinson D, Woerner MG, Alvir JM, *et al*. Predictors of relapse following response from a first episode of schizophrenia or schizoaffective disorder *Archives of General Psychiatry* 1999; **56**: 241–7.

29. Eaton WW, Thara R, Federman E, *et al*. Remission and relapse in schizophrenia: the Madras longitudinal study *Journal of Nervous and Mental Disease* 1998; **186**: 357–63.

30. McGlashan TH. Duration of untreated psychosis in first episode schizophrenia: marker or determinant of course? *Biological Psychiatry* 1999; **46**: 899–907.

31. Larsen TK, Johannessen JO, Opjordsmoen S. First episode schizophrenia with long duration of untreated psychosis – pathways to care *British Journal of Psychiatry* 1998; **172**(Suppl. 33): 45–52.

32. Larsen TK, McGlashen TH, Johannessen JO, *et al*. First episode schizophrenia to pre-morbid patterns by gender *Schizophrenia Bulletin* 1996; **22**: 241–56.

33. Drake RJ, Clifford JH, Akthar S, *et al*. Causes and consequences and duration of untreated psychosis and schizophrenia *British Journal of Psychiatry* 2000; **177**: 511–15.

34. Lincoln CB, McGorry PD. Who cares? Pathways to psychiatric care for young people experiencing a first episode of psychosis *Psychiatric Services* 1995; **46**: 1166–71.

35. Lincoln C, Harrigan S, McGorry PD. Understanding the topography of the early psychosis pathway: an opportunity to reduce delays in treatment *British Journal of Psychiatry* 1998; **172(Suppl. 33)**: 21–5.

36. Norman R, Malla A. Duration of untreated psychosis: a critical examination of the concept and its importance *Psychological Medicine* 2001; **31**: 381–400.

37. Power P. Suicide prevention in first episode psychosis. In: P McGorry and J Gleeson (eds). *Psychological Interventions in Early Psychosis*, pp. 175–90, Chichester: Wiley Press, 2004.

38. Wiersma D, Nienhuis F, Sloof C, *et al*. Natural course of schizophrenic disorders: a 15 year follow-up of a Dutch incidence cohort *Schizophrenia Bulletin* 1998; **24**: 75–85.

39. Almond S, Knapp M, Francois C, *et al*. Relapse in schizophrenia: costs, clinical outcomes and quality of life *British Journal of Psychiatry* 2004; **184**: 346–51.

40. Birchwood M, Todd P, Jackson C. Early intervention in psychosis, the critical period hypothesis *British Journal of Psychiatry* 1998; **172(Suppl. 33)**: 53–9.

41. Department of Health. *Modernising Mental Health Services: safe, secure and supportive* London: DH, 1998.

42. Department of Health. *The National Plan for the NHS* London: DH, 2000.

43. Macmillan F, Ryles D, Shiers D, *et al*. *North Staffordshire Primary Care Exploration and Pilot Research of Pathways to Treatment in Early Psychosis – report to North Staffordshire Health Authority 1998/9*.

44. Cole E, Levy G, King M, *et al*. Pathways to care for patients with a first episode of psychosis: a comparison of ethnic groups *British Journal of Psychiatry* 1995; **167**: 770–6.

45. Burnett R, Mallett R, Bhugra G, *et al*. The first contact of patients with schizophrenia with psychiatric services: social factors and pathways to care in multi-ethnic population *Psychological Medicine* 1999; **29**: 475–83.

46. Hafner H, Nowotny B, Epidemiology of early onset schizophrenia *European Archives of Psychiatry and Clinical Neuroscience* 1995; **245**: 80-92.

47. Lester HE, Tait L, Khera A, *et al*. The development and implementation of an educational intervention on first episode psychosis for primary care *Medical Education* 2005; **39**: 1006–14.

48. Pinfold V, Smith J, Shiers D. Audit of early intervention in psychosis service development in England in 2005 *Psychiatric Bulletin* (in press).

49. Yung AR, Organ BA, Harris MG. Management of early psychosis in a generic adult mental health service *Australian and New Zealand Journal of Psychiatry* 2003; **37(4)**: 429–36.

50. Craig TKJ, Garety P, Power P, *et al*. The Lambeth Early Onset Community Team: a randomised controlled trial of assertive outreach for psychosis *British Medical Journal* 2004; **329**: 1067–73.

51. Garety PA, Craig TK, Dunn G, *et al*. Specialised care for early psychosis: symptoms, social functioning and patient satisfaction: randomised controlled trial *British Journal of Psychiatry* 2006; **188**: 37–45.

52. Almond S, Knapp M, Francois C, *et al*. Relapse in schizophrenia: costs, clinical outcomes and quality of life *British Journal of Psychiatry* 2004; **184**: 346–51.

53. Patrick D, McGorry P, Yung AR, *et al*. Randomized controlled trial of interventions designed to reduce the risk of progression to first-episode psychosis in a clinical sample with subthreshold symptoms *Archives of General Psychiatry* 2002; **59**: 921–8.

54. Morrison AP, French P, Walford L, *et al*. Cognitive therapy for the prevention of psychosis in people at ultra-high risk: randomized controlled trial *British Journal of Psychiatry* 2004; **185**: 291–7.

55. Bines W. *The Health of Single Homeless People* York: Centre for Housing Policy University of York, 1994.

56. World Health Organization. *WHO Guide to Mental and Neurological Health in Primary Care* (second edn) London: RSM Press, 2004.

57. Nazareth I, King M, Haines A. Care of schizophrenia in general practice *British Medical Journal* 1993; **307**: 910.

58. Lang F, Johnstone E, Murray D. Service provision for people with schizophrenia: role of the general practitioner *British Journal of Psychiatry* 1997; **171**: 165–8.

59. Kai J, Crosland A, Drinkwater C. Prevalence of enduring and disabling mental illness in the inner city *British Journal of General Practice*. 2000; **50**: 922–4.

60. Jenkins R, McCulloch A, Friedli L, *et al*. *Developing a National Mental Health Policy* London: Maudsley Monograph, 2002.

61. Department of Health. *The National Service Framework for Mental Health – five years on* London: DH, 2004.

62. Burns T, Greenwood N, Kendrick T, *et al*. Attitudes of general practitioners and community mental health team staff towards the locus of care for people with chronic psychotic disorders *Primary Care Psychiatry* 2000; **6**: 67–71.

63. Brown J, Weich S, Downes-Grainger E, *et al*. Attitudes of inner city GPs to shared care for psychiatric patients in the community *British Journal of General Practice* 1999; **49**: 643–4.

64. Bailey D. What is the way forward for a user-led approach to the delivery of mental health services in primary care? *Journal of Mental Health* 1997; **6**: 101–5.

65. Rogers A, Pilgrim D. *Experiencing Psychiatry: users' views of services* London: Macmillan Press, 1993.

66. Kai J, Crosland A. Perspectives of people with enduring mental ill health from a community-based qualitative study *British Journal of General Practice* 2001; **51**: 730–7.

67. Lester HE, Tritter JQ, Sorohan H. Patients' and health professionals' views on primary care for people with serious mental illness: focus group study *British Medical Journal* 2005; **330**: 1122.

68. Connolly M, Kelly C. Lifestyle and physical health in schizophrenia *Advances in Psychiatric Treatment* 2005; **11**: 125–32.

69. Marder SR, Essock SM, Miller AL, *et al*. Physical health monitoring of patients with schizophrenia *American Journal of Psychiatry* 2004; **161**: 1334–49.

70. Singleton N, Bumpstead R, O'Brien M, *et al*. *Psychiatric Morbidity among Adults Living in Private Households, 2000* London: TSO, 2001.

71. Mukherjee S, Decina P, Bocola V, *et al*. Diabetes mellitus in schizophrenic patients *Comprehensive Psychiatry* 1996; **37(1)**: 68–73.

72. Brown S, Birtwhistle J, Roe L, *et al*. The unhealthy lifestyle of people with schizophrenia *Psychological Medicine* 1999; **29**: 697–701.

73. Chong SA, Mythily S, Mahendran R. Cardiac effects of psychotropic drugs *Annals of the Academy of Medicine, Singapore* 2001; **30(6)**: 625–31.

74. Sernyak MJ, Leslie DL, Alarcon RD, *et al*. Association of diabetes mellitus with use of atypical neuroleptics in the treatment of schizophrenia *American Journal of Psychiatry* 2002; **159**: 561–6.

75. Burns T, Cohen A. Item-of-service payments for GP care of severely mentally ill persons *British Journal of General Practice* 1998; **48**: 1415–16.

76. Kendrick T. Cardiovascular and respiratory risk factors and symptoms among general practice patients with long-term mental illness *British Journal of Psychiatry* 1996; **169**: 733–9.

77. Brown S, Inskip H, Barraclough B. Causes of the excess mortality of schizophrenia *British Journal of Psychiatry* 2000; **177**; 212–17.

78. Sainsbury Centre for Mental Health. *Taking your Partners: using opportunities for inter-agency partnership in mental health* London: Sainsbury Centre for Mental Health, 2000.

79. Preston C, Cheater F, Baker R, *et al*. Left in limbo: patients' views on care across the primary/secondary interface *Quality in Health Care* 1999; **8(1)**: 16–21.

80. Lester HE, Glasby J, Tylee A. Integrated primary care mental health: threat or opportunity in the new NHS? *British Journal of General Practice* 2004; **54**: 282–91.

81. BMA/NHS Confederation. *Investing in General Practice: the new general medical services contract* London: BMA, 2003.

82. Birchwood M, Spencer E, McGovern D. Schizophrenia: early warning signs *Advances in Psychiatric Treatment* 2000; **6**: 93–101.

83. Perkins R, Rinaldi M. Unemployment rates among patients with long-term mental health problems *Psychiatric Bulletin* 2002; **26**: 295–8.

8 | Child and adolescent mental health

Dick Churchill

What this chapter contributes:

the public health impact of child and adolescent mental health

the primary care role in responding to children and adolescents

specific conditions, and their presentation and management.

Introduction

The majority of children and young people with mental health difficulties do not fall neatly into a single diagnostic category. Neither do they present in primary care with well-circumscribed symptoms and signs. Some of the most important features in terms of assessment may be concealed or hidden. Underlying aetiological factors are invariably intertwined with more obvious physical, emotional, educational and social consequences. Simultaneously the child or young person is developing his or her own identity in a way that is strongly influenced both by internal and environmental factors. Meanwhile it is often the case that the frustrations of parents and other adults, unable to fully comprehend or deal with the problems, muddy the water further.

In primary care we have the challenge of disentangling some of this complex web of factors as the first point of contact. Significantly, we influence the way in which a problem is perceived and how it is subsequently acted upon. In doing this, we need to have a clear understanding of the range of normal behaviour, emotions and performance that are to be expected throughout the age spectrum, and to be able to distinguish these from both temporary self-limiting psychological difficulties and from those that are likely to have a permanent impact on the wellbeing of the young person.

Many mental health disorders in adulthood have their origins in youth.[1] Early recognition and intervention may alter the long-term consequences. There are also some types of psychological problems that are unique to young people, but even these can influence later development and be risk factors for other mental health problems in adulthood. However, improving the mental health of young people should be viewed as an endpoint in itself and not merely a means of improving adult functioning.[2]

This chapter covers common mental health problems that affect young people from early childhood to the age of 18. It does not cover learning disability or substance misuse. Within this age range different problems occur at different ages, and alternative approaches are needed as the child develops into adulthood.

The chapter is divided into three sections. The first highlights the public health impact of child and adolescent mental health problems, and the national strategies that are being proposed to address them, with particular reference to primary care. The second describes the roles of primary care in responding to the problem in a general sense, with an emphasis on practical considerations in general practice. The final section briefly describes some specific conditions, highlighting, where appropriate, differences from adult presentations, and briefly presenting, where available, current guidelines on management. It is worth noting at the outset that only limited research has been carried out into child and adolescent mental health in general practice, and so there is a lack of a robust evidence base for providing high-quality care in this setting.[3]

The context

In 2004 the Office of National Statistics conducted its second survey into the mental health of children and young people in Great Britain.[4] Overall nearly one in ten were found to have a clinically diagnosable mental health disorder (see Table 8.1). Conduct disorders were more common than emotional disorders overall, and specifically amongst boys compared with girls. Emotional disorders were most common in older girls.

Table 8.1: Prevalence of mental health disorders in children and young people by age and sex in Great Britain, 2004

All children, Great Britain

Type of disorder	5–10-year-olds			11–16-year-olds			All children		
	Boys	Girls	All	Boys	Girls	All	Boys	Girls	All
	Percentage of children with each disorder								
Emotional disorders	2.2	2.5	2.4	4.0	6.1	5.0	3.1	4.3	3.7
Conduct disorders	6.9	2.8	4.9	8.1	5.1	6.6	7.5	3.9	5.8
Hyperkinetic disorders	2.7	0.4	1.6	2.4	0.4	1.4	2.6	0.4	1.5
Less common disorders	2.2	0.4	1.3	1.6	1.1	1.4	1.9	0.8	1.3
Any disorder	10.2	5.1	7.7	12.6	10.3	11.5	11.4	7.8	9.6
Base (weighted)	2010	1916	3926	2101	1950	4051	4111	3866	7977

Note: prevalence rates are based on the *ICD-10 Classification of Mental and Behavioural Disorders* with strict impairment criteria – the disorder causing distress to the child or having considerable impact on the child's day-to-day life.

Source: adapted from Office of National Statistics (2005).[4]

Mental health problems of all types were significantly more common amongst disadvantaged families. Specifically, rates of mental disorder were higher amongst children who were: living in lone-parent or reconstituted families; in families on low income or in receipt of disability benefits; with parents who were unemployed, not working, or who had no educational qualifications; or who were living in rented as opposed to privately owned accommodation.

There had been no significant change in overall prevalence rates since a previous survey that used identical methodology in 1999.[5] This survey also examined the rates of mental disorders in relation to ethnicity and found that, in comparison with a rate of 10 per cent in white children, 12 per cent of black children, 8 per cent of Pakistani and Bangladeshi children, and 4 per cent of Indian children were assessed as having a mental health problem. Some of the differences may be explained by cultural variation in both presentation and acceptance of mental health problems as well as other protective factors.

The *National Service Framework for Children, Young People and Maternity Services* clearly highlights the potential impact of mental health problems at this age:

> Mental health problems in children are associated with educational failure, family disruption, disability, offending and antisocial behaviour, placing demands on social services, schools and the youth justice system. Untreated mental health problems create distress not only in the children and young people, but also for their families and carers, continuing into adult life, and affecting the next generation.[6]

In recent years the government has initiated strategies to improve the emotional wellbeing of children and young people. Specifically, the green paper *Every Child Matters* lists five intended central outcomes, all of which relate closely to psychological health: being healthy (physically and mentally); staying safe (protected from harm and neglect); enjoying and achieving; making a positive contribution (including not engaging in antisocial or offending behaviour); and economic wellbeing. Whilst the strategy focuses on improving integration of health, education, social and youth justice services for children, it also emphasises the key role of general practice as the cornerstone of family health care.[7]

The *National Service Framework for Children, Young People and Maternity Services* specifically includes a standard for the mental health and wellbeing of children and young people,[8] and highlights the role of primary care professionals (PCPs) in identifying those children and young people at greatest risk of mental health problems.[6] It also emphasises the need for all staff working with children and young people to be trained in the early identification of such problems.

Child and Adolescent Mental Health Services (CAMHS) in England and Wales are organised according to a four-tier model (Table 8.2, p. 160).[9] In 1999 the Audit Commission evaluated provision of services against this model and identified substantial variations in terms of the mix of staff, accessibility, the age of children accepted, and the level of expenditure in relation to need.[10] This has led to increased investment with the expectation that comprehensive mental health services for children and young people should be available in all areas by 2006, and include young people up to their eighteenth birthday. However, demand continues to exceed provision so that waiting times remain excessively long in many areas.[11]

Table 8.2: The four-tier framework for CAMHS in England and Wales

Tier 1	A primary level of care
Tier 2	A service provided by specialist individual professionals relating to services in primary care
Tier 3	A specialised multidisciplinary service for more severe, complex or persistent disorders
Tier 4	Essential tertiary-level services such as day units, highly specialised outpatient teams and inpatient units

Tier 1 of the CAMHS framework includes all professionals who come into regular contact with children – not only members of the primary healthcare team, but also staff in education and social care. Primary care mental health workers are a relatively new group of health professionals that potentially cross the boundary between Tier 1 and Tier 2, sometimes working with general practices and schools either on a referral basis or as a first point of contact.[12,13]

The importance of child and adolescent mental health issues has been acknowledged by the inclusion of relevant topics amongst national evidence-based clinical guidelines (Table 8.3). Initially these guidelines were confined to those that considered childhood disorders in the context of adult disorder, such as those for eating disorders and self-harm. However, they now include some that are specific for children and young people such as the National Institute for Health and Clinical Excellence (NICE) guideline on depression. Guidelines for specific discussions are dealt with later in this chapter (p. 174 ff.).

The role of general practice in child and adolescent mental health

Mental health promotion

Good mental health in children and young people is more than the absence of a disorder – it also requires the presence of normal emotional, psychological, social and intellectual development and functioning.[11] The role of general practice in promoting mental health in children and young people, whilst necessarily limited, should not be

Table 8.3: Recently published guidelines and recommendations for mental health problems that include children and adolescents

Date	Topic	Source	Scope
2001	Attention deficit and hyperactivity disorders[14]	SIGN (NICE Clinical Guideline due 2008)	Management of children and young people presenting with attention deficit hyperactivity disorder (ADHD)/hyperkinetic disorder (HKD)
Updated 2006	Stimulant medication for ADHD[15]	NICE Health Technology Appraisal	Methylphenidate, atomoxetine and dexamfetamine for ADHD in children and adolescents (review)
2003	Autistic spectrum disorder[16]	National Initiative for Autism: Screening & Assessment	
2005	Depression[17]	NICE Clinical Guideline	Children and young people aged up to 18 with depressive disorders
2004	Eating disorders[18]	NICE Clinical Guideline	Adults and children aged eight years and over with anorexia nervosa, bulimia nervosa or related conditions
2006	Obsessive-compulsive disorder (OCD)[19]	NICE Clinical Guideline	Adults and children aged eight years or over who have OCD or body dysmorphic disorder
2005	Post-traumatic stress disorder (PTSD)[20]	NICE Clinical Guideline	Adults and children of all ages who have PTSD
2004	Self-harm[21]	NICE Clinical Guideline	Short-term physical and psychological management of adults and children aged eight years or over who have self-harmed
2006	Self-harm	Mental Health Foundation & Camelot Foundation National Inquiry into Self-Harm	Self-harm amongst children and young people aged 11 to 25 years old including recurrent self-harm
2006	Bipolar disorder[22]	NICE Clinical Guideline	Adults, children and adolescents with bipolar disorder

discounted. Good clinical care should include provision of opportunistic help and advice to families; a holistic approach focused on general wellbeing will have an impact on both physical and mental health. Lifestyle advice that promotes a healthy diet and exercise, and discourages behaviours such as cigarette smoking, substance misuse and excess alcohol intake, can have an impact.

Mental health promotion also includes the identification and modification of risk factors for psychological disorders, ideally at an early stage. In primary care we can often identify such risks from knowledge of other family members; for example, a significant bereavement, illness, or parental disharmony and separation can all impact on the mental health of a young person. In addition certain groups of individuals are known to have a much higher risk of mental health problems. These include children in care, refugees and asylum seekers, young offenders, young people using drugs and alcohol, children of parents who have a mental health disorder, and children with physical illnesses, especially those involving the brain.

The broader primary healthcare team has a key role. Examples include the role of health visitors and Sure Start schemes in providing education on positive parenting, and in identifying and responding to problems at an early stage. School-based interventions also have significant potential, as this is where children spend much of their life. Whole-school approaches that aim to improve self-esteem and to help young people develop generic coping skills can be particularly effective.[23] Primary care services may usefully be involved in the planning and delivery of such schemes on a local basis.

Detecting and recognising mental health disorders

The prevalence of mental health disorders is much higher in young people who attend their general practitioner than in the community. In one sample, 38 per cent of attenders aged 13 to 16 had evidence of a current or recent psychiatric disorder.[24] Despite this, only a small proportion of young people (or parents on their behalf) consult explicitly for psychological or emotional problems.[25]

GPs are often criticised for failing to recognise mental health problems in primary care, with studies showing that less than one quarter of affected children and young people are detected.[24,26,27] GPs are significantly more likely to make a diagnosis if concerns are explicitly presented by the parent or young person, and also in more severe disorders.

There are several possible reasons why mental health disorders are underdiagnosed in general practice:

- key symptoms are not presented or apparent[28]

- GPs lack training, experience or confidence in managing conditions

- parents and/or GPs believe that mental health problems will be transient

- services and treatments are not readily available should identification occur or a diagnosis be made

- the avoidance of potential stigmatisation as a result of a mental health 'label'

- perceived parental resistance to a mental health diagnosis

- problems are incorrectly identified as being part of normal development.

Whilst many disorders *do* resolve spontaneously with time, longer-term persistence is often underestimated, with 62 per cent of conditions still being present 18 months after initial diagnosis.[29] The more persistent the condition, then the more likely it is to have a long-term impact.

Consultations with young people are known to be significantly shorter than those with adults,[30] and part of this reflects the concentration on physical conditions rather than psychological wellbeing. In addition, relatively few GPs have had formal training in child and adolescent psychiatry.[31,32] However, brief training programmes, and the application of systematised rating scales, have been shown to improve detection rates for mental health problems.[27,33-35]

Mental health problems are more likely to be detected if some of the consultation is spent briefly exploring psychosocial issues. In adolescence, one framework for enquiry is the use of HEADSS:[36] Home; Education; Activities; Drugs; Sex; Self-Harm. Young people are more likely to be willing to disclose psychological or emotional problems to their GP if the environment is conducive to do so.[37] Several factors may facilitate this: first, being able to access an appointment easily and at a convenient time without having to disclose personal information in order to do so, and without having to be accompanied by an adult; second, being assured that confidentiality will be preserved (unless they are at significant risk of harm); and, third, by having a GP who demonstrates genuine interest and concern in their problem.[25]

Questions for younger children and their parents or carers can also explore relationships (friends and family), activities and interests, school and performance, food and sleep. The aim is to provide an opening for children and their families to be able to disclose other concerns that might exist, and not an end in itself.

More formal screening tools are available for the detection of mental health problems in children and young people, and they can also be helpful in deciding whether further assessment is necessary:[27,38]

- the Child Functioning Scale – a brief six-item, three-point scale with pictures that explore feelings about relationships at home and school[39]

- the Strengths and Difficulties Questionnaire (SDQ) – a 25-item instrument completed by parents, teachers and older children that can help detect conduct disorder, ADHD and some anxiety disorders in children aged 4–16 years.[40]

- the Paediatric Symptom Checklist (PSC) – a 35-item questionnaire specifically developed for use in paediatric primary care with children aged 6–12 years. Symptoms cover problems in the areas of anxiety, behaviour, attention and school[41]

- the Preschool Feelings Checklist – a 20-item checklist that can help detect depressive disorders in younger children.[42]

Human figure drawing has been proposed as a supplementary method of detecting mood and anxiety disorders in children aged 6 to 12.[43]

Common presentations

Consultations explicitly for mental health problems are commonly initiated by worried parents, sometimes as a result of a crisis, and often when they feel that they can no longer cope with a problem that may have developed over a much longer period of time. Teachers or other adults engaged with a child may suggest that they see their GP, although increasingly there are direct referral pathways to CAMHS that bypass general practice. Consultations for psychological problems that are initiated by children or young people themselves are far less common. Receipt of a hospital or A&E discharge letter following an episode of self-harm may sometimes be the first presentation to primary care.

Some of the commonest ways in which mental health disorders present in children and young people are:

- behaviour problems – conflict with parents; aggression and irritability; eating problems; self-neglect; social withdrawal

- physical symptoms – headaches, recurrent non-specific abdominal pain,[44] fatigue, unexplained pain,[45] sleep problems. The possibility of a mental health disorder should be explored in all children presenting with recurrent or prolonged unexplained physical problems and amongst frequent attenders

- educational problems – school refusal, decline in academic performance[46]

- emotional – mood swings, tearfulness, anxiety

- self-harm – overdose, cutting, repetitive self-harm.

The presentation itself is not necessarily a direct indicator of the real problem. For example, a child who is becoming aggressive and exhibiting behavioural problems at home may actually be doing so because he or she is a victim of bullying at school. In all cases there is therefore a need to spend time assessing the situation fully, and not to take things at face value.

Assessment

A comprehensive mental health assessment of a child or young person can take a significant amount of time and is beyond the remit of the average GP. However, unless the situation is urgent it is worth spending adequate time to gain sufficient understanding of the problem in order to plan appropriate management and follow-up. This is best done over two or three consultations, which also gives the opportunity to determine how the problem is changing with time.

There are several key questions that need to be addressed in the assessment process:

- *What is the real problem?* The presenting problem may only be the consequence of an underlying issue. It is important to spend time trying to understand the whole picture, considering physical, social and emotional aspects

- *How and when did the problem(s) develop?* When were the first signs? Were there any significant life changes at the time, such as starting school or parental conflict? In terms of identifying trigger factors, difficulties that stress children and young people are not necessarily the same as those that stress adults. Factors such as personal appearance and peer acceptance have far greater value in youth, and so care must be taken to avoid applying adult values when assessing the impact of a potential stressor

- *What is the impact of the problem?* Significant changes can include social isolation, poor academic performance at school, physical effects such as poor sleep and loss of appetite, or breakdown of relationships within the family

- *Who is it affecting most?* For example, a child with mild hyperactivity disorder may be coping educationally and socially themselves, but may be causing their parents embarrassment in social situations. Parental stress and anxiety resulting from dealing with their child may need to be dealt with separately

- *How pervasive is the problem?* The persistence of a problem both over time and in different settings is an indicator of a more significant and generalised disorder. In contrast, if the problem is confined to a single setting, such as school, then it is likely that it is linked to a stressor in that setting, such as bullying or undiagnosed learning difficulties

- *What risk factors are present?* Particular groups of children and young people are at much greater risk of significant mental health problems. Key risk factors are listed in Table 8.4 (p. 167). Although the list is not exhaustive, the presence of any of these should lower the threshold of suspicion for the presence of a significant mental health problem

- *Are there undisclosed problems?* Some symptoms may be too distressing or embarrassing to disclose immediately, or a young person may be afraid of the consequences if they are revealed. Sensitive and reassuring direct questioning is often required to uncover such symptoms. Typically, disclosure of recurrent self-harm, abuse, bullying, concerns about weight, obsessional thoughts and compulsive behaviours, or substance misuse, will require such an approach

- *Is the apparent problem part of normal development?* Symptoms that often cause parental concern but may, in fact, fall within the spectrum of 'normal' behaviour include night terrors, conflict with parents, mood swings, imaginary friends, rituals, dieting and experimentation with drugs

- *Is there a physical explanation for the symptoms?* It is important to exclude physical causes or contributory factors such as neurological or endocrine disorders before making a psychiatric diagnosis. There is clearly an overlap between some disorders, such as chronic fatigue syndrome and eating disorders, where both physical and psychological factors are important

- *Is the child or young person at significant risk of harm?* Occasionally the information gathered will indicate that there is an immediate or continuing risk to the welfare of the child or young person to the extent that it will be necessary to institute child protection procedures or an urgent specialist assessment. This may require breach of confidentiality. However, it is also important to avoid over-reaction for problems that have been developing over a long period of time, and where there is time for a more planned and coordinated approach

- *What outcome does the child or young person and their family want?* What are their expectations both in terms of immediate management and also longer-term consequences? Patient and parental beliefs may influence their expectations of treatment and also subsequent engagement with a management plan.[47]

Whenever possible, depending on the age of the young person, they should be interviewed independently of their parents, at least for part of the consultation. In this context, children and young people have the same right to confidentiality as any other patient and this should be explained to them, whilst also emphasising that there are occasions when information must be shared (if they are at risk of harm), and that it is usually ultimately helpful to share their worries or concerns with parents or other adults at some stage.

GPs often feel challenged by consultations with adolescent patients who are in difficulty. They report feeling relatively impotent, afraid of what they might uncover, inadequately trained, and lacking in appropriate resources to deal with any problems. There can be a tendency to avoid exploring sensitive issues, and to make false assumptions about what the young person is seeking.[48] Perhaps as a result of this, young people often report a lack of understanding from their GP and an unwillingness to disclose their problems.[25,49]

Table 8.4: Selected factors that may influence the development of mental illness in children and young people

	Increased risk	Reduced risk
Biological	Genetic risk (family history of disorder) Exposure to toxins in pregnancy (e.g. alcohol) Substance and alcohol misuse Head trauma Chronic illness Malnutrition	Normal development from birth Good physical health
Psychological	Learning difficulties and educational needs Maladaptive personality traits Sexual, physical or emotional abuse or neglect 'Difficult temperament' Poor self-esteem	Normal intellectual functioning Ability to learn from experiences Positive self-esteem Problem-solving skills Social skills
Social		
Family	'Looked-after children' Parental conflict and family discord Poor family discipline including excessive punishment Family bereavement Parents with mental health problems	Family attachment Positive involvement in family Physically and mentally healthy family members Appropriate family discipline
Education	Academic failure Bullying Inadequate support from school	Academic success Positive involvement in school life Good relationships in school environment
Community	Discrimination and marginalisation Exposure to violence Youth offending	Close friendships and peer support Opportunities for leisure Positive role models Connectedness to community

Whilst it is inappropriate to separate younger children from their parents during the assessment process, it is important to engage them in the consultation, to observe their behaviour and reactions, and to see if this is consistent with the story from the parents or carers that are with them. In addition, collateral information can be invaluable, for example from school or other sources.

Whilst gathering information is clearly an important part of the assessment, it is also the start of effective management. Active listening and demonstrating an interest in the concerns of the child or young person are vital steps in acknowledging their importance as an individual and in developing a productive therapeutic relationship.[50]

Management

When deciding on the most appropriate management for mental health problems in children and young people there are two potentially conflicting messages inherent in most of the published guidance. The first is that early intervention can reduce the risk of prolonged disability; the second is that many problems resolve spontaneously and that the role of the GP is to monitor over a period of time (often termed 'watchful waiting'). Several problems, such as hyperkinetic disorders and anxiety states, only reach the threshold for formal psychiatric diagnosis if they have been present for at least six months, during which time they may have been causing significant functional impairment.

'Watchful waiting' should not be considered the passive activity that is frequently implied – GPs have a potentially powerful role in influencing the course of an illness at this stage, providing that they are prepared to engage with the situation. Central to this is the need to develop a relationship of trust with the child or young person and their family by means of active listening, and to provide a non-judgemental, objective but empathic source of support. Families dealing with emotional or behavioural problems require encouragement and a sense of optimism in order to sustain their efforts.

General approaches

- *Dietary advice:* there are established links between diet and mental health, although the therapeutic implications of these have yet to be fully established.[51] Parents may prefer to attribute behavioural or emotional problems to diet rather than a mental health problem. The role of the GP in this case is to promote a balanced diet and to safeguard children from radical dietary manipulations, if necessary, referring for advice from a dietician.

- *Promoting activity:* physical exercise has a range of positive benefits to mental health. Most important is the need to identify, encourage and schedule activities that have been enjoyable or a positive experience in the past.

- *Providing information:* children, young people and their parents can be helped to understand the problems that they are facing, and are often reassured when they realise that these are not unique to them. Leaflets and publications from reliable sources such as the Mental Health Foundation, Young Minds and the Royal College of Psychiatrists can reinforce verbal explanation. Written information for children and young people needs to be appropriate to their age and development. Some self-help materials are also available although these are most appropriately used alongside other support.

- *Involving others:* where appropriate, other members of the primary healthcare team, such as the health visitor, can be recruited to give support, particularly if the problem is affecting members of the family, such as younger siblings. With appropriate consent, communication with the child's school may be helpful in solving practical issues that may have been uncovered.

- *Facilitating problem solving:* families are sometimes so entangled in their problems and emotions that they have difficulty identifying specific problems that could be resolved. At a simple level problem solving involves identification of such issues, examining a range of possible solutions and their potential consequences, and then promoting the implementation and evaluating the chosen course of action.

- *Promoting positive parenting:* some problems, such as conduct disorders, are strongly linked to parenting style. In other disorders, negative parental reactions to the initial problem may serve to potentiate the difficulties. Characteristics of positive parenting include clear and unambiguous communication between the parent and child, consistent messages (especially between parents), reinforcing and rewarding positive behaviour, identifying and applying realistic and appropriate sanctions for non-compliant behaviour, and providing a daily structure for the family that includes constructive shared time.

Referral

A child or young person with a mental health problem does not always need referral to specialist services. Because of the transient nature of many emotional and behavioural conditions they can often be managed in primary care as outlined above. However, the following is a list of situations where referral is definitely recommended:

- repeated or significant self-harm
- persistent and pervasive disabling symptoms
- prolonged absence from school
- self-neglect or social withdrawal
- significant weight loss
- need for a definitive diagnosis
- presence of psychotic symptoms
- complex problems
- significant substance misuse.

Even in the absence of the above, consideration should be given to early referral of individuals at high risk of mental disorder. These include children in care, those exposed to traumatic events or to physical or sexual abuse, those with a strong family history of mental health problems, or where parenting skills are known to be inadequate.

The situation can be complicated if either the child or parent declines the suggestion of a mental health referral at a stage when the GP believes this to be appropriate. Usually the situation can be resolved by continued negotiation over a longer period of time. It may be appropriate to discuss the situation with a CAMHS worker even if it is impossible to engage the young person or their family directly at that time. The wishes of the young person must be taken into account and balanced with the risk to themselves and to others.

A range of psychological therapies can be accessed through specialist referrals that are not usually available in primary care.[52] These include:

- *family therapy* – this works on the premise that a child's difficulties need to be addressed in a social context that may have an impact on precipitating or maintaining behaviours or feelings. It has been shown to be effective in early-onset eating disorders, depression, anxiety, psychosomatic complaints and adjustment reactions. However, there may be difficulty in engaging the whole family to work with the therapist over a sufficient length of time

- *cognitive therapy* – this deals with the thought processes that link to feelings and behaviour, and works on the assumption that the individual has maladaptive or distorted thought processes. It has been found to be effective amongst young people with aggression, anxiety disorders, depression and eating disorders. It is usually provided on an individual basis, mainly in adolescence, but can also be provided in a group format, and with younger children

- *behavioural therapy* – this works on the assumption that any behaviour can be modified by increasing or reducing stimuli that influence it. It can be effective across the age range of child and adolescent disorders in the management of anxiety states, enuresis and encopresis, obsessive-compulsive disorders, conduct disorders, and also in behavioural aspects of psychotic disorders. Therapy involves defining goals, assessing the behaviour and implementing a therapeutic plan

- *other therapies* – include interpersonal therapy, play therapy, music therapy, motivational interviewing, and parenting group interventions.

Prescribing

Most GPs report feeling inadequately trained to prescribe psychotropic drugs for children and adolescents, and would prefer to do so only with specialist support. In addition, less than 50 per cent of drugs used to treat children for *any* condition have been adequately subjected to clinical trials in an appropriate age group. Despite this, the prescribing of psychotropic medication to children and young people has increased significantly until recently.[53,54] The situation has changed recently, particularly with respect to the prescribing of selective serotonin reuptake inhibitors (SSRIs) for young people, with the recognition that the risk-to-benefit ratio of this group of drugs for depression is poor, particularly because of the increased risk of suicidal ideation. As a result, the Committee on Safety of Medicines recommended that only fluoxetine should be used for treating depression in children and young people under the age of 18, and then only if initiated in specialist settings. Prescribing rates for antidepressants by GPs in young people have fallen significantly as a result of this guidance.[55]

For most mental health disorders in children and young people, current clinical guidelines recommend that drug therapies should only be initiated in specialist settings, usually after an adequate trial, or alongside non-pharmacological treatments. However, there may be occasions when, as a result of patient preference, prolonged waiting times for specialist services, or lack of availability of psychological therapies, GPs will still need to initiate drug therapy, although preferably after discussion with a specialist. The use of drug treatment is best established for obsessive-compulsive disorder, tic disorders, and hyperkinetic disorders.[56]

Table 8.5 (p. 172) summarises the indications for psychotropic drugs from the *British National Formulary for Children*, together with comments on their initiation and use. Where psychotropic drug therapy is initiated or prescribed for children or young people in general practice, particular consideration needs to be given to promoting adherence and ensuring safety. Simple dosage regimes, providing adequate explanation of the purpose and side effects of treatment, and involving the young person in planning can all increase adherence.[57] Safety issues include ensuring secure storage, arranging adequate supervision, limiting the quantity prescribed, and organising follow-up to monitor benefits and both short- and long-term risks and side effects.

Follow-up

Whether or not a child or young person is referred to specialist services, continued contact with them and their family can be important to monitor progress, promote continued involvement with any intervention, reassess the needs and problems within the family, and address any physical needs. Because of the potential stigma of mental health disorders, families can sometimes be helped by GPs taking an advocacy role, particularly with other services.

For children with long-term mental health problems, GPs also have a potential key role in facilitating transition from child to adult services. Many young people and their families

Table 8.5: A summary of psychotropic drugs for children and young people[58]

Drug type	Specific drug	Indications and recommendations
Hypnotics Not usually justified except for short-term use such as for night terrors and sleep walking	Zopiclone	Safety and efficacy are uncertain – specialist prescribing only
	Chloral hydrate	Night sedation for children
	Triclofos sodium	Night sedation for children with less gastric irritation than chloral hydrate
	Promethazine hydrochloride	Night sedation and insomnia (short-term use) – not usually justified for use in children
	Melatonin	Sleep disorders in children with autism – specialist initiation only
Anxiolytics Should only be used to relieve acute anxiety (and related insomnia) caused by fear, with dose limited to smallest amount for shortest time	Diazepam	Night terrors and somnambulism
	Buspirone	Safety and efficacy in children have yet to be established
Antipsychotics	Chlorpromazine, haloperidol, levomepromazine, pericyazine, perphenazine, pimozide, sulpiride, trifluoperazine; and atypical antipsychotics (amisulpride, clozapine, olanzapine, quetiapine, risperidone)	Specialist initiation only for childhood psychoses, motor tics, psychomotor agitation, excitement or dangerously impulsive or violent behaviour
Antidepressants	Fluoxetine	Depressive disorders in children aged 12–18, with specialist initiation and close monitoring for suicidal behaviours
	Fluvoxamine	Obsessive-compulsive disorder (ages 8–18)
	Sertraline	Obsessive-compulsive disorder (ages 6–18)
	Tricyclic antidepressants: amitriptyline, amoxapine, nortriptyline	Depression (age 16–18)
Stimulants Longer-acting preparations are usually most effective	Atomoxetine, dexamfetamine sulphate, methylphenidate hydrochloride	Attention deficit hyperactivity disorder – initiated by a specialist physician experienced in managing the condition
Mood stabilisers	Lithium, carbamazepine, valproic acid	Prophylaxis and treatment of mania and bipolar disorder under specialist supervision

report difficulties with transition to services that are completely adult orientated, and GPs can help to build the bridges.

Failure to re-attend is common both amongst young people in general and specifically amongst those with mental health problems. There are numerous reasons why this might occur: crises that triggered the initial consultation may have resolved; the initial consultation may have provided sufficient insight or help that the problem is now under control; the child or its family may have been antagonistic or ambivalent about a potential mental health label; or the problem has deteriorated to such an extent that he or she is too 'disabled' to attend. Alternatively he or she may simply have been unable to get a return appointment at a convenient time.

Several actions can be helpful to maintain contact: first, by facilitating a return visit by actively making an appointment whilst the young person or his or her family is present, and at a time that is convenient to them; second, by avoiding leaving too long before the next contact, in order to maintain momentum; third, by making an agreement with them about how they can be contacted; fourth, by making an explicit decision about how you perceive the current risk and what action you would consider if they do not attend for follow-up; and, finally, if they do not attend, by making provision to identify that this has occurred, and to follow up as planned.

The potential role of GPs with a Special Interest

There is an emerging role for GPs who have a special interest in all areas of general practice (GPwSIs). However, the potential impact is greater in the area of child and adolescent mental health because of the lack of formal training that most GPs have received in this area. Potential roles include acting as local champions for child and adolescent mental health, providing educational input for other primary healthcare professionals, and providing a clinical service for the assessment, management or further referral of young people with such problems. Some may develop more specific expertise in areas such as the management of attention deficit hyperactivity disorders, eating disorders or self-harm.

A GP taking on this role should, as a minimum: be competent in communicating with children, young people and their families about mental health problems; have a good understanding of the range of mental health conditions and how these may present; be able to distinguish normal from abnormal development; be able to manage risk associated with such conditions; and be able to work closely with local specialist services. Although GPwSIs in child and adolescent mental health would be a valuable resource for other GPs, they would not replace the need for improved education and training in this area for all GPs.

An overview of specific mental health conditions affecting children and young people

Anxiety states[48,59–62]

Anxiety states in children commonly present with either somatic symptoms, such as recurrent abdominal pain, or with behavioural problems, such as school refusal. The earliest type of disorder is separation anxiety where a child becomes acutely distressed when placed in a situation away from its parent. Such reactions are common in mild form between the ages of one and four. However, more extreme reactions can inhibit external social interaction. At older ages this can result in school refusal and subsequent school avoidance. Specific phobias are usually maladaptive reactions to normal specific fears, such as the dark or insects. Social anxiety, panic disorder and generalised anxiety can all develop during childhood and be maintained into adulthood.

Management of anxiety states in children and young people requires an understanding of how the problem has developed on an individual basis. Symptom diaries can sometimes be helpful to make a connection between unexplained physical symptoms and anxiety trigger factors. Simple behavioural techniques, such as graded exposure to a trigger factor, may be helpful at an early stage. However, persistent severe and disabling symptoms require referral for formal psychological therapies or occasionally drug treatment. Cognitive behavioural therapy has been shown to be effective in anxiety disorders in children and young people.

Autistic spectrum disorder[16]

Childhood autism crosses the boundary between developmental, educational and psychiatric disorders. It is a complex behavioural disorder with a triad of developmental impairments: communication; social functioning; and play. Its prevalence is up to 1 per cent depending on the definition used, and it is approximately three times more common in boys than girls. There have been numerous theories about its aetiology, most recently, and erroneously, one that attributed it to the MMR vaccine. However, it is likely to be multifactorial in origin with a very strong genetic component and with environmental influences either before birth or in infancy affecting development.

Presentation will depend on severity. In the most severe cases there might be some evidence before the age of 12 months, whilst in milder forms (including higher-functioning autism or Asperger's syndrome) the problems may not be identified until senior school age. Severe autism is associated with a 30 per cent risk of epilepsy in adolescence. There are also associations with obsessive-compulsive disorder, hyperkinetic disorders and dyspraxia.

Primary healthcare professionals need to be aware of early indicators of the disorder in order to make a referral for a multi-agency assessment, particularly if it is likely that the condition will significantly affect development. Key early signs include speech delay, lack of interaction and play with other children, lack of creative play, and inability to cope with changes to routine. A key feature is that the problems are pervasive across a range of settings, and any multi-agency assessment of the child will involve observation in more than one environment. There are no screening tools currently available for use in primary care.

Conduct disorders[62,63]

Conduct disorders are characterised by a pattern of behaviour where the rights of others or social norms are repeatedly violated by aggression (to people or animals), destruction of property, deceitfulness or theft, or other serious violation of rules, such as truancy and staying out at night. By definition the behaviour must have significant social, educational or occupational effects, and must be persistent over at least 12 months for a formal diagnosis.

Oppositional defiant disorder is a related condition, usually in younger children, in which there is persistent non-cooperative, defiant and hostile behaviour towards parents and other authority figures, lasting at least six months, and resulting in significant functional impairment, but not involving major antisocial behaviours.

Both conditions can be associated with learning difficulties, hyperactivity and substance misuse, as well as with poor parenting, depression and a history of abuse. It is therefore important to consider the impact of other causative factors before considering applying such a label.

Depression[62,17,64,65]

Symptoms of depressive disorders in children and young people can be similar to those of adults. Common features include irritability, loss of enjoyment in usual activities, withdrawal from friends, lack of self-care, self-criticism, deterioration in schoolwork, and the presence of somatic symptoms such as tiredness or headaches. For a depressive disorder to be diagnosed the symptoms must be pervasive over time and in different settings. The prevalence of depression is approximately 1 per cent in pre-pubertal children and 3 per cent in post-pubertal young people.

Most major depressive episodes occur in children and young people exposed to long-standing psychosocial difficulties such as parental disharmony, domestic violence or bullying. Less than 5 per cent occur in the absence of such difficulties and these are often precipitated by an acute life event.[66] Around 10 per cent of children and young people with depression recover spontaneously within the first three months, and a further 40 per cent recover by 12 months. However, untreated, 50 per cent remain clinically depressed at one year.[67] There is a 30 per cent risk of recurrence within five years and a 3 per cent risk of suicide in the following 10 years.

NICE recommends a stepped-care approach to the management of children and young people with depression, with a period of 'watchful waiting' being appropriate for those with milder symptoms, followed by non-directive supportive therapy, group CBT or guided self-help. Those with more severe forms should be referred to specialist services for assessment and treatment with a specific psychological therapy. Antidepressant medication is only recommended after these other approaches have failed, with fluoxetine being the first-line treatment, and should not normally be initiated in primary care.

Eating disorders[18,68]

Anorexia nervosa is characterised by low weight, or progressive weight loss, as a result of a preoccupation with body mass. It is formally diagnosed when the body weight is at least 15 per cent below that expected, or below a BMI of 17.5 in a young person who should have achieved adult body mass. The average age of onset is 16 or 17.

Bulimia nervosa is characterised by recurrent episodes of binge eating associated with a subjective feeling of loss of control over eating and sometimes with compensatory behaviour such as self-induced vomiting and laxative abuse. It can often follow an episode of anorexia nervosa and the average age of onset is 18.

In adolescence the prevalence of anorexia nervosa in the population is approximately 0.4 per cent, and for bulimia nervosa 1 per cent, with both conditions being significantly more common in girls. In contrast approximately 35 per cent of young people are dieting because of concerns about weight at any one time, although this may represent the start of an eating disorder in some.

Since the key symptoms of both anorexia nervosa and bulimia nervosa are usually concealed, the diagnosis should be considered in any young person who is underweight, who is requesting information about dieting, who has primary or secondary amenorrhoea, or in whom there are physical signs of malnutrition (such as poor hair growth, dry skin, bradycardia and constipation). Sensitive questioning should be used to elucidate primary symptoms, and co-morbid mood disorders or exposure to abuse need to be excluded.

The challenge for GPs who suspect an eating disorder in a young person is to help them to acknowledge their problem and to accept help. At an early stage simple weight monitoring, feedback and provision of information may be adequate. NICE recommends baseline blood tests, urinalysis and consideration of an electrocardiogram in anyone suspected of having anorexia nervosa. Early referral is recommended for specific evidence-based psychological therapies. Hospital admission is indicated in the presence of very rapid weight loss, very low BMI, high risk of suicide, or signs of physical compromise.

Hyperkinetic disorders[15,69–71]

Hyperkinetic disorder, also known as attention deficit disorder (ADHD/ADD), with or without hyperactivity is a pattern of behaviour that exists at one end of a continuous spectrum within children in the community. The extent to which it is a cause of morbidity is a combination of the severity of the behavioural symptoms, associated impairment, the environment in which it occurs, and the perceptions of the adults who observe it. Although there is still controversy about the extent to which it is a mental health problem and, consequently, how it should be managed, there has been increasing professional consensus about its validity in recent years.

Children with hyperkinetic disorders tend to present in the education system rather than to GPs. A formal diagnosis requires the presence of persistent, pervasive and disabling symptoms that have their onset before the age of 6 or 7 and include inattention (difficulty concentrating or easily distracted), hyperactivity (excessive levels of activity, disorganised, noisy) and impulsivity (interrupts or intrudes, talks constantly). However, children can still have significant impairment if the criteria are not fully met.

The estimated prevalence of hyperkinetic disorder in school-aged children lies between 5 per cent and 10 per cent depending on the criteria used. It is at least four times more common in boys than girls. Hyperactivity symptoms often diminish during adolescence but inattention and associated impairment can persist into adulthood. Despite the prevalence, it has been estimated that only approximately 5 per 1000 boys are currently receiving drug treatment for the condition in the UK.

The impact of ADHD can be widespread – with effects on educational attainment, disrupted family life, antisocial behaviour, and risk of accidents. Persistent negative feedback from adults can result in lowered self-esteem and emotional problems. Children who meet diagnostic criteria therefore merit referral for fuller assessment and decisions on management.

The core symptoms of inattention, hyperactivity and impulsive behaviour can be improved significantly by the use of psychostimulant medication such as methylphenidate or dexamphetamine, or atomoxetine. NICE recommends that treatment should only be initiated by an appropriately qualified healthcare professional with expertise in ADHD based on a comprehensive assessment and diagnosis. Continued prescribing and monitoring of drug therapy may be performed by general practitioners under shared-care arrangements.

Monitoring should include assessment of growth and blood pressure as well as the effectiveness of treatment and presence of any side effects, which include nausea and anorexia, sleep difficulties, rebound behavioural problems, and abnormal movements. Psychosocial and behavioural interventions have limited impact on the core symptoms of hyperkinetic disorder, even when added to medication, but can be used to moderate some of the secondary problems.

Obsessive-compulsive disorder[19,62]

Rituals and repetitive behaviours are common in children, especially between the ages of 3 and 6, and become more evident when the child is under stress or experiencing anxiety. However, these need to be distinguished from obsessions (intrusive repetitive thoughts that usually have a negative content) and compulsions (repetitive actions required to alleviate the thoughts). They are, by nature, distressing and time-consuming.

People who present with symptoms of OCD in adulthood often report that they experienced their first symptoms in childhood or adolescence. The first signs of OCD can be present from as young as 4–5 years of age and the prevalence of OCD in young people is about 1 per cent. There is a four-fold increased risk if a family member is affected, and also an association with the presence of tics. Symptoms of OCD can continue into adulthood in up to 60 per cent of people, but this may underestimate the numbers that recur in later life.

Because of the nature of the thoughts, young people are reluctant to admit to them and sensitive direct questioning is the most useful technique to expose the problem. NICE recommends a stepped-care approach to the management of OCD with guided self-help being the first level for those with mild functional impairment, in conjunction with support and information for the family and carers. For those with more severe disability, an age-appropriate form of CBT is recommended, followed by cautious addition of SSRI with arrangements in place to monitor for adverse effects.

Post-Traumatic Stress Disorder[20]

Children and young people can experience long-term physical and psychological reactions as a result of being exposed to, or witnessing, traumatic or life-threatening events.[72] In the past, such effects have been underestimated but, untreated, symptoms can last for years. PTSD is characterised by re-experiencing the event (by flashbacks or nightmares), avoidance and hyperarousal symptoms (poor concentration and sleep). Symptoms in children can include repetitive re-enactment by play or drawing, sleep disturbance, irritability and sometimes aggressive behaviour.

The prevalence of PTSD in children and young people has been estimated as 1 per cent. NICE recommends that parents of children who are exposed to trauma should be advised to consult their GP if symptoms such as nightmares, sleep disturbance, irritability and poor concentration persist for more than a month. Specialist therapies such as trauma-focused CBT may help if symptoms persist. The use of drug treatment is not endorsed.

Psychoses and bipolar disorder[22,73,74]

Psychotic disorder and bipolar mood disorder are uncommon amongst children and young people, but early recognition and intervention are vitally important as these disorders frequently first present in adolescence (see Chapter 7). Acute symptoms may present with behavioural patterns, such as sleep disturbance, which can be difficult to distinguish from normal adolescence. GPs are sometimes in a position to recognise patterns of change over time, such as gradual social withdrawal, or recurring depressive episodes, which may provide clues to an incipient disorder; more frequent consultation rates in general practice have been shown to be associated with reduced duration of untreated psychosis. The most common cause of acute psychotic symptoms in young people is substance misuse, but even where this has occurred it may only serve to precipitate a latent disorder. Whilst urgent referral of any suspected psychosis or bipolar disorder is important, GPs need to provide continuing support to the young person and his or her family for what may become a chronic illness.

Self-harm[21,75–78]

Whilst not a discrete disorder, incidents of self-harm in adolescence are relatively common, with 13 per cent of young people aged 15–16 reporting having harmed themselves at some point in their lives, with an average age of onset being 12. Self-harm is three times greater amongst girls than boys. The majority of incidents never come to the attention of healthcare services or even parents, because they are concealed. The most common type of self-harm in the community is cutting, whilst self-poisoning is the most frequent cause for presentation to A&E.

Whilst in some cases there is deliberate suicidal intent, self-harm is often an impulsive reaction to an acutely distressing situation, or a recurring method of relieving ongoing emotional distress. There is a strong association between self-harm and mental health disorders such as depression, but also with adverse life events such as physical or sexual abuse.

NICE guidance focuses on the short-term management of self-harm that emphasises the need to address the physical effects first, followed by a formal psychological assessment by professionals trained in the assessment of children and young people. General practitioners are more likely to encounter young people who recurrently self-harm. This was the focus of the National Inquiry into Self-Harm in Young People, which highlighted not only the scale of the problem but also the lack of understanding by many adults including GPs. Recommendations included the need for healthcare professionals to demonstrate empathy and understanding with young people who self-harm, especially at the point of disclosure. Management needs to focus on the underlying causes: identifying alternative methods of coping with distress, problem-solving, and timely help-seeking.

Summary

Historically, mental health problems in children and young people have been poorly recognised and inadequately managed in general practice. This has been partly as a result of the lack of training and experience of most GPs, but also because of poorly developed specialist support services in many areas. GPs can have an important role in the early recognition and assessment of these problems, as well as providing longer-term support for children, young people and their families.

References

1. Maughan B, Brock A, Ladva G. Mental health. In: *The Health of Children & Young People* London: Office of National Statistics, 2004.

2. Black D. Mental health services for children *British Medical Journal* 1992; **305**: 971–2.

3. Jacobson L, Churchill R, Donovan C, *et al.* Tackling teenage turmoil: primary care recognition and management of mental ill health during adolescence *Family Practice* 2002; **19(4)**: 401–9.

4. Green H, McGinnity A, Meltzer H, *et al. Mental Health of Children and Young People in Great Britain, 2004: summary report* London: Office of National Statistics, 2005.

5. Meltzer H, Gatward R, Goodman R, *et al. Mental Health of Children and Adolescents in Great Britain* London: The Stationery Office, 2000.

6. Department of Health. *National Service Framework for Children, Young People and Maternity Services: key issues for primary care* London: DH, 2004.

7. Department for Education and Skills. *Every Child Matters* London: HMSO, 2003.

8. Department of Health. *National Service Framework for Children, Young People and Maternity Services: the mental and psychological well-being of children and young people* London: DH, 2004.

9. NHS Health Advisory Service. *Together We Stand: the commissioning and management of child and adolescent mental health services* London: HMSO, 1995.

10. The Audit Commission for Local Authorities and the National Health Service in England and Wales. *Children in Mind: child and adolescent mental health services* London: Audit Commission, 1999.

11. British Medical Association Board of Science. *Child and Adolescent Mental Health: a guide for healthcare professionals* London: BMA, 2006.

12. Ani C, Garralda E. Developing primary mental healthcare for children and adolescents *Current Opinion in Psychiatry* 2005; **18(4)**: 440–4.

13. Gale F, Vostanis P. The primary mental health worker within Child and Adolescent Mental Health Services *Clinical Child Psychology & Psychiatry* 2003; **8(2)**: 227–40.

14. Scottish Intercollegiate Guidelines Network. *Attention Deficit and Hyperkinetic Disorders in Children and Young People* Edinburgh: SIGN, 2001.

15. National Institute for Health and Clinical Excellence. *Methylphenidate, Atomoxetine and Dexamfetamine for Attention Deficit Hyperactivity Disorder (ADHD) in Children and Adolescents* London: NICE, 2006.

16. National Initiative for Autism: Screening and Assessment. *National Autism Plan for Children* London: The National Autistic Society, 2003.

17. National Institute for Health and Clinical Excellence. *Depression in Children and Young People: identification and management in primary, community and secondary care* London: NICE, 2005.

18. National Institute for Health and Clinical Excellence. *Eating disorders: core interventions in the treatment and management of anorexia nervosa, bulimia nervosa and related eating disorders* London: NICE, 2004.

19. National Institute for Health and Clinical Excellence. *Obsessive Compulsive Disorder: core interventions in the treatment of obsessive compulsive disorder and body dysmorphic disorder* London: The British Psychological Society and the Royal College of Psychiatrists, 2006.

20. National Institute for Health and Clinical Excellence. *Post-Traumatic Stress Disorder (PTSD): the management of PTSD in adults and children in primary and secondary care* London: NICE, 2005.

21. National Institute for Health and Clinical Excellence. *Self-Harm: the short-term physical and psychological management and secondary prevention of self-harm in primary and secondary care* London: NICE, 2004.

22. National Institute for Health and Clinical Excellence. *Bipolar Disorder: the management of bipolar disorder in adults, children and adolescents, in primary and secondary care* London: NICE, 2006.

23. Licence K. Promoting good mental health and positive self-esteem – the evidence. In: Chambers R, Licence K (eds). *Looking after Children in Primary Care: a companion to the Children's National Service Framework* Oxford: Radcliffe, 2005.

24. Kramer T, Garralda M. Psychiatric disorders in adolescents in primary care *British Journal of Psychiatry* 1998; **173**: 508–13.

25. Churchill R, Allen J, Denman S, *et al*. Do the attitudes and beliefs of young teenagers towards general practice influence actual consultation behaviour? *British Journal of General Practice* 2000; **50(461)**: 953–7.

26. Sayal K, Taylor E. Detection of child mental health disorders by general practitioners *British Journal of General Practice* 2004; **54**: 348–52.

27. Cassidy LJ, Jellinek MS. Approaches to recognition and management of childhood psychiatric disorders in pediatric primary care *Pediatric Clinics of North America* 1998; **45(5)**: 1037–52.

28. Sayal K. Annotation: pathways to care for children with mental health problems *Journal of Child Psychology & Psychiatry* 2006; **47(7)**: 649–59.

29. Goodman R, Ford T, Meltzer H. Mental health problems of children in the community: 18 month follow-up *British Medical Journal* 2002; **324**: 1496–7.

30. Jacobson LD, Wilkinson C, Owen PA. Is the potential of teenage consultations being missed? A study of consultation times in primary care *Family Practice* 1994; **11(3)**: 296–9.

31. Weeramanthri T, Keaney F. What do inner city general practitioners want from a child and adolescent mental health service? *Psychiatric Bulletin* 2000; **24(7)**: 258–60.

32. Foreman DM. General practitioners and child and adolescent psychiatry: awareness and training of the new commissioners *Psychiatric Bulletin* 2001; **25(3)**: 101–4.

33. Iliffe S, Gledhill J, da Cunha F, *et al*. The recognition of adolescent depression in general practice: issues in the acquisition of new skills *Primary Care Psychiatry* 2004; **9(2)**: 51–6.

34. Zuckerbrot RA, Jensen PS. Improving recognition of adolescent depression in primary care *Archives of Pediatrics & Adolescent Medicine* 2006; **160(7)**: 694–704.

35. Gledhill J, Kramer T, Iliffe S, *et al.* Training general practitioners in the identification and management of adolescent depression within the consultation: a feasibility study *Journal of Adolescence* 2003; **26(2)**: 245–50.

36. McCabe R. Psychiatric disturbance *Practitioner* 1992; **236**: 1150–4.

37. Churchill D, McPherson A. Getting it right in primary care: creating a child and young person friendly environment. In: Chambers R, Licence K (eds). *Looking after Children in Primary Care* Oxford: Radcliffe, 2005.

38. Ciechomski L, Blashki G, Tonge B. Common psychological disorders in childhood *Australian Family Physician* 2004; **33(12)**: 997–1003.

39. Wildman BG, Kinsman AM, Smucker WD. Use of child reports of daily functioning to facilitate identification of psychosocial problems in children *Archives of Family Medicine* 2000; **9(7)**: 612–16.

40. Goodman R, Ford T, Simmons H, *et al.* Using the Strengths and Difficulties Questionnaire (SDQ) to screen for child psychiatric disorders in a community sample *British Journal of Psychiatry* 2000; **177**: 534–9.

41. Murphy J, Jellinek M. Screening for psychosocial dysfunction in economically disadvantaged and minority group children: further validation of the pediatric symptom checklist *American Journal of Orthopsychiatry* 1998; **58**: 450–6.

42. Luby JL, Heffelfinger A, Koenig-McNaught AL, *et al.* The Preschool Feelings Checklist: a brief and sensitive screening measure for depression in young children *Journal of the American Academy of Child & Adolescent Psychiatry* 2004; **43(6)**: 708–17.

43. Tielsch AH, Allen PJ. Listen to them draw: screening children in primary care through the use of human figure drawings *Pediatric Nursing* 2005; **31(4)**: 320–7.

44. Campo JV, Bridge J, Ehmann M, *et al.* Recurrent abdominal pain, anxiety, and depression in primary care *Pediatrics* 2004; **113(4)**: 817–24.

45. Dilsaver SC, Wu X, Akiskal HS, *et al.* Pain complaints in adolescent patients with affective disorders versus adolescent psychiatric controls *Primary Care Companion to the Journal of Clinical Psychiatry* 2005; **7(4)**: 150–4.

46. Asarnow JR, Jaycox LH, Duan N, *et al.* Depression and role impairment among adolescents in primary care clinics *Journal of Adolescent Health* 2005; **37(6)**: 477–83.

47. Jaycox LH, Asarnow JR, Sherbourne CD, *et al.* Adolescent primary care patients' preferences for depression treatment *Administration & Policy in Mental Health* 2006; **33(2)**: 198–207.

48. Donovan C, Suckling H. *Difficult Consultations with Adolescents* Oxford: Radcliffe, 2004.

49. Jacobson L, Richardson G, Parry-Langdon N, *et al.* How do teenagers and primary healthcare providers view each other? An overview of key themes *British Journal of General Practice* 2001; **51(471)**: 811–16.

50. Wisdom JP, Clarke GN, Green CA. What teens want: barriers to seeking care for depression *Administration & Policy in Mental Health* 2006; **33(2)**: 133–45.

51. Mental Health Foundation. *Feeding Minds: the impact of food on mental health* London: MHF, 2006.

52. Dogra N, Parkin A, Gale F, *et al. Child and Adolescent Mental Health for Front-Line Professionals* London & Philadelphia: Jessica Kingsley Publishers, 2002.

53. Wong IC, Camilleri-Novak D, Stephens P. Rise in psychotropic drug prescribing in children in the UK: an urgent public health issue *Drug Safety* 2003; **26(15)**: 1117–18.

54. Murray ML, De Vries CS, Wong ICK. A drug utilisation study of antidepressants in children and adolescents using the General Practice Research Database *Archives of Disease in Childhood* 2004; **89(12)**: 1098–102.

55. Murray ML, Thompson M, Santosh PJ, *et al*. Effects of the Committee on Safety of Medicines advice on antidepressant prescribing to children and adolescents in the UK *Drug Safety* 2005; **28(12)**: 1151–7.

56. Hazell P. Prescribing psychotropic medication to children in general practice *Australian Prescriber* 2005; **28(5)**: 116–18.

57. Staples B, Bravender T. Drug compliance in adolescents: assessing and managing modifiable risk factors *Paediatric Drugs* 2002; **4(8)**: 503–13.

58. *British National Formulary for Children* London: BMJ Publishing Group Ltd, Royal Pharmaceutical Society, RCPCH Publications Ltd, 2005.

59. Chavira DA, Stein MB, Bailey K, *et al*. Child anxiety in primary care: prevalent but untreated *Depression & Anxiety* 2004; **20(4)**: 155–64.

60. Manassis K. Childhood anxiety disorders. Approach to intervention *Canadian Family Physician* 2004; **50**: 379–84.

61. Castellanos D, Hunter T. Anxiety disorders in children and adolescents *Southern Medical Journal* 1999; **92(10)**: 946–54.

62. Michaud PA, Fombonne E. Common mental health problems *British Medical Journal* 2005; **330**: 835–8.

63. Searight HR, Rottnek F, Abby SL. Conduct disorder: diagnosis and treatment in primary care *American Family Physician* 2001; **63(8)**: 1579–88.

64. Rey J. *More than Just the Blues: understanding serious teenage problems* (second edn) Australia: Simon & Schuster, 2002.

65. Stein REK, Zitner LE, Jensen PS. Interventions for adolescent depression in primary care *Pediatrics* 2006; **118**: 669–82.

66. Goodyer IM, Herbert J, Tamplin A, *et al*. Recent life events, cortisol, dehydroepiandrosterone and the onset of major depression in high-risk adolescents *British Journal of Psychiatry* 2000; **177**: 499–504.

67. Goodyer IM, Herbert J, Tamplin A. Psychoendocrine antecedents of persistent first-episode major depression in adolescents: a community-based longitudinal enquiry *Psychological Medicine* 2003; **33**: 601–10.

68. Nicholls D, Viner R. Eating disorders and weight problems *British Medical Journal* 2005; **330(7497)**: 950–3.

69. Scottish Intercollegiate Guidelines Network. *Attention Deficit and Hyperkinetic Disorders in Children and Young People: a national guideline* Edinburgh: Scottish Intercollegiate Guidelines Network, 2001.

70. Sayal K, Goodman R, Ford T. Barriers to the identification of children with attention deficit/hyperactivity disorder *Journal of Child Psychology & Psychiatry & Allied Disciplines* 2006; **47(7)**: 744–50.

71. Brown TE. *Attention Deficit Disorder: the unfocussed mind in children and adults* New Haven, CT: Yale University Press, 2005.

72. Dirkzwager AJ, Kerssens JJ, Yzermans CJ. Health problems in children and adolescents before and after a man-made disaster *Journal of the American Academy of Child & Adolescent Psychiatry* 2006; **45(1)**: 94–103.

73. Hodgman CH. Psychosis in adolescence *Adolescent Medicine Clinics* 2006; **17(1)**: 131–45.

74. Skeate A, Jackson C, Birchwood M, *et al*. Duration of untreated psychosis and pathways to care in first-episode psychosis. Investigation of help-seeking behaviour in primary care *British Journal of Psychiatry – Supplementum* 2002; **43**: s73–7.

75. Camelot Foundation. *Truth Hurts: report of the National Inquiry into Self-Harm among Young People* London: Camelot Foundation & Mental Health Foundation, 2006.

76. Hawton K, James A. Suicide and deliberate self harm in young people *British Medical Journal* 2005; **330(7496)**: 891–4.

77. Rodham K, Hawton K, Evans E. Reasons for deliberate self-harm: comparison of self-poisoners and self-cutters in a community sample of adolescents *Journal of the American Academy of Child & Adolescent Psychiatry* 2004; **43(1)**: 80–7.

78. Evans E, Hawton K, Rodham K. In what ways are adolescents who engage in self-harm or experience thoughts of self-harm different in terms of help-seeking, communication and coping strategies? *Journal of Adolescence* 2005; **28(4)**: 573–87.

Further reading

British Medical Association Board of Science. *Child and Adolescent Mental Health: a guide for healthcare professionals* London: BMA, 2006.

Brown TE. *Attention Deficit Disorder: the unfocussed mind in children and adults* New Haven, CT: Yale University Press, 2005.

Dogra N, Parkin A, Gale F, *et al*. *Child and Adolescent Mental Health for Front-Line Professionals* London & Philadelphia: Jessica Kingsley Publishers, 2002.

Donovan C, Suckling H. *Difficult Consultations with Adolescents* Oxford: Radcliffe, 2004.

Green H, McGinnity A, Meltzer H, *et al*. *Mental Health of Children and Young People in Great Britain, 2004: summary report* London: Office of National Statistics, 2005.

Rey J. *More than Just the Blues: understanding serious teenage problems* (second edn) Australia: Simon & Schuster, 2002.

Spender, Q, Salt N, Dawkins J, *et al*. *Child Mental Health in Primary Care* Oxford: Radcliffe, 2001.

Stallard, P. *Think Good – Feel Good: using CBT with children and young people* Chichester: John Wiley & Sons, 2005.

9 | Mental health in older people

Chris Drinkwater

> **What this chapter contributes:**
>
> depression and cognitive impairment are more prevalent in older people than in any other age group
>
> the increasing numbers of people over 65 mean that the management of depression and cognitive impairment in older people will need to become a more important part of the role of the general practitioner
>
> understanding what increases the risk of these conditions and what protects against, prevents and ameliorates mental ill health in old age is an important starting point in identifying and managing these conditions
>
> physical and mental ill health commonly coexist in older people, and there is an increased need for a comprehensive biopsychosocial approach in this age group.

Introduction

It is predicted that 2007 will be the year in which there will be more people in the UK who are over pensionable age than aged under 16.[1] This is one illustration of the fact that we live in an ageing society. Providing primary health care to older people will inevitably become an increasingly important part of the role of the GP, and meeting the particular challenges of providing mental health care will be an essential component of that role.

This chapter will focus on the two key challenges, depression and cognitive impairment. The prevalence of depression is higher than it is in the general adult population and evidence suggests that between a fifth and a quarter of older people suffer depression that is likely to cause distress of such severity as to affect their concentration, motivation, functioning and sense of enjoyment with life.[2] In long-term residential and nursing care settings the prevalence of depression rises to 45 per cent.[3] Cognitive impairment also increases with increasing age. The prevalence is 6 per cent in people over 65 but by the age of 80 this rises to 10–20 per cent. It is anticipated that the number of people with dementia in the UK population will double over the next 50 years, largely due to the anticipated increase of people over 80.[4]

Before looking at these two conditions in more detail, it is important to look at mental health in old age in a social and cultural context. The need to assess and manage these conditions in terms of their physical, psychological and social components is essential, and it is difficult to do this without some understanding of the wider social and individual determinants of mental ill health. In order to do this it seems sensible to focus on the concept of successful ageing – free of depression and cognitive impairment. From a GP perspective having an understanding of what protects against, prevents and ameliorates mental ill health in old age is an important starting point.

Successful ageing – a psychosocial perspective

Fifty years ago it was commonly held that ageing was all about inevitable social disengagement resulting in decreased interaction between the ageing person and the society of which they are part.[5] This deterministic and ageist perspective has been increasingly challenged to the extent that it has been turned on its head and replaced by the view that successful ageing is about social and community integration, and the maintenance of, rather than the disengagement from, social networks. A recent model of successful ageing that reflects this perspective has been developed by Godfrey and colleagues in a review of *Prevention and Service Provision: mental health problems in later life*.[6] This review was commissioned by Age Concern and the Mental Health Foundation as part of a UK Inquiry into Mental Health and Well-Being in Later Life.[7] The model outlined in Figure 9.1 is a useful way of thinking through issues of risk, resilience and protective factors in the development of depression in old age. More importantly it helps to identify those most at risk.

The risks to physical health and associated functional ability increase with age, as do the risks of bereavement through loss of a partner or close friends. In the past this perspective has been over-emphasised at the expense of the positive gains of 'more freedom' and 'to be able to do what you want to do, when you want to do it', which can provide the opportunity to extend and deepen family and social networks. These gains and losses are however influenced by an individual's personal resources, their socioeconomic situation and by what the experience means for them.

The relationship between these variables is complex but, to over-simplify, a patient who has suffered from a lifetime of negative events that has damaged his or her self-esteem and who has limited social networks with poor community support is more likely to become depressed if he or she suffers a close bereavement or the onset of disabling ill health than someone with high self-esteem and good social networks. This

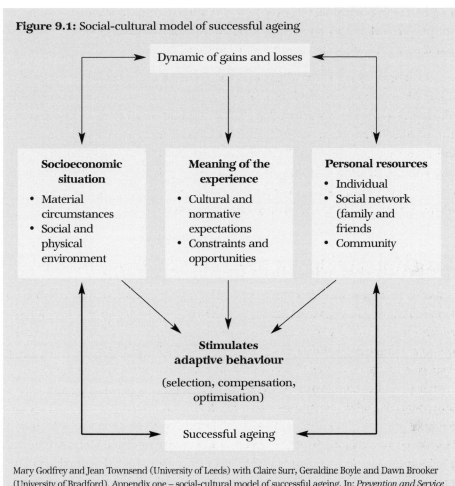

Figure 9.1: Social-cultural model of successful ageing

Dynamic of gains and losses

Socioeconomic situation
- Material circumstances
- Social and physical environment

Meaning of the experience
- Cultural and normative expectations
- Constraints and opportunities

Personal resources
- Individual
- Social network (family and friends
- Community

Stimulates adaptive behaviour

(selection, compensation, optimisation)

Successful ageing

Mary Godfrey and Jean Townsend (University of Leeds) with Claire Surr, Geraldine Boyle and Dawn Brooker (University of Bradford). Appendix one – social-cultural model of successful ageing. In: *Prevention and Service Provision: mental health problems in later life*, p. 397, report commissioned by Age Concern for the UK Inquiry into Mental Health and Well-Being in Later Life, 2005, www.mhilli.org/documents/FinalReport.pdf. Reproduced by permission of Age Concern.

situation is likely to be compounded if this patient is on a low income and lives in an area of deprivation where there is deterioration of the physical fabric, high levels of traffic noise, pollution and crime, and low levels of trust and engagement with neighbours. The GP's role in this situation is to try to stimulate adaptive rather than maladaptive behaviour. This can be difficult if there are entrenched lifelong patterns of behaviour and a risk also of reinforcing dependent illness behaviour.

There are at least two possible ways of addressing these issues. The first would be for GPs to take a more proactive role with the over-50s in promoting the benefits of social engagement through walking groups. There is increasingly robust evidence for the positive effects of exercise in reducing the risk of depression and in reducing depressive symptoms.[8] Arguably the recurrent and timely provision of advice on physical activity needs to become as important a part of the GP's stock in trade as advice to stop smoking. Second, GPs perhaps need to be more aware of support services provided by the local voluntary sector. Carers are a useful example. Most carers are themselves elderly and there is good evidence that they suffer from high levels of depressive symptoms (varies from 29 per cent to 55 per cent, depending on studies).[9] Most areas have voluntary-sector carers' support organisations but these often complain of patchy uptake by local GPs. There is reasonable evidence that carers' support is effective in terms of enhancing coping skills and in some cases reducing depressive symptoms.[10] GPs in their role as practice-based commissioners perhaps need to make more systematic use of these services, not only as a psychosocial intervention for depressed carers, but also perhaps as a means of reducing demand for more expensive hospital and respite care.

Recognising depression in older people

There are innumerable studies that demonstrate that GPs are not always very good at recognising depression.[11,12] This is particularly likely to be the case in people with long-term physical health problems and in older people,[13] who, like their GPs, can sometimes accept depression as part of growing old. Another particular problem of depression in older people is that minor depression and mood disorders that do not reach case level for depression can cause distress that is more persistent, severe and disabling than is the case with younger people.[14]

Rather than repeat what has already been said about depression in adults, the focus of this section is about how depression in older people is different. First, as has already been said, co-morbidity with ill health and physical disability is much commoner and the symptoms of physical conditions may mimic or mesh with mental health problems,[13] making diagnosis more difficult. Stroke is a case in point where a labile mood may be both a result of the stroke and of depression. Difficulties in diagnosis can also be compounded by the fact that older people are more likely to report physical or somatic conditions than psychological ones. Symptoms such as slowing of thought and activity are also relatively common among older people, making it difficult to distinguish between depression and other health problems.[15]

Second, there is some evidence that there is often a real difference in presentation of symptoms between older and younger people. One 13-year follow-up study suggested that sadness may be a less frequent feature of depression in later life.[15] This study also demonstrated that older people with sleep and appetite disturbance but without sadness (hopelessness, worthlessness, thoughts of death and wanting to die) were at increased risk for subsequent functional and cognitive impairment, psychological distress and death.

Bereavement

Effective management of bereavement in general practice has a long history.[16] It is also a major risk factor for depression in later life.[17] It is self-evident that older people, particularly women because they live longer, are more likely to be bereaved. The 2000 General Household Survey showed that around half of older women are currently widowed compared with a fifth of older men, and the rate increases with age.[18] The GP's role in all of this is to try to focus on those at greatest risk. A systematic review of risk in complicated grief following bereavement of older people identified the following risk factors:[19]

- bereaved men are at greater risk of death than women during the first 12 months following bereavement

- younger older people (65–74) are more vulnerable to depressive symptoms in both the short term (12 months) and the longer term (3 years) than people over 75

- the more dependent the bereaved person was on the person that died, the greater the likelihood of complicated grief

- a poor outcome is more likely where bereavement is followed by relocation and loss of or reduction in social contact with family and/or friends.

This review also reported that the impact of these risk factors on poor outcomes was mediated by individual coping strategies and access to, and availability of, social resources both at the personal and community level. This is perhaps part of the explanation of why higher educational status and income levels appear to protect against adverse outcomes.

The quality of pre-death care was not examined in this review. A prospective study comparing hospice care with an acute oncology ward found that the hospice group was significantly less depressed and less anxious than the hospital group at one year after bereavement.[20] In addition none of the hospice group was taking tranquillisers compared with 22 per cent of the hospital group. These conclusions are consistent with an almost universal GP experience that unresolved issues about pre-death care make it difficult for individuals to move on and thus have an adverse effect on outcomes.

Studies looking at the outcome of interventions can be divided into those that look at the impact of individual psychologically based interventions and those that look at the impact of support groups. Most studies suggest beneficial effects but these largely relate to participants' perceptions of benefit, usually with only short-term follow-up.[21] Sadly there do not appear to be any studies looking at the outcome of a structured approach by general practitioners. Proposals have been made by Charlton[22] and by Main[23] for a bereavement protocol for primary care. This would be a sensible approach for GPs to adopt but the next step would be to audit the application of such a protocol and to look at whether it produced better results than standard care.

Suicide in older people

In 1999 the suicide rate in England and Wales was 108 per million for men of all ages, 96 per million for those aged 65–74 and 152 per million for those over 75. The rates for women were 31 per million for all ages, 41 per million for those aged 65–74 and 42 per million for those over 75.[24] Interestingly surveys report low levels of suicidal ideation in older people compared with younger adults[25] and attempted suicide is also less common in this group.[26] However, the rate of committed suicide is proportionately higher, particularly in men, than in any other age group.

Apart from the fact that self-destructive behaviour more often results in death in older people, particular risk factors in this group are lack of social interaction, severity of depressive features and previous attempts.[27] Psychotic illness, personality disorder and an association with drugs or alcohol are uncommon in this age group. The GP response to this needs to be a focus on identifying major depression in socially isolated older men over 75. Having identified them, they need to be treated appropriately and offered programmes that are designed to reduce social isolation. Locally, such programmes, together with befriending services, are most often provided by the voluntary sector.

Managing depression in older people

The National Institute for Health and Clinical Excellence (NICE) produced comprehensive Clinical Guidelines on the management of depression in primary and secondary care in 2004.[28] These guidelines apply to all adults over 18 and, although the guidelines refer to age under patient characteristics, there is a danger that the particular issues of managing depression in older people get overlooked. Based on these guidelines, key points for the GP encountering a depressed older person are:

- in older adults with depression, their physical state, living conditions and social isolation should be assessed. The involvement of more than one agency is recommended where appropriate

- the recommendation that antidepressants are not suggested for the initial treatment of mild depression, because the risk–benefit ratio is poor, is particularly important for older adults. This is because mild depression is more common and more disabling in older adults and because the risks of medication rise with increasing age

- psychosocial interventions are an alternative to medication and NICE recommends that patients, families and carers should be informed of self-help and support groups, and be encouraged to participate in such programmes. In addition it is recommended that Primary Care Trusts and mental health communities should collate information on local self-help groups for practitioners

- encouraging physical activity in depressed older people is important and NICE recommends that patients should be advised of the benefits of following a structured and supervised exercise programme of typically up to three sessions per week of moderate duration (45 minutes to 1 hour) for between 10–12 weeks

- if medication is required then it should be given at an age-appropriate dose for a minimum of six weeks. Careful monitoring of side effects should be undertaken and tricyclics in particular should be used with caution. Practitioners should also be aware of the increased frequency of drug interactions in older adults

- and finally (see next section), depression in patients with dementia should be treated in the same way as depression in other older adults. Practitioners should also be aware that depression responds to antidepressants even in the presence of dementia.

Recognising dementia in older people

Dementia is the other major mental health problem in older people. GPs have a central role in the early identification, diagnosis and management of dementia. However, as with depression, research suggests that dementia remains under-detected and unsatisfactorily managed in primary care.[29] The reasons for this are complex and include older people's reluctance to seek help and perceptions that loss of memory is part of growing old, together with GPs' lack of confidence in making a diagnosis combined with a degree of scepticism about the value of early diagnosis.[30]

There is an emerging consensus that case finding rather than screening is the best way forward.[31] This involves two steps: first, the ability to identify those most at risk and, second, a validated cognitive screening test to confirm or refute the diagnosis. Increasing age is the strongest risk[32] but there is also a genetic component in the development of Alzheimer's disease with evidence of increased risk associated with having a first-degree relative with the disease.[33] There is not a lot that can be done about these risks. The most important group of risks that are capable of being modified are vascular. These include hypertension, type 2 diabetes, high cholesterol levels, stroke and obesity, which not only increase the risk of vascular dementia but also that of Alzheimer's disease.[34] Practice registers of people with hypertension, diabetes, heart disease and stroke could be a useful place to case find for dementia. The other high-risk group are people with depression.[35] Although whether this is causal or the effect of early dementia is difficult to ascertain.

There is a second group of psychosocial and lifestyle factors that appear to protect against dementia. Specifically there is increasing evidence that social engagement, intellectual stimulation and physical activity have a key role in maintaining cognitive health.[36] The strongest evidence relates to physical activity where a recent prospective cohort study demonstrated that exercising regularly for at least 15 minutes three or more times a week reduced the risk of developing dementia by 40 per cent.[37] This suggests that a brief physical activity questionnaire that had been completed opportunistically by older patients attending appointments could be used to identify those who are inactive and at greater risk, and to encourage people to become more active. This would also help in the prevention and treatment of depression.

The best way of objectively confirming the diagnosis once suspicions have been raised is through the use of cognitive screening tests. The most widely used of these is the Mini-Mental State Examination (MMSE).[38] This has been highlighted recently by the revised draft NICE guidance on the use of cholinesterase inhibitors in dementia, which has controversially recommended that treatment should only be initiated by specialists in patients who have an MMSE score of between 10–20 points.[39] This is likely to lead to wider use of this instrument despite continuing concerns about its utility. Specifically, studies have shown high false positive rates when it is used as a screening tool in primary care[40] and there is also evidence that sensitivity is affected by education and ethnicity.[41] Despite these reservations it is still probably the best instrument available and probably one that GPs are going to have to become more familiar with if referral protocols to specialists start to demand inclusion of an MMSE score.

Crossover between dementia and depression

The relationship between dementia and depression is complex. As already indicated older people with depression are more likely to develop dementia. It is difficult to disentangle whether this depression is part of the early development of dementia or whether depression with slowing of thought processes and social withdrawal is in itself likely to trigger dementia as part of a co-morbid process. It is also true that people with dementia suffer from depression. Diagnosing depression in someone with cognitive impairment is difficult and much more reliance has to be placed on information provided by carers in regular contact with the patient and on observation of mood. As NICE guidance indicates, depressed people with dementia respond to appropriate treatment.

Managing dementia in primary care

The GP has three major roles:

- early diagnosis and initial management of the patient

- continuing personal support for the primary carer

- helping to marshal a network of responsive, social, voluntary and health agencies to provide support and respite for people with dementia and their carers. This is possibly a future role for Practice-Based Commissioning.

Initial management has most often been referral to a specialist. Whether revised NICE guidance on use of cholinesterase inhibitors for people with an MMSE above 10 will or should change this pattern is debatable. The key issue for initial management is about maintaining and preserving function for as long as possible. There are now a growing number of psychosocial interventions. Some commentators have expressed the view that dementia care services and memory clinics are now so structured around the pre-scription and monitoring of medicines that this has distracted from the important role of psychosocial interventions.[42]

An increasing body of research provides evidence for the use of activity programmes, reminiscence therapy, cognitive rehabilitation, music and other sensory therapies.[43] These appear to produce benefits both in terms of maintaining function and in improving psychological distress and behaviour. GPs need to work in partnership with specialists and other agencies to agree effective provision of these sorts of services for people with early dementia.

Carers' support is the second important role. Carers have already been discussed in the context of depression and bereavement. Care giving for people with dementia can be par-ticularly demanding; this can also result in bereavement difficulties because of feelings of guilt and ambivalence. Evidence and good practice suggest that early involvement with a local carers' group that includes the use of carer education about dementia is a useful way of providing support.[44] As most GPs will find, there is also a need for continuing one-to-one support and, as may become necessary, the treatment of depression.

Marshalling the network of appropriate services is often the most frustrating and chal-lenging part of the role. Home care, day care, respite care and long-term residential care, despite the rhetoric, still seem more provider- than service user-driven. GPs will be familiar with complaints from carers about inflexibility and about deterioration of behaviour following admission to respite or residential care. The question for the future is whether clusters of local practices can work effectively with specialists and with social services through Practice-Based Commissioning to deliver better services.

The GP's role in residential and nursing home care

The high number of people with depression and dementia in residential and nursing homes make it appropriate to end this chapter with a discussion of the role of the GP in this setting. There is a continuing focus on providing care in community settings rather than in hospitals. Over the last 20 years this has led to a decline in the numbers of older people in low-dependency residential care and an increase in the numbers of frail older people in high-dependency nursing home care. This trend is likely to con-tinue because of the increasing number of people over 80 who will make up the major-ity of people in such care.

Unfortunately the quality of care required for a high-dependency population has not always kept pace with needs. The reasons for this are probably three-fold:

- much day-to-day care is provided by low-paid and undervalued care assistants, often with high turnover rates

- specialist geriatric medicine and old-age psychiatry is less engaged in a structured approach to care in these settings than it was in the past

- primary care has not risen to the challenge of providing a structured and systematic approach to nursing home care.

Community matrons, specialist nurses, GPs with a specialist interest in the care of the elderly, an enhanced role for pharmacists, Practice-Based Commissioning and the development of care pathways that integrate primary care and specialist services provide the opportunity for a better and more integrated approach.

The following suggestions about what needs to be done are based on the recommendations of a joint working party of the Royal College of Physicians, the Royal College of Nursing and the British Geriatric Society.[45]

- There needs to be a more proactive approach to maintaining physical and cognitive functions with regular programmes that should include chair-based exercise and reminiscence therapy.

- Polypharmacy and over-sedation to control behaviour is still a relatively common occurrence. This is sometimes compounded by poor continuity of care and poor inter- and intra-professional communication. There is a need for regular medication review, perhaps involving pharmacists. Drug treatment of disruptive behaviour should only be considered when pain or inter-current illness, the adverse effects of drugs and environmental stressors have been excluded.

- There should be regular reassessment and review of individual care plans.

- There needs to be an integrated approach with GPs with a specialist interest, specialist nurses and care-of-the-elderly specialists agreeing clear roles and responsibilities for nursing home care.

- Just as there are 'teaching general practices' there should be 'teaching nursing homes' that could become a focus for the improvement of quality and for the development of appropriate skills and competencies.

- Providing nursing home care to frail older people, particularly those with dementia, will always be challenging. There is a need to ensure that care in this setting is provided to the same standard and quality as care to terminally ill patients in a hospice.

Conclusion

The key message of this short chapter is that mental health problems in old age need to become a more important part of the role of the GP. There is likely to be increasing demand from increasing numbers of older people and there is evidence that unless older people with mental health problems are treated appropriately they generate increased demand for expensive hospital services.[46] This is often because the mental health problem is not seen to be as important as the commonly associated physical co-morbidity.

As well as being involved in the detection and treatment of mental health problems in older people, there is an increasingly important role to be filled in the prevention of mental ill health in old age. This will involve encouraging people to change their behaviour in order to modify their risk factors for both depression and dementia. Keeping fit, healthy, physically active and socially engaged will reduce the risks of mental ill health.

Dealing with mental health problems in old age perhaps more than any other area of medicine requires a biopsychosocial approach that takes into account the physical, psychological and social components of an illness. It also requires an integrated approach between primary care, care-of-the-elderly specialists, other professionals and agencies. This means that there is a need for the development of integrated care pathways and better shared individual care plans.

Acknowledgements

I am grateful to Age Concern England for allowing me to use Appendix One: Social-cultural model of successful ageing. This is taken from the literature and policy review *Prevention and Service Provision: mental health problems in later life*, October 2005, by Mary Godfrey and Jean Townsend (University of Leeds) with Claire Surr, Geraldine Boyle and Dawn Brooker (University of Bradford). This report was commissioned by Age Concern England for the UK Inquiry into Mental Health and Well-Being in Later Life. The Inquiry Reports, which are available at www.mhilli.org, provide a much more comprehensive overview of mental health in later life than this brief chapter. The final report of the review is due to be published in June 2007.

References

1. Department of Work and Pensions. *Opportunity Age: meeting the challenges of ageing in the 21st century* London: HM Government, 2006, www.dwp.gov.uk/opportunity_age [accessed November 2007].

2. Beekman A, Copeland J, Prince M. Review of community prevalence of depression in later life *British Journal of Psychiatry* 1999; 174(4): 307–11.

3. Godlove Mozley C, Challis D, Sutcliffe C, *et al*. Psychiatric symptomatology in elderly people admitted to nursing and residential homes *Ageing and Mental Health* 2000; 4(2): 136–41.

4. Cooper B. Thinking preventively about dementia: a review *International Journal of Geriatric Psychiatry* 2002; **17**(10): 895–906.

5. Cumming E, Henry WE. *Growing Old: the process of disengagement* New York: Basic Books, 1961.

6. Godfrey M, Townsend J, Surr C, *et al*. *Prevention and Service Provision: mental health problems in later life*. Report for the UK Inquiry into Mental Health and Well-Being in Later Life, 2005, www.mhilli.org/documents/FinalReport.pdf [accessed November 2007].

7. Age Concern and Mental Health Foundation. *UK Inquiry into Mental Health and Well-Being in Later Life*, 2003, www.mhilli.org [accessed November 2007].

8. Lampinen P, Heikkinen R, Ruoppila I. Changes in intensity of physical exercise as predictors of depressive symptoms among older adults: an eight year follow-up *Preventive Medicine* 2000; **30**: 371–80.

9. Alspaugh ME, Zarit SH, Greene R. Longitudinal patterns of risk for depression in dementia care givers: objective and subjective primary stress as predictors *Psychology and Ageing* 1999; **14**(1): 34–43.

10. Cooke DD, McNally L, Mulligan KT, *et al*. Psychosocial interventions for caregivers of people with dementia: a systematic review *Ageing and Mental Health* 2001; **5**(2): 120–35.

11. Crawford M, Prince M, Menezes P, *et al*. The recognition and treatment of depression in older people in primary care *International Journal of Geriatric Psychiatry* 1998; **13**(3): 172–6.

12. Banerjee S, Macdonald A. Mental disorder in an elderly home care population: associations with health and social services use *British Journal of Psychiatry* 1996; **168**(8): 750–6.

13. Blazer D. Psychiatry and the oldest old *American Journal of Psychiatry* 2000; **157**(12): 1915–24.

14. Lyness JM, King DA, Cox C, *et al*. The importance of subsyndromal depression in older primary care patients: prevalence and functional disability *Journal of the American Geriatrics Society* 1999; **47**(6): 647–52.

15. Gallo JJ, Rabins PV, Anthony JC. Sadness in older persons: 13 year follow-up of a community sample in Baltimore, Maryland *Psychological Medicine* 1999; **29**(2): 341–50.

16. Raphael B. The presentation of management of bereavement *Medical Journal of Australia* 1975; **2**: 909–11.

17. Murphy E. Social origins of depression in old age *British Journal of Psychiatry* 1982; **141**(2): 135–42.

18. Office for National Statistics. *Living in Britain: results from the 2000 General Household Survey* London: The Stationery Office, 2001.

19. Long AF, Godfrey M, Randall T, *et al*. *Effectiveness and Outcomes of Preventive Services for Older People: risk factors, coping strategies and outcomes of interventions for bereavement* Leeds: Nuffield Institute for Health, 2002.

20. Ransford HE, Smith ML. Grief resolution among the bereaved in hospice and hospital wards *Social Science and Medicine* 1991; **32**(3): 295–304.

21. Tudiver F, Permaul-Woods JA, Hilditch J, *et al*. Do widowers use the health care system differently? Does intervention make a difference? *Canadian Family Physician* 1995; **41**: 392–400.

22. Charlton R, Dolman E. Bereavement: a protocol for primary care *British Journal of General Practice* 1995; **45**: 427–30.

23. Main J. Improving management of bereavement in general practice based on a survey of recently bereaved subjects in a single general practice *British Journal of General Practice* 2000; **50**(460): 863–6.

24. Pritchard C, Hansen L. Comparison of suicide in people aged 65–74 and 75+ by gender in England and Wales and the major Western countries 1979–1999 *International Journal of Geriatric Psychiatry* 2005; **20(1)**: 17–25.

25. Gallo JJ, Anthony JC, Muthen BO. Age differences in the symptoms of depression: a latent trait analysis *Journal of Gerontology* 1994; **49**: 251–64.

26. Moscicki EK. Identification of suicide risk factors using epidemiologic studies *Psychiatric Clinics of North America* 1997; **3**: 499–517.

27. Waern M, Runeson BS, Allebeck P, *et al*. Mental disorder in elderly suicides *American Journal of Psychiatry* 2002; **159**: 450–5.

28. National Institute for Health and Clinical Excellence. *Clinical Guideline 23, Depression: management of depression in primary and secondary care* London: NICE, 2004, www.nice.org.uk/CG023NICEguideline [accessed November 2007].

29. Iliffe S, Wilcox J, Austin T, *et al*. Dementia diagnosis and management in primary care *Dementia* 2002; **1(1)**: 11–23.

30. Alzheimer's Disease Society. *Right from the Start: primary care and dementia: a report by the Alzheimer's Disease Society on the experiences of GPs and carers of dementia diagnosis* London: Alzheimer's Disease Society, 1995.

31. Database of Abstracts of Reviews of Effects. The primary care management of dementia (structured abstract) *DARE* 2004; 4, Database No. 20008188.

32. Ritchie K, Kildea D, Robine JM. The relationship between age and the prevalence of senile dementia: a meta-analysis of recent data *International Journal of Epidemiology* 1002; **21(4)**: 763–9

33. Abate G, Ferrari-Ramondo V, Di Iorio A. Risk factors for cognitive disorders in the elderly: a review *Archives of Gerontology and Geriatrics* 1998; **Suppl. 6**: 7–15.

34. Haan MN, Wallace R. Can dementia be prevented? Brain ageing in a population-based context *Annual Review of Public Health* 2004; **25**: 1–24.

35. Buntinx F, Kester A, Bergers J, *et al*. Is depression in elderly people followed by dementia? A retrospective cohort study based in general practice *Age and Ageing* 1996; **25(3)**: 231–3.

36. Wang H, Karp A, Winblad B, *et al*. Late-life engagement in social and leisure activities is associated with decreased risk of dementia: a longitudinal study from the Kungsholmen Project *American Journal of Epidemiology* 2002; **155(12)**: 1081–7.

37. Larson EB, Wang L, Bowen J, *et al*. Exercise is associated with reduced risk for incident dementia among persons 65 years of age and older *Annals of Internal Medicine* 2006; **144(2)**: 73–81.

38. Folstein MF, Folstein SE, McHugh PR. Mini-Mental State: a practical method for grading the state of patients for the clinician *Journal of Psychiatric Research* 1975; **12**: 189–98.

39. National Institute for Health and Clinical Excellence. *Dementia: NICE-SCIE guideline DRAFT*, 2006, www.nice.org.uk/page.aspx?o=387300 [accessed November 2007].

40. White N, Scott A, Woods RT, *et al*. The limited utility of the Mini-Mental State Examination in screening people over the age of 75 for dementia in primary care *British Journal of General Practice* 2002; **52(485)**: 1002–3.

41. Dakar-White G, Beattie AM, Gilliard J, *et al*. Minority ethnic groups in dementia care: a review of service needs, service provision and models of good practice *Aging and Mental Health* 2002; **6(2)**: 101–8.

42. Pelosi AJ, McNulty SV, Jackson GA. Role of cholinesterase inhibitors in dementia care needs rethinking *British Medical Journal* 2006; **333**: 491–3.

43. Opie JR, Rosewarne R, O'Connor DW. The efficacy of psychosocial approaches to behaviour disorders in dementia: a systematic literature review *Australian and New Zealand Journal of Psychiatry* 1999; 33(6): 789–99.

44. Simon C. Informal carers and the primary care team *British Journal of General Practice* 2001; 51(472): 920–3.

45. Royal College of Physicians. *Health and Care for Older People in Care Homes. Report of a joint working party of the Royal College of Physicians, the Royal College of Nursing and the British Geriatrics Society* London: Royal College of Physicians, 2000.

46. Simon GE, Von Korf FM, Barlow W. Health care costs of primary care patients with recognized depression *Archives of General Psychiatry* 1995; 52(10): 631–37.

10 | Dual diagnosis

Clare Gerada

What this chapter contributes:

an overview of the association between substance misuse and mental health
  problems

the identification and management of substance misuse in a primary care
  setting.

This chapter draws heavily on the author's 'Drug misuse and co-morbid illness',
published in the *RCGP Guide to the Management of Substance Misuse in Primary Care*.[1]

Definition

Dual diagnosis is a new term to describe a common problem, that of having more than
one diagnosis. General practitioners are well used to patients with dual diagnosis, be they
patients with hypertension and diabetes, or depression and coronary heart disease. When
used in the drug misuse world it is usually taken to mean drug misuse coexisting with a
serious mental health problem – most commonly schizophrenia, though it should include
any co-morbid problem, be that physical (e.g. liver disease, coronary heart disease) or
mental health. The term 'multiple morbidity', suggested by Wright and colleagues,[2] might
more accurately describe the common predicament of patients who have more than one
health problem. With an ageing population of drug users we need to expect that alongside their substance misuse problems we will also find diabetes, hypertension or cancer.

Relationship between addiction and mental health problems

There are many reasons why mental health problems and addiction problems can
coexist and include:[3]

- a primary psychiatric illness, for example schizophrenia, precipitating or leading to substance use

- substance use worsening or altering the course of a psychiatric illness such as when patients with psychotic illness take stimulants

- intoxication and/or substance dependence leading to psychological symptoms, for example cannabis use leading to anxiety

- substances, particularly alcohol, cannabinoids, hallucinogens and stimulants (especially amphetamines and cocaine), can produce psychotic symptoms directly without mental illness.

The relationship between cannabis use and mental health perhaps deserves special mention. Cannabis is the most commonly used illicit drug (with 23.5 per cent of young people reporting use in the past year)[4] and several associations between the use of this drug and psychological problems have been described. These are:

- impairment of psychological and psychomotor performance

- acute intoxication

- relapse in individuals with established schizophrenia

- dependence

- precipitation of psychotic symptoms (including schizophrenia)

- depression and anxiety.

What is the role of the primary care practitioner?

Why should the primary care practitioner need to know anything about patients with dual diagnosis? After all, these patients have complex needs that should place their management outside the normal confines of general practice. It is the author's belief that, the more complex the patient, the greater his or her need for well-organised primary care services to coordinate care. Good primary care services are vital, at the very least to ensure that these patients do not slip through the net of multiple carers and services. It is the very complexity of their problems, requiring many contacts with health, social care and other support professionals, that makes primary care such an important part in their overall management, able to provide continuity throughout their care. This does not of course negate the key working role undertaken by specialist mental health or dual diagnosis services, or the importance of other services in providing valuable input, as ultimately it is through effective shared-care working that these patients are best served.

> **Box 10.1:** What can primary care offer to patients with complex co-morbidities?
>
> Continuity of care.
>
> General medical services.
>
> Enhanced services for coexisting physical problems.
>
> Coordination between services.
>
> Crises intervention.
>
> Containment.
>
> Care to the family.
>
> Advocacy.
>
> Medication review.
>
> Help with housing and benefits issues.
>
> Help with complications of drug use – such as wound dressings.

Prevalence

The prevalence of dual diagnosis has increased in recent years. This may be due to two main factors. First, the general increase in substance use *per se* across the whole country means that patients with mental health problems are as likely (if not more so) to be caught up in general increase in prevalence. The other explanation is that community care means that patients with mental health problems are more exposed to drugs and more likely to use these substances than when resident in long-stay inpatient services. Important epidemiological work has been conducted in the USA. The American Epidemiological Catchments Area (ECA) study[5] surveyed over 20,000 people living in both community and psychiatric settings. Substance use problems were more prevalent among individuals with mental illness than among the general population, with mental illness, on average, doubling the chance of a coexistent substance use problem. On this basis it appears that approximately half of those who experience serious mental illness will have a positive history of substance use.[6] A smaller-scale study of 171 people with psychosis in South London found that the one-year prevalence rate for any substance problem was 36.3 per cent. Broken down further, 31.6 per cent had alcohol problems, while 15.8 per cent had drug problems.[7] Young males were identified as being more likely to have substance use problems and were found to have spent almost twice as long in hospital as those without such problems in the two-year period preceding the study. Significant mental health problems were identified in opiate-dependent patients and amphetamine users in a South Wales drug dependence clinic.[8]

Table 10.1: The proportion of drug users with specific psychiatric conditions found in the National Treatment Outcome Research Study (NTORS)[9]

Psychiatric disorder	Females (%)	Males (%)
Anxiety disorder	32	17
Depression	30	15
Paranoia	27	17
Psychotic	33	20

Box 10.2: The National Treatment Outcome Research Study

The National Treatment Outcome Research Study is a longitudinal (5-year) study of drug users recruited from a variety of treatment and non-treatment settings. The aim of the study is to try and determine the effectiveness of treatment interventions on a number of different outcome measures, including continuing drug use, involvement in criminal behaviour and social outcome measures (such as employment and housing).

Using the General Practice Research Database in work commissioned by the Department of Health, Frischer *et al.* looked at the prevalence of dual diagnosis in primary care in England and Wales from 1993 to 1998. The database recorded 1.4 million patient contacts with 230 practices. They checked for recorded individuals with both substance misuse and a psychiatric disorder, and found that the rate for dual diagnosis increased by 62 per cent during this period, with significant increases in schizophrenic disorder (128 per cent), paranoia (144 per cent) and psychotic disorder (147 per cent). The authors also noted a regional variation, with a 300 per cent increase in the Northern and Yorkshire district and a slow increase in London.[10]

Patterns of drug and alcohol use

Currently cannabis appears to be the most commonly used illicit substance by people with mental illness in the UK, mirroring the high use amongst those without mental health problems. Amongst the general population there is an increase in the availability of cocaine[11,12] and a resurgence in heroin use in some cities.[13] As any drug becomes more readily available we should expect their increasing use to permeate many existing drug cultures including those with which psychiatric patients have contact. Crack cocaine use is also gaining prevalence amongst the general population so there is reason to expect that patients with mental health problems will also show an increase in use.

Patients with schizophrenia have a three-fold greater risk of developing alcohol e compared with individuals without a mental illness.[14] The most common ic disorder amongst injecting drug users is antisocial personality disorder.[15]

Co-morbid mental health and substance use problems are especially prevalent in the homeless and rough sleepers and offenders, including prisoners. There are significant differences between men and women in their patterns of substance use and psychiatric co-morbidity.[16] For example, women:

- who use substances are significantly more likely than other women or men to have been the victim of sexual, physical and /or emotional abuse as children

- are more likely to fund their habit through prostitution and hence are more likely to place themselves at risk of violence, assault and abuse, hence further increasing their risk of mental health problems

- are more likely to present at mental health or primary care services for psychological difficulties rather than for any associated substance use problem

- tend to access alcohol and drug services later than men, which may explain their more severe presentation

- may have children, or want children, and this can deter them from contact with statutory services for fear that their children will be removed from them, meaning that they are likely to present later for care at a time when their use has become more problematic.

Clinical implications

The implications of people with mental health problems who also use drugs and/or alcohol can be serious, and it is important that the primary care practitioner is aware of them. Substance use among individuals with psychiatric disorders is associated with significantly poorer outcomes, including:[17-19]

- worsening psychiatric symptoms

- increased rates of suicidal behaviour

- increased rates of violence[20]

- poor medication adherence

- increased risk of HIV infection

- increased risk of hepatitis C infection and later liver disease

- higher service use

- higher rates of homelessness.

Both mental health problems and substance use are associated with higher rates of physical illness, including complications related to cigarette smoking, poor nutrition and infections, including tuberculosis. The primary care practitioner has an invaluable role in making sure that none of these problems are ignored.

Reasons for substance use

As we have seen, people with mental illness are more likely to be using drugs and/or alcohol than people without. Several theories have been proposed to explain the high rates of substance use among people with schizophrenia.[21]

Treatment approaches (Stages)

Practitioners need to have a realistic and long-term view of treatment, and be aware of the different approaches that may be necessary during different stages of treatment. The following stages of treatment have been described:

- engagement
- motivation for change
- active treatment
- relapse prevention.

Which do you treat first?

Management should of course involve the two problematic elements, namely treating the substance of use and treating any coexisting mental health problem. Three approaches are currently used for delivering services to patients and the choice of course depends on local circumstances. The general practitioner with special interest (GPwSI) may have an important role in determining which service is commissioned. Whatever model is used, a most important aspect of any service is the ability to be flexible and to offer services that meet the needs of that individual patient, at the time he or she presents.

A review of different interventions found little evidence to support the effectiveness of any particular treatment, or to recommend one approach over any other.[22] However, the research[20] does suggest a growing agreement that integrated mental health and substance use services offer a more tolerant, non-confrontational approach for patients and are probably the best and most appropriate way forward for these patients. Whatever the services model, however, a number of steps should be considered to improve the effectiveness of treatment:[23]

Table 10.2: Possible reasons for using drugs and/or alcohol

Possible reasons	Comments
People with schizophrenia often use drugs and/or alcohol to self-medicate and to alleviate the side effects of drugs	Research evidence does not strongly support this view. For example, problematic alcohol use often precedes schizophrenia; specific drugs are not selected in relation to specific symptoms; importantly, various substances of use produce a range of different effects but generally exacerbate rather than relieve symptoms of schizophrenia[24]
Underlying neuropathological abnormalities caused by schizophrenia facilitate the positive reinforcing effects of substance use and hence may predispose people to both conditions	This may explain why people with schizophrenia prefer drugs such as cocaine and nicotine
People with schizophrenia are especially vulnerable to the negative psychosocial effects of substance use because schizophrenia impairs thinking and social judgement, and induces poor impulse control	This would explain why even when using small amounts of drugs and/or alcohol people with schizophrenia are prone to develop significant substance-related problems[25]
People with antisocial personality disorder are at risk of developing substance use problems	The risk factors are the same for both – for example, education failure, poor and inconsistent parenting, lack of support network
The increased availability and acceptance of many substances in society mean that people with schizophrenia are more likely to come into contact with drugs and/or alcohol	People with schizophrenia use substances for the same reasons as the general population, namely to enjoy the experience of intoxication, to escape from emotional distress and as a social activity.[26] Drug dealers can exploit people with an obvious vulnerability

- comprehensive assessments of both mental health and substance use problems
- training for mental health workers in the recognition and management of substance use problems
- training for substance use workers in the recognition and management of mental health problems
- services that are non-judgemental, flexible and take account of the principles of harm minimisation

- assertive outreach with appropriate case loads
- clear understanding of roles and responsibilities
- good liaison between agencies, clearly identifying who has the lead
- development of care pathways
- evaluation of new services using a range of outcome measures.

Whatever model of care is used to deliver services, close communication and effective shared care between all those involved is important. Practitioners with special clinical interest may have a role in supporting patients with dual diagnosis, helping them move across the many interfaces of care, but all primary care practitioners will play an important role.

Particular co-morbid problems that may present to the general practitioner

Depression with alcohol misuse or dependency

Alcohol dependency and depression often coexist and doctors often wonder which to treat first, the depression or the alcohol dependency. Though in practice each case needs to be taken on its own merit, the first line of treatment would be, ideally, to assist the patient to withdraw from alcohol and then to reassess his or her mental state. It is in fact difficult to accurately assess a patient's mental state when he or she is drinking heavily – as we know that alcohol can both cause and mask underlying mental health problems. In all events, it is likely that alcohol misuse has contributed to the depressive features and, once abstinence has been achieved, that the depressive symptoms will significantly reduce. Overall, antidepressants may improve mood but not necessarily alcohol-drinking behaviour in depressed alcohol-dependent patients. The prescribing of antidepressants needs to be done with caution where drinking continues, as there are potentially serious interactions between antidepressants and alcohol, including cardiac toxicity and death in overdose.

Depression with opioid dependence

As with alcohol dependence, opioid use is a risk factor for the development of depression and may persist even when the patient is abstinent. Patients withdrawing from opioids, especially methadone, often report dysthymia and depressed mood, as do patients on buprenorphine. For long-term users, the loss of not just the drug but also of the lifestyle involved in taking drugs (which, after all, can be a full-time occupation) leaves them feeling empty and deflated. Coming off drugs also exposes the losses associated with a lifetime of drug taking: the years spent seeking and using illicit substances rather than pursuing relationships, education and employment. There are limited studies from which to derive recommendations, though antidepressants may improve mood but not necessarily drug behaviour in depressed opioid addicts. Perhaps the most important impact the primary care practitioner can make is 'being there' and continuing to provide regular support, certainly for the first six months following abstinence.

Cocaine and depression

Depression is a common feature of cocaine use and can be so severe as to risk deliberate self-harm. Clearly, as with other drugs of misuse, achieving abstinence or minimising misuse of cocaine is critical in trying to improve mood.

Anxiety and alcohol/drug dependence

Since anxiety is a feature of alcohol withdrawal, waiting until the acute withdrawal period is over for a clearer assessment is important. On the whole prescribing anxiolytics to patients who currently misuse alcohol, or have done so previously, is not generally recommended. Abstinent alcohol-dependent patients may be at greater risk of benzodiazepine misuse and dependence due to greater rewarding effects. Those patients who are severely dependent, with antisocial personality disorder or with polysubstance misuse, are most at risk of misusing benzodiazepines. However, there is evidence to suggest that, for those who are less severely dependent, benzodiazepine prescribing may not result in misuse.[27] How then should anxiety in substance-misusing patients be treated? Deny them benzodiazepines and risk under-treatment, or prescribe benzodiazepines for the anxiolytic effect and risk contributing to addiction? There is no definitive answer and, though most benzodiazepine prescriptions are not misused,[28] a history of alcohol and drug misuse suggests high potential for benzodiazepine misuse. Alcohol and substance misusers tend to ingest benzodiazepines for recreational purposes. Thirty to 50 per cent of alcoholics undergoing detoxification and 44 per cent of IV drug misusers also may be misusing benzodiazepines.[29] Benzodiazepines are cross-tolerant with alcohol, and alcoholics may use them with alcohol or as a substitute when alcohol is unavailable. They also may self-medicate with benzodiazepines to ease alcohol's withdrawal symptoms. Opiate, amphetamine and cocaine abusers may use benzodiazepines with their drugs of choice, as may younger abusers of 'ecstasy'. Even patients who begin taking benzodiazepines for legitimate reasons may end up misusing them. In one study of 2600 patients prescribed diazepam, up to 60 per cent had misused and/or become dependent on it.[30] Long-term users of prescribed benzodiazepines often develop tolerance and may escalate their doses to get the same desired effects. If their supply is threatened, these patients may seek benzodiazepines illicitly. Benzodiazepines may enhance or prolong the elation ('high') associated with other drugs or mitigate the depression ('crash') that follows a stimulant 'high'. Sometimes benzodiazepines are the drug of choice, as high doses of potent, short-acting agents may provide a stimulant 'high'.

Non-pharmacological treatments have been shown to reduce substance use and control anxiety in some studies. These include cognitive behavioural therapy, motivational enhancement therapy, interpersonal therapy, and brief dynamic therapy, among others. Their use requires specific training or referral to more experienced colleagues.

Conclusion

Patients with coexisting serious mental/physical problems and substance use problems place great challenges on treatment services, including primary care services. As a group they are more difficult to treat and manage due to their higher level of physical, social and psychological impairment. Gaining compliance with taking medication can also be a problem and reduce the chance of improvement. Keeping these patients engaged is perhaps the greatest impact that primary care can make, such that in partnership with their specialist colleagues these patients can receive effective care. Too many dual-diagnosis patients fall through the net as treatment services pass responsibility to each other. A primary care practitioner is in the obvious position to stop this happening.

References

1. Gerada C. Drug misuse and co-morbid illness: 'dual diagnosis'. In: Gerada C (ed.). *RCGP Guide to the Management of Substance Misuse in Primary Care*, pp. 317–31, London: RCGP.

2. Wright N, Smeeth L, Health I. Moving beyond single and dual diagnosis in general practice *British Medical Journal* 2003; **326**: 512–14.

3. Crome I. *Psychiatric Disorder and Psychoactive Substance Use Disorder: towards improved service provision* London: Centre for Research into Drugs and Health Behaviour, 1996.

4. Home Office. *Drug Misuse Declared: findings from the 2004/2005 British Crime Survey. Home Office statistical bulletin* London: Home Office.

5. Regier D, Farmer M, Rae D, *et al*. Comorbidity of mental disorders with alcohol and other drug use *Journal of the American Medical Association* 1990; **264**: 2511–18.

6. Mueser K, Bennett M, Kushner M. Epidemiology of substance use disorders among persons with chronic mental illness. In: Lehman A, Dixon L (eds). *Double Jeopardy: chronic mental illness and substance use disorders* Chur, Switzerland: Harwood Academic, 1995.

7. Menezes P, Johnson S, Thornicroft G, *et al*. Drug and alcohol problems among individuals with severe mental illnesses in South London *British Journal of Psychiatry* 1996; **168**: 612–19.

8. Barrowcliff A, Champney-Smith J, McBride A. The opiate treatment index OTI. Treatment assessment with Welsh samples of opiate prescribed or amphetamine prescribed clients *Journal of Substance Use* 1999; **4(4)**: 98–103.

9. Marsden J, Gossop J, Stewart D, *et al*. Psychiatric symptoms amongst clients seeking treatment for drug dependence: intake data from the National Treatment Outcome Research Study *British Journal of Psychiatry* 2000; **176**: 285–9.

10. Frischer M, Hickman M, Kraus L, *et al*. A comparison of the different methods for estimating problematic drug use in Great Britain *Addiction* 2000; **96**: 1465–76.

11. Corkery J. *Drug Seizure and Offender Statistics, United Kingdom 1998: Home Office statistical bulletin 3/00* London: Home Office Research Development and Statistics Directorate, 2000.

12. Boys A, Marsden J, Griffiths P. Reading between the lines: is cocaine becoming the stimulant of choice for urban youth? *Druglink* 1999: **14(1)**: 20–3.

13. Eggington R, Parker H, Bury C. Heroin still screws you up: responding to new heroin outbreaks *Druglink* 1998; **13(5)**: 17–20.

14. Crawford V. Comorbidity of substance use and psychiatric disorders *Current Opinion in Psychiatry* 1996; **9**: 231–4.

15. Drake R, Noordsy D. Case management for people with co-existing severe mental disorder and substance abuse disorder *Psychiatric Annals* 1994; **24**: 427–31.

16. Department of Health. *Mental Health Policy Implementation Guide: dual diagnosis good practice guide* London: HMSO, 2002.

17. Carey M, Carey K, Meisler A. Psychiatric symptoms in mentally ill chemical abusers *Journal of Nervous and Mental Disease* 1991; **179**: 136–8.

18. Drake R, Wallach M. Substance abuse among the chronic mentally ill *Hospital and Community Psychiatry* 1989; **40**: 1041–6.

19. Kelly J, Heckman T, Helfrich S, *et al*. HIV risk factors and behaviours among men in a Milwaukee homeless shelter *American Journal of Public Health* 1995; **85**: 465–8.

20. Smith J, Frazer S, Boer H. Dangerous dual diagnosis patients *Hospital and Community Psychiatry* 1994; **45**: 280–1.

21. Siegfried N. A review of comorbidity: major mental illness and problematic substance use *Australian and New Zealand Journal of Psychiatry* 1998; **32**: 707–17.

22. Ley A, Jeffrey DP, McLaren S, *et al*. Treatment programmes for people with both severe mental illness and substance use (Cochrane Review), in *The Cochrane Library* 1, Oxford: Update Software, 2000.

23. Champney-Smith J. Dual diagnosis. In: Petersen T and McBride A (eds). *Working with Substance Users: a guide to theory and practice*, pp. 267–74, London: Routledge, 2002.

24. Chambers A, Krystal JH, Self DW. A neurobiological basis for substance abuse comorbidity in schizophrenia *Biological Psychiatry* 2001; **50**: 71–83.

25. Mueser KT, Drake RE, Wallach MA. Dual diagnosis: a review of etiological theories *Addictive Behaviours* 1998; **23**: 717–34.

26. Lamb HR, Bachrach L. Some perspectives on deinstitution *Psychiatric Services* 2001; **52**: 1039–45.

27. Ciraulo DA, Sands BK, Shader RI. Critical review of liability for benzodiazepine abuse among alcoholics *American Journal of Psychiatry* 1988; **145(12)**: 1501–6.

28. Woods JH, Katz JL, Winger G. Use and abuse of benzodiazepines. Issues relevant to prescribing *Journal of the American Medical Association* 1988; **260(23)**: 3476–80.

29. Shaw M, Brabbins C, Ruben S. Misuse of benzodiazepines. Specify the formulation when prescribing *British Medical Journal* 1994; **308(6945)**: 1709.

30. Woody GE, O'Brien CP, Greenstein R. Misuse and abuse of diazepam: an increasingly common medical problem *International Journal of the Addictions* 1975; **10(5)**: 843–8.

11 | Talking therapies

Ian McPherson and Alan Cohen

What this chapter contributes:

an accessible introduction to talking therapies and their contribution to treating commonly occurring mental health problems in primary care

an outline of recent innovations in practice and the Department of Health's (DH) programme for improving access to psychological therapies.

Introduction

The idea that, when we are experiencing severe emotional distress, talking to a skilled and sensitive listener who can use different approaches to help us clarify what may be contributing to our feelings, and consider alternative means of addressing these, does not seem particularly radical. However, until recently, talking therapies – also referred to as psychological therapies – were often viewed within the NHS with some suspicion and continue to be available only to a relatively small number of those who want and would benefit from this type of approach. While this may have been a function of limited resources and appropriately skilled therapists, it may also have reflected the combination of an implicit biological model of mental health and a deep-seated cultural attitude in the UK that talking about feelings was, at best, indulgent and, at worst, harmful.

Within the last few years there has been a radical change reflecting:

- growing demand from people wanting access to talking therapies as alternatives to other forms of intervention, particularly medication. The Mental Health Foundation, together with some of the other main UK mental health charities, recently published *We Need to Talk*. It quotes an online survey which found that, while 82 per cent of people seeking help in primary care for depression would have been willing to try talking therapies, it was only available to 42 per cent[1]

- support for talking therapies from the National Institute for Health and Clinical Excellence (NICE) in all of its guidance on mental disorders

- support from public figures and politicians, notably Lord Richard Layard, Emeritus Professor of Economics at the London School of Economics, who is widely credited with getting this issue on to the Cabinet Office agenda and becoming a manifesto commitment by the Labour Party in the 2005 election.[2]

The combined impact of the above has resulted in psychological therapies featuring in the latest white paper for Health and Social Care, *Our Health, Our Care, Our Say*,[3] and the launch of a DH-sponsored programme, 'Improving Access to Psychological Therapies'.

Despite this heightened profile, there remains significant confusion among many people, including those working in primary care and who deal with 90 per cent of those seeking help for these conditions, about what exactly talking therapies are, who they might benefit, and where they fit in the range of interventions available to support people experiencing symptoms of mental and/or physical distress. What follows is an attempt to help clarify this and to consider how talking therapies can be used most effectively in primary care.

What are talking therapies?

One of the difficulties facing anyone trying to understand this area is the plethora of therapies, often with similar titles reflecting variations and offshoots from different schools of thought. Twenty years ago Kazdin suggested that there were over 400 different therapies, and there have been significant additions since then, though in practice the differences between these may not be as important to those who use or commission these services than they are to adherents of competing models or methods.[4]

A useful synopsis of the main therapies available in the UK is provided in a DH publication *Treatment Choice in Psychological Therapies and Counselling*.[5] This identifies two main traditions in talking therapies, psychotherapy and counselling. These are in no sense distinct entities but rather lie on a continuum. In psychotherapy the focus tends to be on the remediation of mental health problems and symptoms by structured interventions, whereas in counselling the emphasis is more on the individual's resources rather than psychopathology, with a focus on a reflective, experiential process. This DH publication defines the main therapies commonly practised in the UK as follows.

Psychotherapies
Cognitive behavioural therapy

This refers to the pragmatic combination of concepts and techniques from cognitive and behavioural therapies, common in clinical practice. *Behavioural therapy* is a structured therapy originally derived from learning theory, which seeks to solve problems and relieve symptoms by changing behaviour and the environmental factors that control behaviour. Graded exposure to feared situations is one of the commonest behavioural treatment methods and is used in a range of anxiety disorders. *Cognitive therapy* is a structured treatment approach derived from cognitive theories. Cognitive techniques (such as challenging negative automatic thoughts) and behavioural techniques (such as activity scheduling and behavioural experiments) are used with the main aim of relieving symptoms by changing maladaptive thoughts and beliefs.

Psychoanalytic therapies

A number of different therapies draw on psychoanalytic theories, although they differ in terms of technique. *Focal psychodynamic therapy* identifies a central conflict arising from early experience that is being re-enacted in adult life producing mental health problems. It aims to resolve this through the vehicle of the relationship with the therapist giving new opportunities for emotional assimilation and insight. This form of therapy is often time-limited, with anxiety aroused by the ending of therapy being used to illustrate how reawakened feelings about earlier losses, separations and disappointments may be experienced differently. *Psychoanalytic psychotherapy* is a longer-term process (usually a year or more) of allowing unconscious conflicts opportunity to be re-enacted in the relationship with the therapist and, through interpretation, worked through in a developmental process.

Systemic therapy

Systemic and family therapists understand individual problems by considering the relevance of family relationships and the impact of the wider social and economic context on people's lives, their wellbeing and their mental health. Therapeutic work is undertaken with individuals, couples or families, and may include consultation to wider networks such as other professionals working with the individual or the family. Therapy aims to identify and explore patterns of belief and behaviour in roles and relationships. Therapists actively intervene to enable people to decide where change would be desirable and to facilitate the process of establishing new, more fulfilling and useful patterns. Therapists may work in teams using live consultation or as sole practitioners using retrospective consultation. Therapy is often relatively short term.

Eclectic therapies

Many NHS therapists formulate the patient's difficulties using more than one theoretical framework and choose a mix of techniques from more than one therapy approach. The resulting therapy is pragmatic, tailored to the individual. These generic therapies often emphasise important non-specific factors (such as building the therapeutic alliance and engendering hope). By their nature, they are more idiosyncratic and difficult to standardise for the purposes of randomised controlled trials research.

Integrative therapy

An integrative therapy differs from eclectic approaches, as it is a formal theoretical and methodological integration of, for example, behavioural, cognitive, humanistic or psychodynamic approaches. These therapies are therefore amenable to research. One such approach is cognitive analytic therapy.

Other psychotherapies

The above list is by no means comprehensive. Other types of therapy include interpersonal, existential, humanistic, process-experiential (client-centred), feminist, personal construct, art therapy, drama therapy, transactional analysis and group analysis. Further information about psychotherapy can be obtained from the UK Council for Psychotherapy (www.psychotherapy.org.uk) and the British Association of Behavioural and Cognitive Psychotherapies (www.babcp.org.uk).

Counselling

Counselling is a systematic process that gives individuals an opportunity to explore, discover and clarify ways of living more resourcefully, with a greater sense of wellbeing. Counselling may be concerned with addressing and resolving specific problems, making decisions, coping with crises, working through conflict, or improving relationships with others.

Counsellors may practise within any of the therapeutic approaches listed above, using psychodynamic counselling, cognitive behavioural counselling, systemic counselling and so on. However, most are influenced by humanistic, process-experiential and psychodynamic principles.

The work of most counsellors is generalist (analogous to general practice) and is not necessarily linked to diagnostic categories. Many counsellors work in primary care, but they are increasingly found in secondary care settings. A broad distinction can be made between generic and specific counselling. The latter may be specific to a therapeutic model (for example psychodynamic counselling) or a life crisis (for example bereavement counselling).

More information about counselling can be found on the British Association of Counselling and Psychotherapy website (www.bacp.co.uk).

Who could benefit from talking therapy?

Like most apparently simple questions, the answer to this one is not straightforward. Probably the best overview of this topic has been provided by Roth and Fonagy in *What Works for Whom? A critical review of psychotherapy research*.[6] This highlights just how complex the issues are and the challenges not only of conducting evaluative research on psychological therapies in comparison with other types of intervention, but also of extrapolating from research findings to evidence-based practice and from there to decisions about commissioning services for patient populations and for individuals.

Among the key issues are:

- certain types of talking therapy are more readily adapted to more robust types of evaluation such as randomised controlled trials than others

- the way in which therapies is applied in research trials is likely to be much more systematic than in normal practice

- in research it is customary to tightly specify the inclusion criteria for the condition being studied. In everyday practice, however, many commonly occurring clinical conditions such as anxiety and depression are difficult to differentiate and co-occur with other problems such as substance misuse and physical conditions, which can impact on people's wellbeing and vice versa.

As a result of the above, research in talking therapies has tended to be conducted more on some procedures and on more selected populations by people practising in ways that are more 'textbook' than would be found in typical clinical practice.

Fortunately most primary care professionals will not need to get into the intricacies of this, rather relying on the detailed NICE clinical guidelines for particular conditions. However, in doing so it is important to be aware that factors such as the above may influence the research evidence that NICE expert panels have available to them and the weighting this is given. NICE is well aware of these limitations and takes a balanced approach, but overly simplistic interpretations sometimes appear in media coverage suggesting that, because NICE has recommended it, a particular form of talking therapy 'works', with the implication that others do not and as a result should not be made available. With this proviso, NICE guidance provides the most accessible introduction to the potential contribution of talking therapies for particular conditions and has the added advantage of putting this in the context of other types of intervention in both primary and secondary care. Of particular value is the use of the Stepped-Care Model discussed in chapters on commissioning and patients with common mental health conditions.

NICE has produced clinical guidelines on a range of mental health problems commonly dealt with in primary care, and the implications for talking therapies are summarised below. Chapter 20 describes how NICE guidelines can be implemented. Full details of all of the guidelines referred to below are available at www.nice.org.uk.

Anxiety and panic disorder

Anxiety is a normal protective reaction to stress; however, if the symptoms of anxiety appear either at inappropriate times or in inappropriate situations, then it may be that there is an 'anxiety disorder' present. Panic disorder and generalised anxiety disorder (GAD) together represent the largest category of common mental health conditions. However, the clinical picture is often less clear, since anxiety frequently coexists with depression, with individuals suffering from both conditions. Such 'mixed anxiety and depression' is an extremely common and disabling condition. The diagnosis of panic disorder (PD) – to be distinguished from a 'panic attack' – is characterised by the presence of recurrent, unexpected panic attacks followed by at least one month of persistent concern about having another panic attack, worry about the possible implications or consequences of the panic attacks, or a significant behavioural change related to the attacks.

GAD is diagnosed after a person has on most days for at least six months experienced prominent tension (increased fatigue, trembling, restlessness, muscle tension), worry, and feelings of apprehension about everyday problems. The person is anxious in most situations, and there is no particular trigger for anxiety. The NICE guidelines for the management of GAD and PD, also published in December 2004, recommended that effective interventions were medication, CBT or bibliotherapy (use of written self-help material).[7] Computerised CBT (see below) may be an appropriate way to deliver the CBT option.

Phobias are another form of 'anxiety disorder'. They are characterised by the presence of anxiety, and panic in relation to specific and focused external stimuli, e.g. spiders.

NICE guidelines recommend:

- cognitive behavioural therapy
- medication
- bibliotherapy – and other forms of self-help.

Depression

Depression is a common mental health condition, which according to the World Health Organization will be the second most common long-term condition worldwide by 2020. The diagnosis of depression is based on the presence of a number of symptoms and signs described in the 10th version of the International Classification of Diseases.[8] A depressive episode is diagnosed if at least two out of three core symptoms have been experienced for most of the day, nearly every day for at least two weeks. These core symptoms are:

- low mood (feeling low, unhappy, sad or miserable)
- fatigue (feeling tired or having little energy)
- anhedonia (lack of interest or enjoyment in things).

The disorder is further subclassified into mild, moderate, severe and depression with psychosis, depending on the number of symptoms and signs present. The NICE guidelines for the management of depression were published in December 2004, and recommended a 'stepped care' approach.[9] This stepped-care approach recommends different interventions depending on the severity of the depression. Thus, as an example, the guidelines recommend that medication is not usually prescribed for people with mild depression. The 2006 review of the nGMS contract introduced a new domain for depression, and a specific indicator that incentivises the use of approved questionnaires to assess severity.[10]

Recommendations of the NICE guidelines

A stepped-care approach is recommended by NICE, having assessed the severity of the depression first. For people with mild depression, the following is recommended:

- counselling
- computerised CBT
- exercise
- active review.

For people with moderate and moderately severe depression:

- CBT and/or
- medication.

For people with severe depression, psychotic depression and resistant depression, referral to a community mental health team is appropriate.

Eating disorders

Eating disorders take many forms, but the most common are anorexia nervosa and bulimia. In anorexia nervosa people refuse to eat sufficient to maintain their physical health in the mistaken belief that they are already overweight. In bulimia people do eat, frequently bingeing, but use vomiting and/or laxatives to control their weight.

Recommendations of the NICE guidelines

For people with anorexia nervosa:

- most people with anorexia nervosa should be managed by a specialist team in an outpatient setting, which provides specialist psychological and physical support.

For people with bulimia nervosa:

- as a first-line treatment, people should be offered self-help and bibliotherapy

- as an alternative, or additional intervention, people should be offered antidepressants

- adults should be offered CBT specifically tailored to bulimia

- adolescents should be offered CBT tailored both to bulimia and the needs of adolescents.

For people with atypical eating disorders:

- CBT specifically tailored for binge eating should be available.

Obsessive-compulsive disorder

Obsessive-compulsive disorder (OCD) is a common form of anxiety characterised by obsessive thinking and compulsive behaviour. Obsessions are distressing, repetitive thoughts that may be seen as irrational, but cannot be ignored. Compulsions are ritual actions that people feel compelled to repeat in order to relieve anxiety or to stop obsessive thoughts.

Recommendations of the NICE guidelines

Adults with OCD should initially be offered:

- brief CBT (delivered individually or by telephone)

- group CBT.

Adults with OCD should subsequently be offered (if appropriate)

- more intensive CBT (more than 10 sessions) or

- SSRI antidepressants.

Post-traumatic stress disorder

Post-traumatic stress disorder (PTSD) is the name given to the psychological and physical problems that can sometimes follow particular threatening or distressing events. These events might include a major disaster, rape or sexual, physical or emotional abuse, witnessing a violent death or a serious accident, or other situations in which a person was very afraid, horrified, helpless, or felt that his or her life was in danger. The trauma can be a single event or a series of events taking place over many months or even years. One of the most common symptoms of PTSD is having repeated and intrusive distressing memories of the event. There may also be a feeling of reliving (or 're-experiencing') the event through 'flashbacks' or nightmares, which can be very distressing and disorientating. There can also be physical reactions, such as shaking and sweating.

Recommendations of the NICE guidelines

- Adults who have experienced a traumatic event should NOT be offered debriefing.

- In the short term (four weeks) people who have experienced a traumatic event should be supported with 'watchful waiting' and reviewed at the end of that time to assess their mental state.

- If symptoms persist, trauma-focused CBT should be available.

Other conditions

NICE has also produced clinical guidelines indicating the potential value of psychological interventions in schizophrenia[11] and bipolar disorder[12] where clinical management is normally led by specialist services but where the interface with primary care is crucial (see Chapter 7).

Talking therapies and primary care

The previous section covered talking therapies by conditions commonly treated in primary care. However, another approach is to look at whether certain types of talking therapy are particularly suited to primary care and some innovations that may make these more accessible.

Counselling

Currently the most commonly available form of talking therapy in primary care is counselling. Counselling can be provided by counsellors based in GP practices either by individuals or on a central site provided by the Primary Care Trust (PCT) or contracted from a local agency or NHS trust. Most counselling sessions last for 50 minutes; a course for mild to moderate problems would generally be six to eight sessions though this may be extended for people with more complex problems.

Counselling expanded significantly during the period of GP Fund Holding. This fact reflects both the awareness of GPs that there was a need for additional support for people who would not normally meet the criteria for referral to specialist mental health services, and the availability of counsellors who were previously mainly self-employed or working for voluntary agencies.

Notwithstanding its popularity with both patients and primary care professionals, the evidence for the impact of counselling is not as robust as for some other talking therapies. A Cochrane Review in 2006 assessed both the efficacy and the cost-effectiveness of counselling in primary care based on cost and outcome data in randomised controlled trials, controlled clinical trials and patient preference trials.[13] They found that, while there was significantly greater clinical effectiveness in counselling groups compared with standard care in the short term and that satisfaction with counselling was high, there were no significant clinical differences between the two groups in the longer term.

While this may seem to indicate that counselling in primary care is not particularly effective, similar findings emerged from a review of input by different mental health professions working in primary care when compared with standard care.[6] It may to some degree reflect the limitations of the studies, which typically had heterogeneous samples and did not clearly specify the interventions conducted in either the counselling or standard practice groups. The challenge, therefore, may be for counsellors to consider how they can engage in more robust evaluations of their work in which the benefits for particular client groups of particular approaches to counselling can be more adequately assessed.

Computerised cognitive behavioural therapy

The idea that talking therapies can be delivered via a computer at first may seem counterintuitive – not least because there is no therapist present to whom the individual can talk. However, there is evidence that for certain conditions the principles of cognitive behavioural therapy can be applied via interactive computer programs, which the individual uses with minimal professional support. In 2006 NICE produced a Technology Appraisal[14] in which it recommended two computerised cognitive behavioural therapy (cCBT) programmes, FearFighter for anxiety and Beating the Blues for mild and moderate depression. These should have been available in all PCTs by March 2007.

Mental health conditions for which computerised CBT may be indicated

Depression
Computerised delivery of CBT is recommended for people with mild and moderate depression.

Panic and anxiety disorders
The NICE guidelines did not make any specific recommendations about cCBT as an effective intervention for the anxiety disorders.

Obsessive-compulsive disorder
The NICE Technology Appraisal was unable to recommend OCFighter for general use in the NHS. This is the specific cCBT program for people with OCD.

Severe mental illness
Bipolar disorder
The recently published guidelines recommend the use of cCBT for pregnant women with bipolar disorder, who have a mild depressive disorder.

Schizophrenia
Whilst the NICE guidelines for the management of people with schizophrenia recommend CBT as a treatment option, computerised delivery is not mentioned. The absence of any quoted papers on cCBT implies that there is little evidence in this area, and that, until there is, it is probably not appropriate for general use in the NHS.

Using computerised CBT

cCBT has been used by a number of organisations within the NHS already, as part of research programmes, 'return to work' programmes, or talking therapy service within a PCT.

There is no single model for using cCBT that is suitable for all situations. However, some of the issues that need to be considered include the following.

Referrals, assessment and booking appointments

Who can make a referral?

- The user/patient – self-referral.

- Only the GP – after undertaking an assessment.

- By other mental health professionals working in primary or secondary care services.

- By employment advisers, education workers, prison services, etc.

- By employers' occupational health service.

- By employers.

Assessment of the mental state, including risk assessment, could/should be carried out by:

- the patient's GP

- those who are responsible for commissioning the cCBT service.

Process for booking appointments can involve:

- the PCT-commissioned service managing the booking process

- the GP receptionist/administrator managing the process

- the librarian/employment service managing the process

- an independent organisation managing the process

- booking incorporated into the overall service provided by an intermediate therapy team (Improving Access to Psychological Therapies Programme [IAPT]) programme.

Location of the service can be:

- remote – home, library, office, etc.

- the GP surgery

- the Psychological Therapies Service

- a Community Mental Health Team (CMHT) service centre

- a library or employment centre

- a leisure centre or charity café.

Would it be appropriate for there to be a service in a prison?

Whatever the location it is appropriate to have:

- multiple computers in one room
- investment in lots of single computers distributed at a variety of locations within the PCT area (as an alternative to investing in multiple computers in one centre), although providing support may be a problem
- provision for CD-ROMs/internet access so that users/clients can access the service at a location convenient to them, e.g. their own home. Support may be a problem, and keeping track of CD-ROMs may also become an administrative burden.

Support for the user of the programmes

Experience suggests that most users of the programmes need access to some sort of support, both technological support for software failure, and occasionally psychological support. Support can be provided through three routes:

- telephone access
- face-to-face access
- email support.

Technological support is usually provided by the software provider as part of the support and upgrade package.

Psychological support can be provided by the following:

- graduate mental health worker
- practice nurse
- GP
- assistant psychologist
- care worker
- other mental health professionals.

Level of psychological support

- Support could be provided at the beginning and end of every session or
- Support could be provided at the first and the last session, and at times that are known to have a high dropout rate, e.g. session 4 or 5.

The above is a list of alternatives, generated through consultation with professionals who have used cCBT. Some of the alternatives will work for your particular set of circumstances, while others may be entirely inappropriate – you will generate your own way of delivering cCBT.

What is abundantly clear is that there is no evidence that demonstrates that one set of alternatives is superior to another, given a particular configuration within a PCT or community service. This means that the commissioner of the service has to ensure that good clinical records including outcome measures are recorded for every client/user of the system, so that the set of circumstances that deliver the best results can be described accurately. Details of who is responsible for recording the clinical outcomes need to be explicit.

Improving access to psychological therapies

In December 2004 Lord Layard presented a paper at a Downing Street seminar that described some of the data concerning unemployment and mental health.

The premise that Lord Layard proposed was that there was a strong economic case for providing cognitive behavioural therapy to people who are off work with a mental health problem, as the benefit to the country of those people returning to work would far exceed the cost of delivering the improved service (see Layard *et al.* for a summary of his arguments).[2]

He proposed that 200 new psychological treatment services, each covering about 250,000 people, should be created over the next five years; each service would consist of senior and junior psychologists who would offer evidence-based psychological interventions to people with common mental health problems. The service or team would have about 40 new therapists, a GP with a special interest (GPwSI) in mental health, and employment and accommodation advisers. In total some 10,000 new posts would be created.

As a result of that seminar, the Labour Party manifesto made reference to the need for increased psychological therapies (and in particular CBT), and the white paper *Our Health, Our Care, Our Say* described in more detail the DH programme that is now putting that programme in place. That programme is called Improving Access to Psychological Therapies (IAPT), and currently represents one of the major policy initiatives for the mental health branch of the DH.

> Almost a third of people attending GP surgeries have mental health problems and mental health occupies approximately one third of a GP's time. So we will continue to invest in and improve our services for people with mental health problems at primary and secondary levels, including behavioural as well as drug therapies. (Labour Party manifesto, 2005)

Key Layard statistics

- 3 in 10 working age people have sick leave in any one year due to mental illness.
- 91 million working days are lost each year.
- There are more people on incapacity benefit for mental illness than there are unemployed (about 1 million people).
- <10 per cent are in contact with specialist mental health services; the vast majority of people off work with mental health problems have depression and/or anxiety.
- The proportion returning to employment, after having been on incapacity benefit for 12 months or more, is less than 5 per cent.

The evidence base

The evidence base for the majority of Lord Layard's proposals are based on NICE guidelines for depression and anxiety, and he has been extensively supported by senior academic clinical psychologists. He makes the point that there is ample evidence of effectiveness of psychological treatments in the management of depression and anxiety, but that there is no priority to deliver this service amongst PCTs. Comparing this lack of interest in CBT with the debate over the availability of herceptin for the treatment of cancer makes for an interesting discussion.

The Department of Work and Pensions (DWP) has also been running a number of programmes offering CBT (or similar programmes called conditioned management programmes) to people who are unable to work. It has achieved return-to-work rates of up to 40 per cent.

The IAPT programme

The IAPT programme aims to implement the Layard proposal in two demonstration sites, Newham and Doncaster. There are some differences in the style of the two PCTs being developed in the pilot sites. Other parts of the IAPT programme include eight smaller projects in Care Services Improvement Partnership (CSIP) regional development centres, and a contribution to the National Primary Care Development Team Collaborative on Common Mental Health Conditions. The whole programme is being evaluated externally through a formal research programme.

Primary care engagement

Both pilots have been successful in engaging GPs in the programme. The pilots have been running for four months, and in both sites there is a clear understanding that the programme is about delivering a service that would not otherwise be available. GPs are clear that the programme is about providing high-quality evidence-based CBT to a group of people who otherwise would not have received treatment.

The population group at risk are identified by the characteristics of:

- having a common mental health condition (usually anxiety and/or depression) and
- whose physical health is at risk because of their mental health condition or
- whose employment or accommodation is at risk because of their mental health condition.

The programme aims to make CBT available widely through a care pathway initiated by general practice. It does not require GPs to provide more care than other practices; it does ask GPs to provide a primary care level of management for anxiety and depression in line with NICE guidelines, and in line with the Depression QOF clinical domain. The completion of PHQ-9 (as described in DEP2) is requested as part of the referral process.

Evaluation

The programme is being evaluated in the short term by the London School of Economics, and over three years by a Service Delivery and Organisation Programme (SDO)-funded project.

Conclusions

The potential contribution of talking therapies to addressing the needs of people presenting with mental health problems in primary care has now been accepted by the public, by NICE and by politicians. The challenge is how best to deliver this in a way that reflects the developing evidence base and the available resources. There is the potential that the IAPT programme will produce results that persuade the government to invest heavily in this area. However, in the current financial climate in the NHS, it would not necessarily follow that having a good case will lead to new investment. Further, it is important to realise that NICE guidelines and technology appraisals require that PCTs make available the therapies they have recommended now, not at some time in the future if the money becomes available, and this applies to mental health problems as much as physical ones.

Within primary care, therefore, clinicians, practitioners and managers need to consider how they currently provide or commission psychological therapies and how this can be done more effectively in the context of their overall approach to mental health care. In doing so they may benefit from a new resource pack, *Improving Primary Care Mental Health Services*, launched in 2006 by the National Institute for Mental Health in England – part of the Care Services Improvement Partnership.[15] This contains material designed to help address some of the practical challenges that face people in primary care who do not consider themselves expert in mental health. It helps them in making practical service changes to meet their particular circumstances.

Like the NICE guidelines this reinforces that talking therapies, while an important option, cannot be considered in isolation from the range of other options that assist people with mental health problems. To implement the stepped-care approach a shared understanding is needed of what can be provided in primary care and what may need to be provided by other agencies.

Update on Improving Access to Psychological Therapies programme

In August 2007, 11 new psychological therapy sites were announced. In October 2007 the Secretary of State announced funding for a national programme of training and implementation of psychological therapies in the NHS in England – £30m in 2008, £100m in 2009, and £170m in 2010. The new resources were identified to provide training for 3600 new psychological posts, treatment of up to 900,000 people, and the development of 20 new psychological sites in the first year. This three-year programme of funding is seen as the first half of a six-year programme that will ultimately deliver a step change in access to psychological therapies for patients in primary care. The programme of funding and development is seen to be the opportunity to implement NICE guidelines for common mental health problems in primary care, by the provision of a significant number of new professionals who can deliver evidence-based interventions. The impact of this programme on primary care will be a major advance on what is currently available.

References

1. Mental Health Foundation, Mind, Rethink, Sainsbury Centre for Mental Health, Young Minds. *We Need to Talk* London: Mental Health Foundation, 2006.

2. Layard R, Bell S, Clark D, *et al. The Depression Report: a new deal for depression and anxiety disorders* London: London School of Economics, 2006.

3. Department of Health. *Our Health, Our Care, Our Say: a new direction for community services* London: DH, 2006, www.dh.gov.uk/assetRoot/04/12/74/59/04127459.pdf [accessed November 2007].

4. Kazdin AE. Comparative outcome studies in psychotherapy: methodological issues and strategies *Journal of Consulting and Clinical Psychology* 1986; 54: 95–105.

5. Department of Health. *Treatment Choice in Psychological Therapies and Counselling* London: DH, 2001.

6. Roth A, Fonagy P. *What Works for Whom? A critical review of psychotherapy research* (second edn) New York: Guilford, 2005.

7. National Institute for Health and Clinical Guidance. *Clinical Guideline 22, Anxiety: management of anxiety (panic disorder, with or without agoraphobia, and generalised anxiety disorder) in adults in primary, secondary and community care* London: NICE, 2004, www.nice.org.uk/nicemedia/pdf/CG022NICEguidelineamended.pdf [accessed November 2007].

8. World Health Organization. *ICD-10 Classification of Mental and Behavioral Disorders* Geneva: WHO, 1992.

9. National Institute for Health and Clinical Excellence. *Clinical Guideline 23, Depression: management of depression in primary and secondary care* London: NICE, 2004, www.nice.org.uk/CG023NICEguideline [accessed November 2007].

10. British Medical Association and NHS Employers. *Revisions to the GMS Contract 2006/2007: delivering investment in general practice* London: BMA, 2006.

11. National Institute for Health and Clinical Excellence. *Clinical Guideline 1, Schizophrenia: core interventions in the treatment and management of schizophrenia in primary and secondary care* London: NICE, 2002, www.nice.org.uk/nicemedia/pdf/CG1NICEguideline.pdf [accessed November 2007].

12. National Institute for Health and Clinical Excellence. *Clinical Guideline 38, Bipolar Disorder: the management of bipolar disorder in adults, children and adolescents, in primary and secondary care* London: NICE, 2006, www.nice.org.uk/nicemedia/pdf/CG38niceguideline.pdf [accessed November 2007].

13. Bower P, Rowland N. Effectiveness and cost effectiveness of counselling in primary care. Cochrane Database of Systematic Reviews 2006, Issue 3.

14. National Institute for Health and Clinical Excellence. *Information about NICE Technology Appraisal 97, Computerised Cognitive Behaviour Therapy for Depression and Anxiety: understanding NICE guidance – information for people with depression and anxiety, their families and carers, and the public* London: NICE, 2006, www.nice.org.uk/nicemedia/pdf/TA097publicinfo.pdf [accessed November 2007].

15. National Institute for Mental Health in England. *Improving Primary Care Mental Health Services* London: DH, 2006.

12 | Medication

Alan Cohen

What this chapter contributes:

provides information on the national trends of psychotropic prescribing

provides a clinical overview on the use of psychotropic medication including:

    benzodiazepines

    antidepressants

    antipsychotic agents

    mood-stabilising drugs.

Medication

The prescribing of drugs used to help people with mental health problems is widespread and increasing (see Figure 12.1).[1,2]

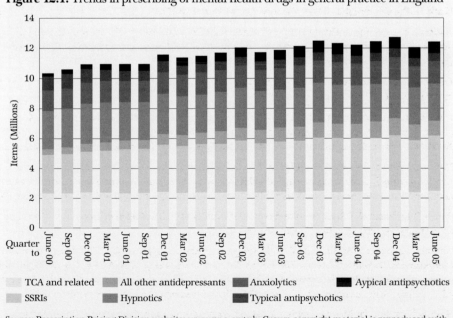

Figure 12.1: Trends in prescribing of mental health drugs in general practice in England

Source: Prescription Pricing Division website: www.ppa.org.uk. Crown copyright material is reproduced with the permission of the Controller of OPSI.

The overall number of items prescribed in the five years from June 2000 has risen from 10 million to 12 million items per year, an increase of 20 per cent in five years. Similar increases are found in all other prescribing groups.

The costs associated with the prescribing of drugs related to mental health conditions have increased significantly (see Figure 12.2), an increase that is not matched in other clinical areas. Costs over the five years from June 2000 have increased from £105 million to a little over £140 million, the majority of the increase being represented by atypical antipsychotics, and some of the newer antidepressants such as selective noradrenergic reuptake inhibitors (SNRIs).

Figure 12.2: Trends in spending on mental health drugs in general practice in England

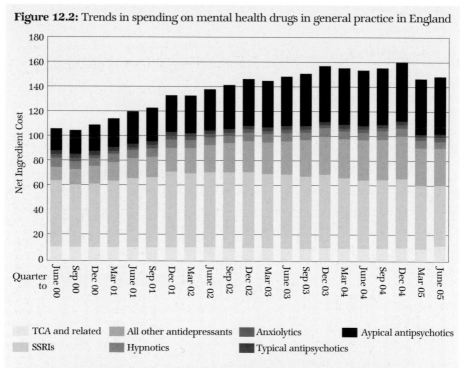

Source: Prescription Pricing Division website: www.ppa.org.uk. Crown copyright material is reproduced with the permission of the Controller of OPSI.

Overall prescribing costs over the last 2–3 years have slowed considerably, which relate to both changing prescribing habits and the use of generic drugs (see Figure 12.3).

Figure 12.4 demonstrates how variable the costs of different drugs can be, and how this accounts for the nearly 40 per cent increase in total costs associated with prescribing mental health drugs over the last five years.

Figure 12.3: Change in the rate of growth of prescription costs

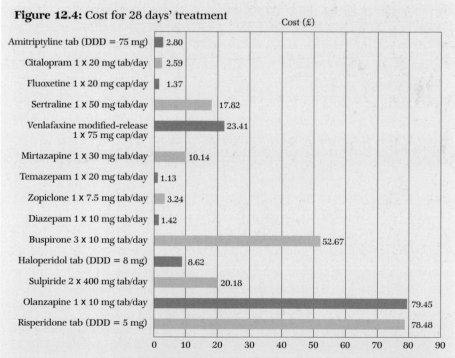

Source: Prescription Pricing Division website: www.ppa.org.uk. Crown copyright material is reproduced with the permission of the Controller of OPSI.

Figure 12.4: Cost for 28 days' treatment

Cost (£)

Amitriptyline tab (DDD = 75 mg)	2.80
Citalopram 1 x 20 mg tab/day	2.59
Fluoxetine 1 x 20 mg cap/day	1.37
Sertraline 1 x 50 mg tab/day	17.82
Venlafaxine modified-release 1 x 75 mg cap/day	23.41
Mirtazapine 1 x 30 mg tab/day	10.14
Temazepam 1 x 20 mg tab/day	1.13
Zopiclone 1 x 7.5 mg tab/day	3.24
Diazepam 1 x 10 mg tab/day	1.42
Buspirone 3 x 10 mg tab/day	52.67
Haloperidol tab (DDD = 8 mg)	8.62
Sulpiride 2 x 400 mg tab/day	20.18
Olanzapine 1 x 10 mg tab/day	79.45
Risperidone tab (DDD = 5 mg)	78.48

0   10   20   30   40   50   60   70   80   90

Note: the prices are based on the *Drug Tariff*, November 2005. The dose is based on the World Health Organization's Defined Daily Dose (DDD) where possible, and otherwise the *British National Formulary* (BNF)-stated dose. The DDD is a unit of measurement based on the assumed average maintenance dose in adults. It may not necessarily reflect the actual dose used.

Source: Prescription Pricing Division website: www.ppa.org.uk. Crown copyright material is reproduced with the permission of the Controller of OPSI.

The costs associated with the SNRIs (venlafaxine and mirtazapine) are considerably more than generic fluoxetine or citalopram, and with little evidence that there is a significant difference in their ability to improve depression. The costs associated with risperidone and olanzapine are also highly significant, although the overall number of items prescribed in this group are much smaller than for the antidepressant group. In the year June 2003 to June 2004, the number of items of antipsychotics increased by 5.9 per cent, but the increase in cost of this group was a massive 16.3 per cent. The impact on prescribing budgets, and the NHS as a whole, is significant.

Terms used in drug medication

Medications, especially those that relate to the management of mental health conditions, are frequently labelled as being 'addictive' or causing 'withdrawal effects'. In fact the terms tend to be used to mean different things by different people. For the sake of clarity the following WHO definitions will be used.[3]

Addiction, drug or alcohol

This is the repeated use of a psychoactive substance or substances, to the extent that the user (referred to as an addict) is periodically or chronically intoxicated, shows a compulsion to take the preferred substance (or substances), has great difficulty in voluntarily ceasing or modifying substance use, and exhibits determination to obtain psychoactive substances by almost any means. Typically, tolerance is prominent and a withdrawal syndrome frequently occurs when substance use is interrupted. The life of the addict may be dominated by substance use to the virtual exclusion of all other activities and responsibilities. The term addiction also conveys the sense that such substance use has a detrimental effect on society, as well as on the individual; when applied to the use of alcohol, it is equivalent to alcoholism. Addiction is a term of long standing and variable usage. It is regarded by many as a discrete disease entity, a debilitating disorder rooted in the pharmacological effects of the drug, which is remorselessly progressive. From the 1920s to the 1960s attempts were made to differentiate between addiction and 'habituation', a less severe form of psychological adaptation. In the 1960s the World Health Organization recommended that both terms be abandoned in favour of dependence, which can exist in various degrees of severity. Addiction is not a diagnostic term in ICD-10, but continues to be very widely employed by professionals and the general public alike.

Craving

This is a very strong desire for a psychoactive substance or for the intoxicating effects of that substance. Craving is a term in popular use for the mechanism presumed to underlie impaired control. It is thought by some to develop, at least partly, as a result of conditioned associations that evoke conditioned withdrawal responses. Craving may also be induced by the provocation of any physiological arousal state resembling an alcohol or drug withdrawal syndrome.

Dependence

As a general term this is the state of needing or depending on something or someone for support or to function or survive. As applied to alcohol and other drugs, the term implies a need for repeated doses of the drug to feel good or to avoid feeling bad. In DSM-IIIR, dependence is defined as 'a cluster of cognitive, behavioural and physiologic symptoms that indicate a person has impaired control of psychoactive substance use and continues use of the substance despite adverse consequences'. It is roughly equivalent to the dependence syndrome of ICD-10. In the ICD-I0 context, the term dependence could refer generally to any of the elements in the syndrome. The term is often used interchangeably with addiction and alcoholism. In 1964 a WHO Expert Committee introduced 'dependence' to replace addiction and habituation. The term can be used generally with reference to the whole range of psychoactive drugs (drug dependence, chemical dependence, substance use dependence), or with specific reference to a particular drug or class of drugs (e.g. alcohol dependence, opioid dependence). While ICD-I0 describes dependence in terms applicable across drug classes, there are differences in the characteristic dependence symptoms for different drugs. In unqualified form, dependence refers to both physical and psychological elements. Psychological or psychic dependence refers to the experience of impaired control over drinking or drug use, while physiological or physical dependence refers to tolerance and withdrawal symptoms. In biologically orientated discussion, dependence is often used to refer only to physical dependence. Dependence or physical dependence is also used in the psychopharmacological context in a still narrower sense, referring solely to the development of withdrawal symptoms on cessation of drug use. In this restricted sense, cross-dependence is seen as complementary to cross-tolerance, with both referring only to physical symptomatology (neuroadaptation).

Detoxification

This is, first, the process by which an individual is withdrawn from the effects of a psychoactive substance.

Second, as a clinical procedure, this is the withdrawal process carried out in a safe and effective manner, such that withdrawal symptoms are minimised. The facility in which this takes place may be variously termed a detoxification centre, detox centre, or sobering-up station.

Typically, the individual is clinically intoxicated or already in withdrawal at the outset of detoxification. Detoxification may or may not involve the administration of medication. When it does, the medication given is usually a drug that shows cross-tolerance and cross-dependence to the substance(s) taken by the patient. The dose is calculated to relieve the withdrawal syndrome without inducing intoxication, and is gradually tapered off as the patient recovers. Detoxification as a clinical procedure implies that the individual is supervised until recovery from intoxication or the physical withdrawal syndrome is complete. The term 'self-detoxification' is sometimes used to denote unassisted recovery from a bout of intoxication or withdrawal symptoms.

Habituation

This is becoming accustomed to any behaviour or condition, including psychoactive substance use. In the context of drugs, the term has overtones of dependence. In 1957, a WHO Expert Committee distinguished drug habituation from drug addiction on the basis of the absence of physical dependence, desire rather than compulsion to take the drug, and little or no tendency to increase the dose (see 'tolerance', below). In 1964 another WHO Expert Committee replaced both terms with drug dependence.

Misuse, drug or alcohol

This is use of a substance for a purpose not consistent with legal or medical guidelines, as in the non-medical use of prescription medications. The term is preferred by some to abuse in the belief that it is less judgemental.

Tolerance

This is a decrease in response to a drug dose that occurs with continued use. Increased doses of alcohol or other drugs are required to achieve the effects originally produced by lower doses. Both physiological and psychosocial factors may contribute to the development of tolerance, which may be physical, behavioural or psychological. With respect to physiological factors, both metabolic and/or functional tolerance may develop. By increasing the rate of metabolism of the substance, the body may be able to eliminate the substance more readily. Functional tolerance is defined as a decrease in sensitivity of the central nervous system to the substance. Behavioural tolerance is a change in the effect of a drug as a result of learning or alteration of environmental constraints. Acute tolerance is rapid, temporary accommodation to the effect of a substance following a single dose. Reverse tolerance, also known as sensitisation, refers to a condition in which the response to a substance increases with repeated use. Tolerance is one of the criteria for the dependence syndrome.

Withdrawal syndrome

This is a group of symptoms of variable clustering and degree of severity that occur on cessation or reduction of use of a psychoactive substance that has been taken repeatedly, usually for a prolonged period and/or in high doses. The syndrome may be accompanied by signs of physiological disturbance. A withdrawal syndrome is one of the indicators of a dependence syndrome. It is also the defining characteristic of the narrower psychopharmacological meaning of dependence.

The onset and course of the withdrawal syndrome are time-limited and are related to the type of substance and dose being taken immediately before cessation or reduction of use. Typically, the features of a withdrawal syndrome are the opposite of those of acute intoxication.

The alcohol withdrawal syndrome is characterised by tremor, sweating, anxiety, agitation, depression, nausea and malaise. It occurs 6–48 hours after cessation of alcohol consumption and, when uncomplicated, abates after 2–5 days. It may be complicated by grand mal seizures and may progress to delirium (known as delirium tremens).

Sedative withdrawal syndromes have many features in common with alcohol withdrawal, but may also include muscle aches and twitches, perceptual distortions, and distortions of body image.

Opioid withdrawal is accompanied by rhinorrhoea (running nose), lacrimation (excessive tear formation), aching muscles, chills, gooseflesh and, after 24–48 hours, muscle and abdominal cramps. Drug-seeking behaviour is prominent and continues after the physical symptoms have abated.

Stimulant withdrawal (the 'crash') is less well defined than syndromes of withdrawal from central nervous system depressant substances; depression is prominent and is accompanied by malaise, inertia and instability.

Source: www.who.int/substance_abuse/terminology/who_lexicon/en/index.html. The preceding section is used with the permission of the World Health Organization.

For up-to-date prescribing information consult the latest addition of the British National Formulary.[4]

Benzodiazepines
How do they work?
Benzodiazepines work at the level of neuroreceptors in the brain to increase the amount of available gamma-aminobutyric acid (GABA). The consequence of increasing levels of GABA is a reduction in anxiety, a reduction in convulsions and an increase in feelings of relaxation. Other groups of drugs that work on the GABA receptors include alcohol, zolpidem (used for sleep disturbance), carbamazepine, gabapentin and valproic acid, all used in epilepsy, but also used as mood stabilisers in bipolar disorder.

There are a number of different benzodiazepines, which fall into two broad categories: hypnotics (BNF 4.1.1) and anxiolytics (BNF 4.1.2). The distinction between hypnotics, intended to sedate at night, and anxiolytics, intended to reduce anxiety during the day, is not great, and certainly there are at times an overlap between night-time sedation and reduction in daytime arousal for both groups of drugs.

Hypnotics include nitrazepam and flurazepam, both of which have a relatively long half-life, and loprazolam, lormetazepam and temazepam, which have much shorter half-lives.

Anxiolytics include diazepam, alprazolam, lorazepam and oxazepam. Diazepam and alprazolam have longer half-lives than lorazepam and oxazepam.

What are the indications for their use?

Hypnotics are indicated for the management of sleep disturbances. Short-term sleep disturbance (jet lag, for example) rarely requires medication. In those few cases where medication is justified, a short-acting drug such as temazepam, given only for 2–3 days, should be sufficient. Where the sleep disturbance is part of an underlying disturbance, e.g. pain associated with osteoarthritis, then it is appropriate to first treat the underlying condition. If medication is to be prescribed, it should be for no longer than 14 days, since tolerance occurs after 2–3 weeks of continued use. Finally for those few individuals who suffer from chronic and severe insomnia, then referral to a sleep disorder service may be more appropriate than the long-term prescribing of a hypnotic, to which the patient rapidly becomes both tolerant of the effects and addicted to the medication.

Anxiolytics are indicated for the management of short-term relief of severe anxiety. NICE guidelines[5] recommend the use of benzodiazepines for the short-term management of generalised anxiety disorder (GAD), but not for panic disorder (PD). There is some evidence that the use of benzodiazepines to manage panic disorder produces worse outcomes; in particular the use of benzodiazepines as a 'token' is associated with poor outcomes. A 'token' is a medication that is kept 'just in case' and is never actually consumed. It is perceived to be a crutch or a support, and whilst patients maintain that they need such a support they will be unable to develop new ways of managing the restrictions that the panic disorder imposes on their life.

Like hypnotics, diazepam and other anxiolytics cause tolerance within 2–3 weeks, and addiction. There may be a need to control severe anxiety symptoms in the short term, but there is no indication for the long-term prescribing of anxiolytics.

Other uses of this group of drugs include the management of status epilepticus, as part of an alcohol detoxification programme, for febrile convulsions, and pre-operatively. They may also be used for a short duration in the management of a manic episode,[6] whilst the correct dose of lithium is being titrated. In such a circumstance, however, the patient should be managed as an inpatient and will be being supervised by a psychiatrist and his or her team.

Cautions using benzodiazepines

Use of benzodiazepines is associated with addiction, dependence, tolerance, overdose, sedation and drowsiness. Therefore benzodiazepines should not be prescribed for longer than 2–3 weeks, and advice should be provided on the caution needed to drive and in the use of machinery, and also on the potentiation of side effects such as drowsiness due to alcohol consumption. Benzodiazepines also cause slowing of reactions and impaired perception so that driving becomes significantly more hazardous. This advice should be recorded in the clinical record.

Benzodiazepines can also cause a paradoxical effect; rather than the relaxation and anti-anxiety effects for which they are usually prescribed, they can cause aggression, hostility, excessive talking or over-activity. The effects can be attenuated by manipulation of the dose (either increasing or decreasing the dose).

Benzodiazepines should be used with caution in the elderly, as they are more likely to cause confusion and falls. In 2001 Pierfitte *et al.* published a paper that described no association between single use of benzodiazepine and hip fractures,[7] but there was some debate subsequently as to the accurate analysis of the data.

Benzodiazepines generally should not be used in children for the management of mental health problems. Clearly there may be other clinical reasons for prescribing in children, e.g. management of epilepsy, pre-operatively, etc.

Managing dependence of benzodiazepines

The management of benzodiazepine dependence is time consuming and difficult. The BNF recommends a regime for the planned reduction in prescribing – see below – but the management of such patients requires more than a prescribing plan.

The identification of people who are dependent on prescribed benzodiazepines can be identified in practices by undertaking the appropriate search of the practice prescribing system. The identification of those who are purchasing the drugs on the black market is much harder, and usually comes about as part of a wider consultation, in which medication misuse is a part. In either case, ensuring that the patient really wants to stop the medication is absolutely essential.

There is a group of relatively older patients who have been taking night sedation, such as nitrazepam, for many years, and are addicted to the drug. This group in particular have often no motivation to stop taking their 'nightly fix', and a pragmatic solution needs to be negotiated that is acceptable both to prescribing physicians and the patients themselves.

The BNF recommends the following regime for the planned reduction in prescribing of benzodiazepines:

1. Transfer the patient to an equivalent daily dose of diazepam

2. Reduce the daily dose of diazepam by 2.0–2.5 mg daily every two or three weeks. If withdrawal symptoms develop, maintain the current dose until symptoms resolve

3. Continue to reduce the dose of diazepam at a slow pace – it is better to reduce the dose slowly than too quickly

4. Stop completely; withdrawal symptoms can continue for up to one year.

As well as the planned reduction in prescribing, other support may be necessary, such as counselling. The use of antidepressants may be appropriate if depression is present, and if they are prescribed in line with the NICE guidelines on depression.[8] Beta blockers to manage some of the more physical symptoms may be appropriate if the symptoms are severe. Antipsychotic medication tends to cause agitation and should be avoided.

Other hypnotics

There are a number of other hypnotics that are used commonly in primary care: zaleplon, zolpidem and zopiclone. All three are very similar.

How do they work?

They are GABA neurotransmitter agonists, and have a short half-life. They have a rapid onset of action, but an abrupt cessation of effect, ensuring that there is little hangover effect the following day.

What are the indications for their use?

The indications are for their use in the short-term management of sleep disturbance, including those causes related to the external environment, e.g. jet lag, or night shift workers, as well as sleep disturbance associated with an underlying physical condition that needs other treatment. The long-term management of insomnia or other sleep disorder is not an indication for their use.

Cautions, contraindications and side effects

Caution should be exercised when prescribing for people with liver impairment, respiratory failure, drug or alcohol addiction, or for a pregnant woman. Absolute contraindications include sleep apnoea syndrome and myasthenia gravis. Breastfeeding is also a contraindication.

Side effects include drowsiness, confusion and impaired concentration.

Other anxiolytics

The other anxiolytic that is sometimes used in primary care is buspirone. Older tricyclic antidepressants such as clomipramine have a role in managing people with anxiety, but the use is 'off licence' – further information and advice is provided in the NICE anxiety guidelines.[5]

How do they work?

Buspirone is thought to act at the specific serotonin $5HT_{1A}$ receptor sites.

What are the indications for their use?

Buspirone is indicated for the short-term management of anxiety. There has been a question as to whether buspirone can be used to alleviate the withdrawal effects of benzodiazepines. The BNF is clear that buspirone cannot be used for this reason. The NICE guidelines for the management of anxiety found that the evidence for its use was equivocal.[5]

Buspirone takes up to two weeks to work. It is recommended that, if prescribed, it should only be for short periods, although some psychiatrists do prescribe it for longer periods.

Cautions, contraindications and side effects

Like other drugs in this group, it can impair driving, and the medication can cause drowsiness, impaired concentration and sometimes confusion. It should be avoided in epilepsy, severe liver or renal impairment and in women who are pregnant or breastfeeding.

Drugs used in psychoses and related disorders

This group of drugs includes the traditional neuroleptic medications, such as chlorpromazine and haloperidol, the newer atypical antipsychotics such as olanzapine and risperidone, and finally the antimanic drugs such as lithium and sodium valproate.

How do the neuroleptic medications work?

The cause, or causes, of schizophrenia are not well understood. There are a number of different ideas as to the cause of this disorder, including the concept that it represents the endpoint of a number of different disease processes that include biochemical, genetic or environmental potential insults. Some of the evidence for a biochemical approach to schizophrenia lies with the effectiveness of neuroleptic medication.

The primary pharmacological action of antipsychotic medication lies at the dopamine receptor sites, and in particular at the D2 receptor site, which it blocks. Snyder et al.[9] and later Kapur et al.[10] were able to demonstrate that the potency of a specific antipsychotic medication was related to its affinity to the D2 site, and this finding is in part responsible for the emerging dopamine theory for schizophrenia. A similar explanation can be applied to other psychoses, in which the neuroleptics are effective.

The D2 receptor sites that are blocked are also involved in the control of fine movement, and hence the side effect of this group of medications is uncontrolled fine movement, also known as extrapyramidal side effects, similar to Parkinson's syndrome. Other side effects include dystonia and dyskinesia, which are linked to its mode of action at the D2 receptor site. However, although antipsychotic medication has a strong affinity for D2 receptors, they also have an affinity for other types of receptors such as serotonin, histamine and alpha-adrenergic sites, all of which can influence the overall profile of individual drugs.

In the 1970s, a drug called clozapine was introduced that had a strong affinity for the D4 receptor site. Whilst this meant that the extrapyramidal symptoms associated with traditional neuroleptics were significantly reduced, an unrelated but serious problem with blood dyscrasia was noted, and led to its withdrawal. Subsequent research led to its reintroduction for the management of treatment-resistant schizophrenia, and the development of other drugs that block the D4 receptor site. These drugs have a different side effect profile, with the most marked benefit being a significant reduction in extrapyramidal symptoms and signs, whilst retaining effective control of the psychosis. This group of drugs is known as atypical antipsychotic medication and includes drugs such as amisulpride and quetiapine.

What are the indications for their use?

Neuroleptic medication, either traditional or atypical, is indicated for use in people who have florid psychotic symptoms such as hallucinations, delusions, thought disorder, and for the prevention of relapse. Medication can be in an oral preparation that needs to be administered daily, or in an intramuscular preparation that is administered once every two to four weeks.

Since thought disorder, hallucinations and delusions occur in conditions other than schizophrenia, these drugs can be used in conditions such as bipolar disorder and other psychoses.

The indication and use of medication in the first episode of schizophrenia is dealt with in more detail in Chapter 7.

Compliance with medication

Management with medication tends to be long term, and people usually end up being prescribed these types of medication for many months or years. The issue of patients taking the medication that has been prescribed for them is complex; indeed there is even debate as to what to call this process. A letter in the *British Medical Journal* from Dickinson describes the difference between concordance and compliance.[11] 'Concordance is a new approach to the prescribing and taking of medicines. It is an agreement reached after negotiation between a patient and a healthcare professional that respects the beliefs and wishes of the patient in determining whether, when, and how medicines are to be taken.' Compliance 'implies taking orders from a health professional'. A review of the literature associated with compliance in psychotic conditions by Carter *et al*. in 2005 is helpful in summarising some of the complex issues.[12]

Compliance with prescribed medication in schizophrenia is generally poor. A study in 2003 by Dolder *et al*. found a compliance rate of 41 per cent.[13] This means that 59 per cent of people were not taking their prescribed medication. Factors related to poor compliance have been categorised by Carter *et al*. into four areas:

- patient-related factors
  - lack of insight into the illness
  - co-morbid alcohol or substance abuse
  - poor social functioning
  - youth
  - male sex
  - presence or severity of symptoms

- environment-related factors
  - lack of social support
  - stigma of illness
  - living alone

- healthcare professional-related factors
  - poor therapeutic relationship

- treatment-related factors
  - presence or severity of side effects
  - delayed onset of therapeutic effects
  - complex treatment regimen.

Fenton and colleagues estimated that non-compliant patients had a six month to two year risk of relapse that was 3.7 times greater than the compliant patient.[14] However, it should be remembered that improved compliance may be an indicator of improved psychological wellbeing, rather than being the result of the medication itself.

Nosé *et al.* undertook a survey of published papers to assess what techniques improved compliance.[15] They found that educational interventions repeated frequently (less than six-monthly) were effective. Kemp *et al.* had earlier developed a programme called Compliance Therapy, which had some beneficial effects.[16] It is worth pointing out, though, that the programme was financed by the pharmaceutical industry.

Side effects and cautions

The side effects of neuroleptic medication are well known; indeed much research has been focused on ameliorating some of the side effects. The mode of action of neuroleptics is to block D2 receptor sites – one of the dopamine neurotransmitters. Although dopamine is involved in aspects of psychotic illness, it is also involved in the fine control of movement, and that, as a consequence of its blockade by neuroleptics, fine control is lost, and coarse involuntary movements develop. These are known as extrapyramidal symptoms, as it is the extrapyramidal tracts of the spinal cord that ensure control of fine movements.

The use of neuroleptics produces extrapyramidal symptoms that includes:

- Parkinsonian symptoms – including bradykinesia, pill-rolling tremor and rigidity

- dystonia – abnormal face and/or body movement

- akathisia – abnormal restlessness, a need to keep constantly moving

- tardive dyskinesia – rhythmic involuntary movements usually of the tongue, jaw or face, and trunk

Extrapyramidal symptoms occur most frequently with piperazine phenothiazines (e.g. fluphenazine and prochlorperazine) the butyrophenones (such as haloperidol) and the depot preparations.

Extrapyramidal symptoms occur less frequently with the newer atypical antipsychotic medications such as olanzapine or risperidone, as they block the D4 receptor site; it is for this reason that they are the first-line drug of choice recommended by NICE in its guidelines on schizophrenia.[17] The newer atypicals are not more effective than their traditional counterparts; they just cause fewer side effects. The consequence is that concordance with treatment plans is improved – as the previous section showed, unpleasant side effects are a significant cause of poor compliance and concordance.

Managing the extrapyramidal side effects

The management of the side effects is changing rapidly as more and more new cases are started on the atypical antipsychotics that cause far fewer side effects. However, for those who remain on the more traditional medication groups there are a number of ways of managing the effects.

Parkinsonian side effects

These are usually managed by using the antimuscarinic type of drugs such as benzhexol or procyclidine. These should only be prescribed if there are Parkinsonian symptoms present – and should not be prescribed to prevent the development of symptoms. Caution must be used as these drugs can worsen tardive dyskinesia, or even unmask it.

Tardive dyskinesia

This is an extremely unpleasant condition that has no treatment. Withdrawing the medication that caused the tardive dyskinesia makes the symptoms worse, so that maintaining the medication seems to be the only way of preventing the deterioration of the symptoms. Since the changes were irreversible, and a consequence of drugs administered by doctors, there was a time before the wider availability of atypical antipsychotics when the medication review included the careful assessment of a patient's tongue looking for the very earliest signs of tardive dyskinesia – called vermiculation.

Other side effects

Hypotension and interference with temperature regulation

These occur with all types of neuroleptic medication. The symptoms are worse in the elderly, and can cause falls, hypothermia or hyperthermia.

Neuroleptic malignant syndrome

This is a rare condition where any neuroleptic drug can cause a potentially fatal condition characterised by hyperpyrexia and fluctuation in levels of consciousness. The early signs are rigidity or mental status changes; other early signs include obtundation, catatonia, tachycardia, tachypnoea, labile blood pressure, dysarthria, dysphagia, diaphoresis, sialorrhea, incontinence, rigidity, myoclonus, tremors, low-grade fevers or serum creatine kinase elevations. As the illness develops it is characterised by a fever in excess of 38°C, profuse sweating, changes in level of consciousness, tachycardia or tachypnoea, and enzyme changes such as raised levels of creatine phosphokinase (CPK). It usually starts within days of commencing neuroleptic medication, and is treated by withdrawal of the medication, together with appropriate supportive measures.

Cardiac arrhythmias

The Quality and Outcomes Framework (QOF) of the GMS contract, in describing the content of the checks that should be carried out on people who are taking neuroleptic medication, makes particular mention of the arrhythmias caused by these drugs, and quotes the article by Hennessy et al. as a reference source.[18] The authors make clear that neuroleptics prolong the QT interval, and that people who are taking neuroleptic medication are more likely to die from cardiac arrest or other arrhythmias, but they also make clear that they are unable to say if the prolongation of the QT interval is the cause of the increased mortality. Elsewhere in this book (Chapter 1) there is an extensive section on the physical health of people with severe mental illness, including coronary heart disease, and the association with deprivation and smoking, all of which will contribute significantly to the increased mortality in this group of very vulnerable people. It may be too simple to ascribe the increased mortality purely to the increase in QT interval, and not acknowledge the more complex other factors that contribute to the four-fold increase in mortality experienced by people with a severe mental illness.

Hyperprolactinaemia

This is a recognised effect of neuroleptic medication that GPs should be aware of, as it can cause a range of gynaecological complaints that are significant. The Disability Rights Commission Formal Investigation[19] into the physical health needs of people with mental illness discusses in some detail the fact that many patients with mental health problems perceive that GPs explain all their symptoms as being a consequence of the disordered mental state – and irregular vaginal bleeding is a frequently quoted example of this. In fact irregular vaginal bleeding in women and galactorrhoea and gynaecomastia in men are real side effects caused by the hyperprolactinaemia – not hallucinations or delusions caused by the underlying psychotic illness.

Weight gain and diabetes

Diabetes is more common in people with schizophrenia – up to five times as common. However, whilst the newer atypical antipsychotic medications without doubt cause weight gain, and increase the chance of developing diabetes, it is worth noting that the first papers that recognised the association between diabetes and schizophrenia were published in the 1920s prior to the development of chlorpromazine, let alone the development of atypical antipsychotic medication.[20]

Antidepressant medication

Prescribing antidepressant medication is a common activity in primary care. Table 12.1 illustrates the numbers of items of antidepressants prescribed in England in June 2000 and June 2005.[1,2]

Table 12.1: Prescribing antidepressants in England (millions of items prescribed)

	June 2000	*June 2005*
TCAs	2.2 (22%)	2.2 (17.7%)
SSRIs	2.2 (22%)	3.9 (31.4%)
Others including MAOIs and SNRIs	0.2 (2%)	0.6 (4%)
All categories of mental health drugs	10.2 (100%)	12.4 (100%)

Notes: TCAs: tricyclic antidepressants; SSRIs: selective serotonin reuptake inhibitors; SNRIs: selective noradrenergic reuptake inhibitors; MAOIs: monoamine oxidase inhibitors.

Source: Prescription Pricing Division website: www.ppa.org.uk. Crown copyright material is reproduced with the permission of the Controller of OPSI.

In 2005, there were about 60 million items of all types of drugs prescribed by English GPs. There is about a 5 per cent increase, year on year, across all prescribing groups in the volume of prescription items.

There are four main categories of antidepressants, the tricyclic antidepressants (TCAs), the selective serotonin reuptake inhibitors (SSRIs), the monoamine oxidase inhibitors (MAOIs) and a heterogeneous group that does not fall neatly into one of the other three groups. This includes drugs such as the selective noradrenergic reuptake inhibitors (SNRIs) such as venlafaxine.

How do antidepressants work?

There are different views as to the cause of mental health problems and mental illness. This section will look at the pharmacology of antidepressants in relation to neurotransmitters, and does not address the much wider, complex and philosophical debate as to the different causes of mental illness.

Antidepressants influence different neurotransmitters to varying degrees. The increasing knowledge about what neurotransmitters are, how they behave, and what effects they have is reflected in the increasing sophistication in the specificity of antidepressant medication.

The three main neurotransmitters influencing mood are noradrenaline, dopamine and serotonin. When these neurotransmitters are released into the synapse, they have an effect on the post-synaptic neuron, and are then inactivated. All the antidepressant medications have an effect by prolonging the post-synaptic response by preventing the inactivation (or reuptake) of the neurotransmitter.

Monoamine oxidase inhibitors increase levels of all three neurotransmitters by inhibiting the enzyme monoamine oxidase, which metabolises these chemicals. However, it can also affect other neurotransmitters, and hence has a number of potentially serious side effects. Tricyclic antidepressants also influence all three neurotransmitters, whilst the SSRIs, as the name implies, influence only serotonin, and the newer SNRIs influence only the noradrenergic receptors.

The neurotransmitters are also responsible for effects other than mood; pain is mediated through these transmitters, and antidepressants can therefore also be used to manage people with chronic pain.

If it is accepted that neurotransmitters play a role in mood disorders (and there are some people that do not accept this), then it becomes logical to consider if there is a genetic basis to the changing levels and effectiveness of neurotransmitters – in fact is there a genetic basis to depression? A recent review by Ebmeier and colleagues looked at some of the evidence.[21] They felt that 'without doubt' genetic factors play an important role in depression. They report that heritability as calculated from twin studies has been estimated to be between 31 per cent and 42 per cent. However, further and more detailed analysis of specific genes, candidate genes, and specific sites for antidepressant activity revealed that there is no concordance amongst the variety of results – at least none that will deliver a coherent explanation. Their conclusion was that practical applications of the current knowledge were some time away – although there was some early helpful information available.

What are the indications for using antidepressants?

The indications for the use of antidepressants are a consequence of their mode of action; they influence the neurotransmitters that mediate mood. However, since some antidepressants are non-specific in their action they also have an effect on neurotransmitters that mediate other actions such as pain.

They are indicated for the management of depression, anxiety and panic attacks, and for the management of chronic pain.

Antidepressants in the management of depression

NICE guidelines recommend the use of antidepressants for the treatment of people with moderate or severe depression.[8] The guidelines do not recommend the use of antidepressants for people with mild depression. The *Lancet* summary by Ebmeier and colleagues points out how these recommendations are at odds with guidelines and advice elsewhere:[21]

- the NICE guidelines go much further than those of the American Psychiatric Association[20]

- the evidence on which these recommendations are based is derived from a small number of studies

- mood-related cognitive impairment can make engaging with talking therapies difficult or ineffective

- the lack of sufficient skills or individuals to deliver appropriate quantity and quality of talking therapies.

Given these difficulties, and in particular the lack of a universally available effective talking therapy service such as cognitive behavioural therapy (CBT), it is not surprising that implementation of this recommendation is slow, and has met with some resistance. Further, there has been no demonstrable reduction in antidepressant prescribing as a consequence of the guidelines.

Risk assessment

When starting an antidepressant, it is important to undertake a risk assessment for suicide. A detailed discussion on risk assessment is found in Chapter 15. Current regulatory advice is clear that the use of antidepressants in children and young people increases the likelihood of suicidal ideas and self-harm. If treatment is considered necessary in this age group (18–30 years), then the health professional should monitor the effects of the medication and the progress of the patient, closely and frequently.

When discussing with a patient about commencing a course of treatment some of the issues that may be helpful to consider are:

- antidepressants generally take at least 10 days, and usually 14 days, to start having a pharmacological effect

- antidepressants need to be taken for at least six to eight weeks to assess the full impact of the medication

- antidepressants should be continued for at least six months following remission of the depression, to prevent further relapse

- common concerns should be addressed about medication, e.g. fear of addiction, using medication is a sign of weakness

- as with all other drugs, the patient should be informed of potential side effects, and potential effects of discontinuation or withdrawal of the medication.

The continued monitoring and follow-up of patients with depression is discussed in more detail in Chapter 6, which includes advice for the duration of treatment, likely time to see an effect, etc.

The choice of antidepressant has been reviewed in the NICE guidelines, and some of its recommendations are repeated in Box 12.1.[8]

Box 12.1: NICE guidelines on choice of antidepressant

- When an antidepressant is to be prescribed in routine care, it should be an SSRI.

- When prescribing an SSRI, consideration should be given to prescribing a generic form.

- Dosulepin, phenelzine, combined antidepressants and lithium augmentation should be prescribed by either specialist mental health professionals or general practitioners with a special interest (GPwSIs) in mental health.

There are further detailed recommendations in the guidelines, to which the interested reader is directed.

If the patient fails to respond to antidepressant medication it is appropriate to consider the following:

- is the patient taking the medication correctly?

- the dose of the antidepressant can be increased slowly if the response is unsatisfactory over four weeks, in line with the Summary of Product Characteristics

- the medication can be switched to another drug after 4–6 weeks if there has been no response, and the patient wishes to continue with an antidepressant

- suggested second-line medication includes another SSRI, or mirtazapine, but there are others such as moclobemide, reboxetine and tricyclic antidepressants that may be appropriate.

There is value to some patients who show clear clinical response in maintaining them on low-dose tricyclic antidepressants.

The 2006 changes to the QOF of the nGMS contract recommend case-finding people with depression who also have cardiovascular disease and diabetes. Their subsequent management should be considered in the light of the following:

- sertraline has the best evidence that it is safe in people who have had a recent myocardial infarction, or unstable angina

- there are increased risks of using a tricyclic antidepressant in people with cardiovascular disease

- for patients with pre-existing cardiovascular disease, venlafaxine should not be used.

There are no recorded drug interactions or effects for antidepressants and people using diabetic medications, although there is some evidence that antihypertensive medication can have an increased effect when taken with MAOIs.

When a course of antidepressant medication has been completed, consideration should be given to the gradual withdrawal of the drug over 2–4 weeks. Patients should be told that neither craving nor tolerance occurs with antidepressant medications in the same way that it does with opiate drugs. If withdrawal symptoms do occur, then increasing the medication back to the therapeutic level, and a slower reduction in the dose, should manage the symptoms. Drugs with a very long half-life such as fluoxetine can be stopped more quickly, as it takes a very long time for the drug level to decline. In contrast, stopping paroxetine, which has a relatively short half-life, must be done with some caution and over a prolonged period, so that the change in drug level is equally gradual.

Antidepressants in the management of anxiety disorders

Antidepressants are indicated for managing both GAD and PD. For people who have mixed anxiety and depression, the depression should be managed and treated first.

In GAD, for those patients who have elected to take an antidepressant, an SSRI is appropriate. Paroxetine has been licensed specifically for the management of GAD, but experience suggests that any SSRI may be appropriate. Like depression, if the first-line medication does not provide an adequate therapeutic effect, then substituting a different SSRI may well show some benefit. Unlike depression, it is recommended that a full three months' trial is allowed prior to making a change. Also, the dose needed to produce significant benefits in GAD are likely to be at the upper end of the therapeutic range.

For people with panic disorder, who have elected to take an antidepressant, an SSRI is an appropriate first-line drug, and paroxetine has a licence for this condition. For those who do not respond to an SSRI as a first-line drug, and wish to try another medication, it is appropriate to consider imipramine or clomipramine. It is worth noting that neither of these two tricyclic antidepressants have a licence for the treatment of panic disorder, but have extensive published evidence for their effectiveness. Like GAD, long-term treatment and doses at the upper therapeutic range may be necessary.

General considerations about appropriate information, choice, warnings about adverse effects, etc. that apply to the administration of antidepressant medication in depression apply equally to the management of people with anxiety disorders.

Indications for other mental health conditions

Bipolar disorder

For patients who are experiencing a manic episode as part of a bipolar disorder,[6] the antidepressant should be stopped. Whether or not the antidepressant should be stopped suddenly or gradually will depend on the clinical situation, and experience of the individual who may have suffered from discontinuation effects previously.

Managing the depressive cycle of a person with bipolar disorder is not the same as managing a person with unipolar depression. The antidepressant can encourage 'switching' to the manic phase of the disorder, and so care must be taken to ensure that an antimanic drug is prescribed at the same time. Long-term prophylaxis with antidepressants is not recommended. An SSRI is appropriate where an antidepressant is indicated.

The management of people with bipolar disorder involves not only prescribing antimanic drugs, and often antidepressants, but also mood stabilisers such as lithium or sodium valproate. In such circumstances, where physical illness is also significant, close working with specialist mental health teams is essential to ensure that a complete and effective care plan is developed that describes the responsibilities of both specialist and primary care services.

Post-traumatic stress disorder

For people who have both post-traumatic stress disorder (PTSD)[22] and depression, the PTSD should be managed first, providing that the depression is not so severe as to make the sufferer suicidal – in which case managing the depression first is appropriate.

Generally psychological interventions for PTSD are to be preferred to medication. However, in some limited situations, for example where the trauma is continuing (domestic violence for example), an antidepressant may be appropriate. Evidence suggests that mirtazapine, amitriptyline and phenelzine are all effective, but the former would be the most appropriate considering the side effect profile. Particular attention needs to be paid to the side effect profile of phenelzine, which should generally not be prescribed by a GP. Paroxetine may be a suitable alternative to mirtazapine.

If an antidepressant does produce a beneficial effect, it should be continued for at least 12 months. If the effect is only partial, the dose can be increased, or olanzapine added. In most cases, an individual needing such support would benefit from a specialist opinion.

Obsessive-compulsive disorder

People with mild or moderate functional impairment who have not responded to low-intensity CBT should be offered treatment with an SSRI.[23] People with severe functional impairment should be offered SSRI treatment together with higher-intensity CBT. The SSRIs recommended are fluoxetine, paroxetine, citalopram, fluvoxamine or sertraline. For people with BDD (body dysmorphic disorder) fluoxetine is indicated (although it does not have a UK licence for this use). Treatment should generally be continued for 12 months beyond remission. Although the NICE guidelines describe a stepped-care approach to the management of these conditions, primary care physicians should consider seeking a specialist opinion on the management of these people, as their care can often be complex and long term.

Side effects and cautions when using antidepressants

Antidepressants have a range of side effects that need to be monitored regularly. The possibility of side effects needs to be discussed with the patient at the onset of treatment, together with symptoms associated with stopping the drug, known either as withdrawal or discontinuation symptoms.

Tricyclic antidepressants

Arrhythmias and heart block can occur with antidepressants, and may be a cause of sudden death in patients with heart disease. Convulsions can also occur, as can hepatic and haematological reactions – particularly well-recorded for mianserin.

Other side effects include those related to its antimuscarinic effects, e.g. dry mouth, sweating, drowsiness and blurred vision. It is reported that tolerance to these effects can develop, and that they can be minimised by slowly increasing the dose of the medication over a number of weeks to the recommended adult dose. Other side effects that are marked in older people are low blood pressure, syncope and hyponatraemia.

Overdose of any tricyclic is dangerous, as there are significant cardiac effects, and fatality rates are higher than for other groups of antidepressants. It is for this reason, the risk benefits, that NICE recommended SSRIs over tricyclics, rather than an improved effect at improving depression.

Selective serotonin reuptake inhibitors

SSRIs should be used with caution in people with epilepsy, especially if it is poorly controlled. If the patient is receiving ECT, or has a history of mania, cardiac disease or diabetes, caution should be used in the prescribing of SSRIs. Caution should also be exercised if the patient has renal or hepatic impairment, or is a pregnant or breastfeeding woman.

Side effects include fairly common gastrointestinal reactions, including nausea, vomiting and diarrhoea. A dry mouth and headache can occur as well. Some drugs are more likely to cause gastric bleeding, and if these are being taken by the elderly, who also are taking a non-steroidal anti-inflammatory agent, then real consideration should be given to prescribing a gastro-protective agent such as lansoperazole. Hyponatraemia is also more common as a side effect in elderly people taking an SSRI. In some cases, usually soon after starting the SSRI, akathisia or agitation can develop. If the symptoms are severe, the use of that medication should be reviewed.

Monoamine oxidase inhibitors

The principle and major concern with using this group of medications is a consequence of its mode of action. As described above, MAOIs act by inhibiting the enzyme that destroys amine neurotransmitters. As a consequence, other agents that contain these proteins or their precursors can have a potentiated effect. Drugs that contain indirectly acting sympathomimetic agents, such as are found in over-the-counter cough and cold preparations, can have their pressor action potentiated. In the same way there are a large number of food groups that also contain vaso-active amines whose effects are also potentiated by MAOIs. Such foodstuffs include strong cheese, pickled herring, broad beans and yeast extracts, such as Marmite. An early symptom of such a potential occurrence is a throbbing headache. Patients should be warned that the effects of MAOIs can last for up to two weeks after the cessation of treatment, and, for the same reason, other antidepressants should not be started until there has been a similar period of washout. Using a MAOI at the same time as another antidepressant is very hazardous. Patients should wait one week after stopping any other antidepressant before starting an MAOI.

Other antidepressants

Included in this group are drugs such as venlafaxine and reboxetine. Each drug has its own mode of action and pharmacological profile. For details of specific drugs, the reader is directed to an up-to-date BNF.[4]

Lithium and anticonvulsants

Lithium and drugs such as sodium valproate, carbamazepine or lamotrigine are used as 'mood stabilisers'. It is not clear how these drugs work, although there are some emerging theories about the role of inositol, which Belmaker *et al*. describe in more detail.[24]

The use of mood stabilisers

These drugs are used to supplement other treatments being provided to people either with bipolar disorder or with relapsing unipolar depression. It is clear that the management decision to start any of these medications should lie with a specialist mental health professional, but that the longer-term monitoring is a shared responsibility of both primary and specialist care teams. This is recognised in the QOF, which incentivises the structured supervision of people who are currently on lithium.

There are four major drugs that are used in this fashion: lithium, sodium valproate, lamotrigine and carbamazepine. There are some specific indications for individual drugs, depending on an individual's presentation and longer-term previous history. The decisions are complex, and depend in part on what other treatment (including psychological treatments) are available, so that the decision as to which medication to use in which circumstance should lie with the consultant psychiatrist. Valproate should not be used in women who are pregnant (or of childbearing age) because of its teratogenicity.

Cautions

The major caution that needs to be exercised when supporting a patient who is taking lithium is the accurate monitoring of both the blood lithium level and the renal and thyroid function, as these can be compromised by continued lithium use.

The therapeutic range of lithium is narrow: 0.6 mm/l and 0.8 mm/l. Recent experience with the QOF of the nGMS, which originally specified the therapeutic range of lithium as an incentive, demonstrated that some laboratories had a different therapeutic range for lithium. Individual clinicians, based on their knowledge of the local laboratory facilities, are supervising their patient appropriately, including monitoring of locally appropriate blood levels.

It is recommended that at the initiation of lithium by the mental health specialist the following physical assessment is done:

- the patient is advised that adequate fluid intake is maintained, and that the medication should be taken regularly

- baseline height, weight, renal and thyroid function tests should be taken, and the results shared with the patient's GP

- an ECG performed for those people who are at risk of, or who suffer from, cardiovascular disease and the results shared with the patient's GP.

The monitoring of lithium should include the following:

- serum lithium levels should be measured every THREE months

- renal and thyroid function tests should be measured every SIX months.

As well as the biochemical monitoring described above, there should be a clinical review to assess for symptoms of neurotoxicity, and to assess the mental state of the patient.

The clinical signs that occur when the serum lithium level lies above the narrow therapeutic window are increasing confusion leading to drowsiness and coma. These effects can also be seen as a consequence of several important drug interactions, most noticeably non-steroidal anti-inflammatory drugs (NSAIDs) and diuretics. Both alter the excretion of sodium, which competes at the nephron with lithium, resulting in excessively raised lithium levels. Since NSAIDs can now be bought over-the-counter, particular care must be given to this potential interaction.

There are cards available from the pharmacist for the patient to carry, which records the dose of lithium that the patient is taking.

Bioavailability varies significantly between preparations; it is important that the medication is prescribed by brand and not generically, so that the bioavailability and serum levels are measured against a consistent drug input.

Valproate can also be used as a mood stabiliser but does have certain drawbacks. It is significantly teratogenic, and therefore should not be used in women who are of child-bearing age, or unless there has been an appropriate discussion about contraception. Valproate can also cause liver damage and blood dyscrasias, but these are likely to develop as a drug sensitivity reaction, rather than from prolonged use – so blood tests to assess for these changes should be undertaken six months after starting treatment, but do not need to be repeated at regular intervals.

Lamotrigine, which is better known as an anticonvulsant, has as its major cautions Stevens–Johnson syndrome and reduced effectiveness of oral contraception. There is no need for regular monitoring of serum lamotrigine levels.

Carbamazepine can cause liver damage and blood dyscrasias. Like lithium it has a narrow therapeutic range, and so patients should have their carbamazepine level measured every six months. At the same time, renal function should be measured, as hyponatraemia can occur. Like valproate there is only a need to measure liver function and a full blood count, six months after starting treatment.

Hypericum perforatum

Hypericum perforatum or St John's wort has been used as a treatment for depression for many years. Its attraction to some people is, first, the fact that it is both available without a prescription, and hence available without the 'interference' or medicalisation by a doctor, and, second, it is considered to be a natural product, and therefore 'better' than manufactured antidepressant drugs.

There have also been a number of studies[25,26] and a *British Medical Journal* editorial[27] that considers in what circumstances hypericum could be used. There is also increasing information as to the potential for significant drug interactions with hypericum.

Indications for the use of hypericum

Hypericum is indicated for the treatment of mild to moderate depression. A study by the National Center for Complementary and Alternative Medicine (part of the National Institutes of Health) in the USA compared the use of hypericum and sertraline, together with a placebo arm. There was no statistical difference in response between hypericum and the placebo, but, as the authors point out, neither was there a statistical difference between placebo and sertraline (included as an active control). Linde and colleagues carried out a systematic review of hypericum.[26] They concluded that, combining results, hypericum was significantly better than placebo, and that it was as effective as antidepressants. The subsequent *British Medical Journal* editorial weighed up the evidence provided by Linde and concluded that further research was needed.[27]

Cautions

Whether or not hypericum is effective remains open to debate, but the fact that there are significant interactions is clear. The BNF lists the various drugs that interact with hypericum, and makes the point that, if hypericum is withdrawn, the concentration of the interacting drug may increase, leading to toxicity and potentially death. The joint administration of hypericum and an antidepressant is also hazardous and should be avoided. It is therefore essential as part of the assessment of an individual who is depressed to enquire about over-the-counter medication including hypericum.

References

1.   Prescription Pricing Authority Pharmaceutical Directorate. *Update on Growth in Prescription Volume and Cost Year to June 2004* Newcastle upon Tyne: PPA, www.ppa.org.uk/pdfs/publications/ volume_cost_year_jun04.pdf [accessed November 2007].

2.   Prescription Pricing Division. *Prescribing Review: drugs used in mental health*, 2005, www.ppa.org.uk/news/pact-092005.htm [accessed November 2007].

3.   World Health Organization. *Lexicon of Alcohol and Drug Terms Published by the World Health Organization*, www.who.int/substance_abuse/terminology/who_lexicon/en/ [accessed November 2007].

4.   *British National Formulary*, www.bnf.org.uk.

5.   National Institute for Health and Clinical Guidance. *Clinical Guideline 22, Anxiety: management of anxiety (panic disorder, with or without agoraphobia, and generalised anxiety disorder) in adults in primary, secondary and community care* London: NICE, 2004, www.nice.org.uk/nicemedia/pdf/CG022NICEguidelineamended.pdf [accessed November 2007].

6.   National Institute for Health and Clinical Excellence. *Clinical Guideline 38, Bipolar Disorder: the management of bipolar disorder in adults, children and adolescents, in primary and secondary care* London: NICE, 2006, www.nice.org.uk/nicemedia/pdf/CG38niceguideline.pdf [accessed November 2007].

7.   Pierfitte C, Macouillard G, Thicoïpe M, *et al*. Benzodiazepine and hip fractures in elderly people; case control study *British Medical Journal* 2001; **322**; 704–8.

8.   National Institute for Health and Clinical Excellence. *Clinical Guideline 23, Depression: management of depression in primary and secondary care* London: NICE, 2004, www.nice.org.uk/CG023NICEguideline [accessed November 2007].

9.   Snyder SH, Greenberg D, Yamumura HI. Antischizophrenic drugs: affinity for muscarinic cholinergic receptor sites in the brain predicts extrapyramidal effects *Journal of Psychiatric Research* 1974; **11**: 91–5.

10. Kapur S, Remington G. Dopamine. D(2) receptors and their role in atypical antipsychotic action: still necessary and may even be sufficient *Biological Psychiatry* 2001; **50**: 873–83.

11. Dickinson D, Wilkie P, Harris M. Taking medicines: concordance is not compliance *British Medical Journal* 1999; **319**: 787.

12. Carter S, Taylor D, Levenson R. *Supplementary Chapter: compliance in psychotic conditions* Medicine Partnerships, 2005, www.npc.co.uk/med_partnership/assets/research-qoc-psychotic-condns.pdf [accessed November 2007].

13. Dolder CR, Lacro JP, Leckband S, *et al*. Interventions to improve antipsychotic medication adherence: review of recent literature *Journal of Clinical Psychopharmacology* 2003; 23(4): 389–99.

14. Fenton WS, Blyler CR, Heinssen RK. Determinants of medication compliance in schizophrenia: empirical and clinical findings *Schizophrenia Bulletin* 1997; 23(4): 637–51.

15. Nosé M, Barbui C, Gray R, *et al*. Clinical interventions for treatment non-adherence in psychosis: meta-analysis *British Journal of Psychiatry* 2003; 183: 197–206.

16. Kemp R, David A, Hayward P. Compliance therapy: an intervention targeting insight and treatment adherence in psychotic patients *Behavioural and Cognitive Psychotherapy* 1996; 24: 331–50.

17. National Institute for Health and Clinical Excellence. *Clinical Guideline 1, Schizophrenia: core interventions in the treatment and management of schizophrenia in primary and secondary care* London: NICE, 2002, www.nice.org.uk/nicemedia/pdf/CG1NICEguideline.pdf [accessed November 2007].

18. Hennessy S, Bilker WB, Knauss JS, *et al*. Cardiac arrest and ventricular arrhythmia in patients taking antipsychotic drugs: cohort study using administrative data *British Medical Journal* 2002; 325; 1070.

19. Disability Rights Commission. *Equal Treatment: closing the gap*, www.drc-gb.org/library/publications/health_and_independent_living/health_formal_investigation.aspx [accessed November 2007].

20. Meyer JM, Nasrallah HA (eds). *Medical Illness and Schizophrenia* Washington, DC: APA, 2003.

21. Ebmeier K, Donaghey C, Steele JD. Recent developments and current controversies in depression *Lancet* 2006; 367: 153–67.

22. National Institute for Health and Clinical Guidance. *Clinical Guideline 26, Post-Traumatic Stress Disorder (PTSD): the management of PTSD in adults and children in primary and secondary care* London: NICE, 2005, www.nice.org.uk/nicemedia/pdf/cg026niceguideline.pdf [accessed November 2007].

23. National Institute for Health and Clinical Guidance. *Clinical Guideline 31, Obsessive-Compulsive Disorder: core interventions in the treatment of obsessive-compulsive disorder and body dysmorphic disorder* London: NICE, 2006, www.nice.org.uk/nicemedia/pdf/cg031niceguideline.pdf [accessed November 2007].

24. Belmaker RH, Bersudsky Y, Agam G, *et al*. How does lithium work on manic depression? Clinical and psychological correlates of the inositol theory *Annual Review of Medicine* 1996; 47: 47–56.

25. National Center for Complementary and Alternative Medicine. *A Trial of St John's Wort (Hypericum Perforatum) in the Treatment of Major Depression*, 2004, www.nih.gov/news/pr/apr2002/nccam-09a.doc [accessed November 2007].

26. Linde K, Ramirez G, Mulrow CD, *et al*. St John's wort for depression – an overview and meta-analysis of randomised controlled trials *British Medical Journal* 1996; 313: 253–8.

27. De Smet PAGM. Editorial *British Medical Journal* 1996; 313; 241–2.

13 | Simple yet effective
Challenging the traditional approach

Denise Fisher

What this chapter contributes:

indications for the use of:

- bibliotherapy
- guided self-help
- relaxation
- sleep hygiene
- diet and exercise.

This chapter examines alternatives to the traditional view of addressing common mental health problems, be they pharmacological care or referral to a *specialist*.

Having spent 30 years working in the field of mental health I have observed many changes in practice. Patients with common mental health problems are increasingly receiving treatment in primary care settings, yet many colleagues (in both primary and secondary services) continue to promote the view that patients with these problems require specialist help in the form of counselling or therapy from qualified mental health professionals. Many primary care colleagues continue to consider that mental health *is somebody else's business*. However, as can be seen in Chapter 6, advocating a stepped-care model places common mental health problems firmly not only in primary care but also in care delivery by primary care staff.

Dealing with common mental health problems has now become *everybody's business* and there is an emerging evidence base for more innovative approaches.[1] What follows is an exploration of some of these approaches based on psychoeducation and facilitated self-help, such as:

- bibliotherapy
- guided self-help
- relaxation
- sleep hygiene
- lifestyle changes, such as diet and exercise.

Within primary care many mental health problems have traditionally been dealt with using a pharmacological approach. Whilst medication can be effective, for example as a first step to dealing with a moderate to severe depression, it is not recommended in milder cases.[2] There is also the question of compliance, which we know to be poor[3,4] for a variety of reasons such as side effects, early discontinuation, sub-therapeutic doses, etc. Also patients are expressing a preference for *talking therapies* and there is evidence of the effectiveness of cognitive behavioural therapy (CBT) in the treatment of both anxiety and depression. However, a demand for this type of intervention will only serve to increase the already long waiting lists.

The rationale for the introduction of 1000 graduate primary mental health workers, identified in the NHS Plan,[5] was to support primary care colleagues in the provision of low-key interventions for common mental health problems. However, the reality is that the introduction of these workers across England has been 'patchy'. In some areas there are no graduate primary mental health workers although, where these workers have been introduced, they are beginning to have an impact on service provision, and some PCTs (for example across Cumbria and Lancashire) are employing over-the-baseline numbers.

However, bearing in mind the prevalence of common mental health problems in primary care, they are not in a position to 'mop up' all these problems. Psychoeducation and facilitated self-help can be, and, I would argue, should be, delivered by primary care staff with minimum, if any, training requirements, and there is evidence of the positive impact not only on mental health but also on co-morbid physical health problems as well.[6,7,8] It should also be noted that the public are increasingly in favour of self-help interventions and approaches.[1]

Bibliotherapy

Increasingly there are available a number of self-help books dealing with common mental health problems, written in everyday, easy to understand language, that provide the reader with practical suggestions on how to tackle and deal with the problems. Dr Neil Frude first introduced a book prescription scheme in Cardiff and this approach has now been adopted by Primary Care Trusts (PCTs) across the country with PCTs collaborating with local libraries to stock a selection of self-help material readily available for patients to access. Knowsley PCT is one example of a trust adopting bibliotherapy (see Figures 13.1 and 13.2).[9]

Most of this material is based on a CBT approach, which is a short-term, problem-focused psychosocial intervention. CBT has a significant evidence base for effectiveness across a wide range of mental health difficulties. The basis of CBT is that what people think affects how they feel emotionally also alters what they do.[1]

However, when recommending a self-help book to patients it is important that the chosen material reflects the problems experienced by the individual. Williams suggests that individual clinical assessment should precede any recommendation in order to ensure that the material is suitable and acceptable to the patient.[10]

Figure 13.1: Knowsley book prescription scheme – booklist 2006

Knowsley Book Prescription Scheme - Booklist 2006

Problem Issue	Title	Author(s)	Year	Publisher	ISBN	Price
Anger	Overcoming Irritability and Anger	Will Davies	2000	Robinson	1854875957	£9.99
Anxiety	Overcoming Anxiety	Helen Kennerley	1997	Robinson	1854874225	£9.99
Bereavement / Loss	Life After Loss – A Practical Guide to Renewing Your Life After a Major Loss	Bob Deits	2004	De Capo Press	0306813149	£8.25
	On Grief and Grieving – Finding the Meaning of Grief Through the Five Stages of Loss	Elisabeth Kubler-Ross, David Kessler	2005	Simon & Schuster Ltd	0743263448	£7.25
Depression	Overcoming Depression	Paul Gilbert	2000	Robinson	1841191256	£9.99
	Mind Over Mood	Dennis Greenberger, Christine Padesky	1995	Guilford	0898621283	£16.99
	The Feeling Good Handbook	David Burns	2000	Plume Books	0452281326	£12.99
Eating Disorder	Getting Better Bit(e) by Bit(e)	Ulrike Shmidt, Janet Treasure	1993	Psychology Press	0863773222	£11.35
	Breaking Free – Anorexia Nervosa – A Survival Guide for Families, Friends and Sufferers	Janet Treasure	1997	Psychology Press	0863777600	£12.99
Health Anxiety	It's Not All in Your Head	Gordon J G Asmundson & Steven Taylor	2005	Guilford Press	1572309938	£11.99
Mood Swings	Overcoming Mood Swings	Jan Scott	2001	Constable & Robinson	1841190179	£11.99
Obsessions and Compulsions	The Angry Heart – Overcoming Borderline and Addictive Disorders – An Interactive Self Help Guide	Joseph Santoro, PhD Ronald Cohen, PhD	1997	Joseph Santoro	1572240806	£8.97
	Overcoming Obsession Compulsive Disorder – A Behavioural and Cognitive Protocol for the Treatment (Client Manual)	Gail Steketee	1999	New Harbinger Publications	1572241292	£8.91
Panic	Overcoming Panic	Derrick Silove	1997	Constable & Robinson	1854877011	£9.99
Self Esteem	Overcoming Low Esteem	Melanie Fennel	1999	Constable & Robinson	1854877259	£9.99
	Self Esteem for Women	Lynda Field	2001	Vermillion	009187632X	£6.99
Social Anxiety / Social Phobia	Overcoming Social Anxiety and Shyness	Gillian Butler	1999	Constable & Robinson	1854877038	£9.99
Stress	Managing Stress – Teach Yourself	Terry Looker, Olga Gragson	2003	Teach Yourself	0340860073	£8.99
Trauma	Overcoming Childhood Trauma – Self Help Guide using CB Techniques	Helen Kennerley	2000	Constable & Robinson	1841190810	£9.99

Figure 13.2: Knowsley book prescription scheme – leaflet

Patient Information Leaflet

This leaflet tells you about a new scheme that has been set up by Knowsley Primary Care Trust and Knowsley Library Service. It is about using books to help people who suffer from stress or other emotional problems.

If you take part in the scheme, it means that your GP or other health professional has prescribed a book to help with your specific problem.

How the Scheme Works

If your doctor has decided that you suffer from stress or have other emotional problems, they might prescribe you some medication, or refer you to someone else with expertise in this area. This scheme will give you and your doctor a further treatment option.

This Scheme will give you a further treatment option.

If your doctor feels that a book may be helpful to you, they will give you a prescription for the book that they think is most likely to help. You can then take this prescription along to one of the libraries in Knowsley where the library will loan you the book.

The doctor or health professional will also make a follow-up appointment with you to talk about how useful the book has been to you.

The kind of books your doctor may prescribe

The books your doctor might ask you to read will give up-to-date information about the specific problem that you have. The book will suggest things that you might try or think about which will help you deal with your problem and hopefully help you to feel better.

The book that your doctor prescribes will be chosen from a list of the best books available. Local doctors and specialists have worked together on making this list. The books on the list are known to be effective and have been useful to other people.

Please treat the book as you would any other library book. Please don't mark or write on the book but make your own copy and use this to write on. This way the book can be used again for other people with similar problems.

Some other Questions you might have

Can books really help?

Yes! There is some very good evidence showing that books can help people who have emotional problems. Of course, not everyone will be helped in this way. Self-help books need you to make an effort for it to work best. It would be useful if you could set aside some regular time to yourself to read the book and then try to follow any advice suggested.

What kind of emotional problems can be helped using self-help books?

The current recommended booklist contains books to help with:

- Anger
- Anxiety
- Bereavement and Loss
- Compulsions
- Depression
- Eating Disorder
- Health Anxiety
- Insomnia
- Mood Swings
- Obsessions
- Panic
- Self Esteem
- Social Anxiety
- Social Phobia
- Stress
- Trauma

A recommended title will be identified by your doctor or health professional for your particular problem using the current booklist. The booklist will be reviewed on a regular basis to ensure that the best books become available as recommended by the specialist.

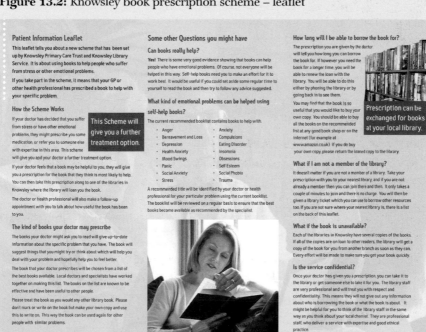

How long will I be able to borrow the book for?

The prescription you are given by the doctor will tell you how long you can borrow the book for. If however you need the book for a longer time, you will be able to renew the loan with the library. You will be able to do this either by phoning the library or by going back in to see them.

You may find that the book is so useful that you would like to buy your own copy. You should be able to buy all the books on the recommended list at any good book shop or on the internet (for example at www.amazon.co.uk) if you do buy your own copy, please return the loaned copy to the library.

Prescription can be exchanged for books at your local library.

What if I am not a member of the library?

It doesn't matter if you are not a member of a library. Take your prescription with you to your nearest library, and if you are not already a member then you can join there and then. It only takes a couple of minutes to join and there is no charge. You will then be given a library ticket which you can use to borrow other resources too. If you are not sure where your nearest library is, there is a list on the back of this leaflet.

What if the book is unavailable?

Each of the libraries in Knowsley have several copies of the books. If all of the copies are on loan to other readers, the library will get a copy of the book for you from another branch as soon as they can. Every effort will be made to make sure you get your book quickly.

Is the service confidential?

Once your doctor has given you a prescription, you can take it to the library or get someone else to take it for you. The library staff are very professional and will treat you with respect and confidentiality. This means they will not give out any information about who is borrowing the book or what the book is about. It might be helpful for you to think of the library staff in the same way as you think about your local chemist. They are professional staff, who deliver a service with expertise and good ethical practice.

Source: Sanderson (2006).[9] Reproduced by permission of Knowsley Primary Care Trust.

The *Overcoming* series of books empower patients to deal with their mental health problems using a structured approach. Each book is developed by a clinician trained in CBT and written in everyday language. Further information about this series of books can be found at publisher Constable Robinson's website: www.constablerobinson.com. Another useful site for information on self-help materials is the Oxford Stress and Trauma Centre: www.oxdev.co.uk.

Guided self-help

Another approach to helping patients is by guided self-help activities such as *behavioural activation* (BA) and *problem solving*. Both of these interventions are low key but are effective in dealing with anxiety and depression. Three universities in the northwest, Liverpool John Moores University, Manchester and the University of Central Lancashire (UCLan), use the Self-Help for Anxiety and Depression (SHADE) manual developed by Dr Karina Lovell in the training for graduate primary mental health workers. This manual can be used by the patient or as part of the brief interventions delivered by these new workers. As such, the approaches (BA and problem solving) are also a useful tool for primary care staff in delivering care to their patients.

BA is very useful for patients who, due to a diagnosis of depression, have lost their motivation. Whilst this approach has been used as part of a CBT programme there is evidence to suggest that this can be used as a low-key intervention in its own right.[11]

BA works on the principle that when individuals are depressed they do not perform normal everyday tasks or follow other activities as they normally would.[12]

BA works from the premise that part of a depressed behaviour pattern therefore is practising avoidance, such as a social situation or dealing with everyday tasks such as opening the mail. Therefore the gradual and steady reintroduction or increase of these normal activities encourages individuals to re-establish their normal routine, which in turn will have a positive impact on their mood.

Box 13.1: Stages of BA

1. Establish a baseline by monitoring current activity levels (see Table 13.1).
2. Draw up a schedule of achievable activities/tasks, such as:
   a) taking a short walk
   b) introducing concentration tasks, such as reading a newspaper
   c) focusing on a life problem, such as dealing with an unpaid bill.
3. Keep a diary of achievement (Tables 13.2 and 13.3).
4. Focus on an external event such as a social activity or work.
5. Gradually withdraw the diary.

Source: CCAWI (2006).[12]

Table 13.1: Behavioural activation diary

	Monday	Tuesday	Wednesday	Thursday	Friday	Saturday	Sunday
9–10							
10–11							
11–12							
12–1							
1–2							
2–3							
3–4							
4–5							
5–6							
6–7							
7–8							
8–9							

Notes: On the chart write the activities you aim to do in the next week. Write them on the day and time that you aim to do them. To begin with, write down one or two things a day. On completing each activity score your feeling of achievement and pleasure using the following scales:

Achievement (the sense of achievement you felt)

```
0——————2——————4——————6——————8
None           moderate          complete
```

Pleasure (the amount of pleasure you gained)

```
0——————2——————4——————6——————8
None           moderate          complete
```

Source: Lovell (2000).[11] Reproduced by permission of Dr Karina Lovell, University of Manchester.

Table 13.2: Behavioural activation diary – achievement

	Monday	Tuesday	Wednesday	Thursday	Friday	Saturday	Sunday
9–10	Work	Work	Work	Read paper for 30 minutes A=5 P=3	Read paper for 30 minutes A=5 P=3	Read paper for 30 minutes A=5 P=4	Read paper for 30 minutes A=5 P=4
10–11	Work	Work	Work	Library A=5 P=5			
11–12	Work	Work	Work				
12–1	Work	Work	Work				
1–2	Work	Work	Work				
2–3	Work	Work	Work				
3–4	Work	Work	Work				
4–5	Work	Work	Work				
5–6				Ring a friend A=6 P=6			
6–7							
7–8							
8–9							

Source: Lovell (2000).[11] Reproduced by permission of Dr Karina Lovell, University of Manchester.

Table 13.3: Behavioural activation diary – achievement (six weeks later)

	Monday	Tuesday	Wednesday	Thursday	Friday	Saturday	Sunday
9–10	Work	Work	Work	Read paper for 30 minutes A=4 P=4	Read paper for 30 minutes A=4 P=4	Read paper for 30 minutes A=5 P=4	Coach outing with friend all day
10–11	Work	Work	Work				As above
11–12	Work	Work	Work			Shopping A=3 P=2	As above
12–1	Work	Work	Work				As above
1–2	Work	Work	Work				As above
2–3	Work	Work	Work	Library A=6 P=5	Enquired re. nightschool A=8 P=8		As above
3–4	Work	Work	Work			Gardening	As above
4–5	Work	Work	Work			Gardening	As above
5–6	Read paper A=4 P=4	Read paper A=4 P=4	Read paper A=4 P=4		Read novel A=6 P=5	Gardening A=6 P=7	As above A=7 P=7
6–7	Cinema				Read novel A=6 P=5		
7–8	Cinema						
8–9	Cinema A=7 P=7						

Note: by about week 12 Anne was beginning to feel like her normal self. She felt it had been difficult to do some of the tasks she set herself, particularly in the first four weeks but very much worthwhile the effort.

Source: Lovell (2000).[11] Reproduced by permission of Dr Karina Lovell, University of Manchester.

Problem solving

Patients experiencing depression often complain that they turn problems over and over in their minds, and these problems gradually appear insurmountable. By attempting to deal with these problems in a systematic way, the patient is helped to feel more empowered through the identification of realistic and practical solutions. Again there is evidence to support the effectiveness of this type of intervention.[11]

Box 13.2: Stages of problem solving

- Identifying the problem, assess whether this needs to be broken down into separate parts.

- Write down as many solutions as possible, no matter how silly they sound.

- Consider the pros and cons of each possible solution.

- Select the best/most promising solution.

- Plan how to carry out the chosen solution – what resources might be necessary, what problems need to be overcome, what steps need to be taken. All need to be realistic and a time scale must be set for achievement.

Source: CCAWI (2006).[12]

Relaxation

Acquiring the ability to relax is not only necessary when an individual is experiencing anxiety but can also be effective in helping to deal with other types of mental health issues. However, it will not be useful if a patient is experiencing the hallucinations and delusions common in schizophrenia since preoccupation with these symptoms will affect the ability to learn to relax.

It can be very difficult to relax if feeling depressed. Feeling stressed results in complaints of physical problems such as muscular tension in the neck, legs, shoulders, etc., tension headaches and so on. Worrying about the symptoms will make those same symptoms worse and the individual becomes trapped in what we call a 'vicious circle'. Learning relaxation skills will enable the individual to reduce these symptoms. Relaxation techniques are therefore very useful for anyone having difficulty *unwinding*. However, it should be noted that relaxation is contraindicated if the patient is complaining of phobias or panic disorders.[12]

Learning to relax is a skill,[13] which is only acquired through consistent practice. In my clinical experience I have found that beginning with systematic relaxation, learning to tense and relax muscles, and working from head to toe have a greater success rate than simply suggesting to the patient that he or she listens to soothing music, since it is important to understand what tension means and how it feels. There are instruction tapes that can be purchased which demonstrate systematic relaxation. It can take between 4–6 weeks, practising on a daily basis, before an individual acquires the knack of deep muscle relaxation, so patients should not expect to acquire this skill quickly. Such tapes may be available through bibliotherapy; it is worth checking if this is available in your own area.

Box 13.3: Some general guidelines for suggesting to a patient how to begin to relax

- Decide in advance when you are going to practise, so as to develop a routine.

- Make sure the chosen area is quiet and you will not be disturbed.

- Do not attempt the exercise if you feel hungry, have just eaten, feel too hot/cold.

- Try to adopt a passive attitude – *have a go, let it happen.*

- Breathe through your nose, keep your breathing regular.

Note: there is a steady increase in activity coupled with a sense of achievement and pleasure over a period of weeks.

Source: Powell (2003).[13]

Sleep hygiene

It can be difficult to assess to what extent an individual has sleep difficulties without first exploring what to them is *normal*. We all have different sleep patterns, which will also be affected by age, and we tend to need less as we grow older.[13] Encouraging individuals to practise good sleep hygiene will have a positive knock-on effect on their mood, since they will awake feeling more rested and able to cope with the day.

When individuals are depressed they may sleep poorly but stay in bed beyond their normal wake-up time, especially if they are not working, and it is important to re-establish a routine of waking up at a regular time.[12]

Box 13.4: Advice on sleep hygiene

- Establish a routine wake-up time.

- Go to bed only when sleepy.

- Avoid napping during the day.

- Avoid stimulants late at night such as caffeine and smoking.

- Avoid using alcohol – this is a depressant but it can also develop into a negative coping strategy.

- Take physical exercise, but before 6 p.m. where possible.

- Eat a light supper – this can be helpful, so long as it does not include items such as chocolate or sugar. Alternatively, have a milky drink (e.g. Horlicks).

- Establish a bedtime routine; a warm bath before bed can help.

Source: CCAWI (2006).[12]

Ensuring that the bed is comfortable is also another practical way to address sleep difficulties; a mattress that is too hard or too soft can impact on the quality of sleep. With the exception of sexual intercourse, individuals should be encouraged to view the bedroom as somewhere to sleep rather that to watch television or to read.[13] Once in bed if the problem is waking due to worrying thoughts it can be useful to keep a notepad by the bed and to use it to jot down how this worry will be addressed the next day. In this way the problem has been dealt with as far as it can be in the early hours of the morning.[13]

If the problem is that the patient is waking up during the night and then experiencing difficulties getting back to sleep the best approach is to advise him or her not to lie there since this could create further tension. Instead, encourage the patient to get up, use the bathroom, maybe go downstairs for a milky drink, and then return to bed, in an attempt to fool the body into thinking this is the first attempt to go to bed.

Diet

Diet can aggravate a whole range of mental health illnesses including common mental health problems such as anxiety and depression.[14] Therefore, by the same token, addressing this problem through a sensible diet regime will have a positive effect on mental health. There is a growing interest in nutrition and its effect on mental health[15] and Professor Andre Tyleé, of the National Institute for Mental Health in England (NIMHE), describes the benefits of nutritional therapy as 'the breakthrough we have been waiting for'.[15]

Two informative documents have been published by the Mental Health Foundation on nutrition and mental health: *Feeding Minds: the impact of food on mental health*[16] and *Changing Diets, Changing Minds: how food affects mental well being and behaviour*.[17]

Andrew McCulloch, Chief Executive of the Mental Health Foundation, states, 'The time is now right for nutrition to become a mainstream, everyday component of mental health care, and a regular factor in mental health promotion.'[16]

Cornah suggests that the brain is no different from other organs in the body that are affected by the food and drink we consume. Studies have shown the benefits of including folic acid, Omega-3 and selenium in the diet, which have a positive impact on levels of depression.[17] Fish, especially oily varieties, are known to contain Omega-3; therefore introducing more fish into a diet can have a beneficial impact on mood. Yet people in the UK consume 59 per cent less fish than they did 60 years ago[16] whilst two Brazil nuts each day will provide the necessary levels of selenium, which in turn assists in building the immune system.

Cornah's report suggests that patients are encouraged to include complex carbohydrates, folic acid, Omega-3, selenium, tryptophan, zinc and vitamins B1, B2 and C in their diets since doing so can provide relief from the symptoms of depression by up to 50 per cent.[16]

It has been suggested that primary care professionals should have:

- ready access to information on the link between diet and mental health
- a working knowledge of the information
- expertise available to support patients through dietary change.[17]

It is important that all maintain a healthy balanced diet yet when unwell this may seem like too much effort. The Food Standards Agency (www.food.gov.uk) recommends the following:

- 30 per cent fruit and vegetables
- 30 per cent bread, potatoes, rice or pasta
- 15 per cent milk and dairy products
- 15 per cent meat and fish
- 10 per cent fat and sugary foods.

Frequently patients with common mental health problems complain of poor appetite and a reliance on *snacking*. This should be discouraged as it can be difficult to keep track of how much has been consumed.[12] Another issue can be *comfort eating* and usually this is done due to boredom or negative feelings about self and usually involves food high in sugar or carbohydrates. This should be discouraged and instead the individual encouraged to turn his or her thoughts away from food and into some form of activity.[12]

Exercise

Primary care with its knowledge and understanding of the patient's physical health is in a unique position to recommend appropriate forms of physical exercise. There has been an evidence base for the use of exercise particularly in the treatment of depression for several years now. Babyak *et al*. found exercise to be more beneficial in the long term for older adults with major depression than sertraline.[18] This is further supported by the research carried out by Callaghan,[19] who concluded that exercise is beneficial in the treatment of anxiety and depression, having a positive impact on cognitive functioning and self-esteem. He went on to state that mental health services seldom recognise the benefits of the therapeutic use of exercise.

The concept of *Exercise by Prescription* is not a new one and was first recommended by the Department of Health in 2001 with the publication of national standards for GP exercise referral schemes. These acknowledged the benefits of exercise not only for depression but also for a variety of physical health problems.[20]

The benefits of exercise are also emphasised in the NICE guidelines on the management of depression, which advises that:[2]

> Patients of all ages with mild depression should be advised of the benefits of following a structured and supervised exercise programme of typically up to 3 sessions per week of moderate duration (45 minutes to 1 hour) for between 10 and 12 weeks.

At the same time as the above publication the Department of Health produced evidence which suggested that exercise is as effective as psychotherapy or medication in the treatment of clinical depression. The Department of Health concluded that:[21]

- physical activity helps people feel better, as reflected in improved mood and reduced state and trait anxiety. It can also help people feel better about themselves through improved physical self-perceptions, and can improve self-esteem, particularly in those with initial low self-esteem

- physical activity can help reduce physiological reactions to stress. It may also improve sleep. Those who do not have good quality of sleep are particularly likely to benefit

- rhythmic, aerobic forms of exercise – such a brisk walking, jogging, cycling, swimming or dancing – appear to be effective in achieving mental health benefits.

This approach to dealing with mild to moderate mental health problems has been further supported by the Mental Health Foundation in *Up and Running*,[22] which focuses on the benefits of exercise therapy in primary care.

Box 13.5: Supporting theories on the benefits of exercise

Biological/chemical: by releasing endorphins and enkephalins, which promote feelings of wellbeing.

Social: exercise can promote increased social interaction thus building relationships.

Esteem boosting: the positive impact of acquiring new skills and achieving goals enhances self-esteem.

Distraction: exercise can be used to divert negative thoughts common in individuals who are depressed.

Source: adapted from Halliwell (2005).[22]

Halliwell also goes on to describe the advantages of exercise therapy, in that exercise is:

- a more cost-effective intervention than traditional methods of treating anxiety and depression
- 'low-risk' in terms of side effects
- not a *passive* treatment given to the patient but rather an informed choice
- normalising and non-stigmatising
- cited by patients as an important part in their recovery programme.[22]

In many areas of the country PCTs working in conjunction with local leisure centres offer Exercise by Prescription where patients can access facilities at minimum costs.

However, if individuals are not keen on attending gyms, there are alternatives. Halliwell describes the 'Green Gym' concept set up by an Oxfordshire GP and the British Trust for Conservation Volunteers.[22] There are now more than 60 such groups around the UK, which meet weekly and undertake local conservation projects. This form of interaction promotes health, fitness and wellbeing through physical work. This not only benefits the local community but also helps improve the individual's sense of self-esteem and self-worth (http://sonningcommon.btcv.org.uk/).

Exercise does not have to be time consuming or intensive. It is recommended that individuals exercise in some form between 20 minutes each day[12] or 45–60 minutes three times each week, for 10–12 weeks, as recommended by the Green Gym.[2]

Conclusion

It can be seen therefore that successful alternatives exist that may be more effective in the long term than the more traditional approaches using pharmacology and/or talking therapy.

None of these forms of intervention is complex, they do not require the primary care professional to undertake intensive training and they are cost-effective in terms of service delivery. The benefits for the patients cannot be underestimated. All of the interventions described involve the patient as an active partner rather than a passive/powerless recipient of 'treatment'. This alone has an impact on their self-confidence and self-esteem, enabling them to feel more in control of their situation/surroundings. Facilitated self-help works from the premise that patients have inner resources and abilities, which can be enhanced through support and/or guidance from the primary care professional.[12]

Each low-key intervention described can be used alone or in combination, for example, as has been described, exercise can have a beneficial impact on the quality of sleep.

Table 13.4: When to use which approach?

Therapeutic strategy	Problem area
BA	Depression
Problem solving	All problems
Relaxation	Anger problems, generalised anxiety disorder (GAD), sleep problems, stress
Sleep hygiene	Insomnia
Diet	All problems
Exercise	All problems

Source: adapted from CCAWI (2006).[12]

The evidence of the current extent of common mental health problems in the community means that in order for us to offer support to as many individuals as possible we have to start thinking *outside the box* and challenge the more traditional approaches. This will enable us to use the finite resources of the NHS more effectively and to the greater benefit of more patients.

Acknowledgements

The author would like to gratefully thank Knowsley Primary Care Trust for permission to reproduce the bibliotherapy leaflets (Figures 13.1 and 13.2) and Dr Karina Lovell, University of Manchester, for permission to reproduce documents from SHADE (Tables 13.1, 13.2 and 13.3).

References

1. NIMHE. *Expert Briefing: self-help interventions for mental health problems* London: Department of Health, 2003.

2. National Institute for Health and Clinical Excellence. *Clinical Guideline 23, Depression: management of depression in primary and secondary care* London: NICE, 2004, www.nice.org.uk/CG023NICEguideline [accessed November 2007].

3. Gardner DM, Murphy AL, Woodman AK, *et al*. Community pharmacy services for antidepressant users *International Journal of Pharmacy Practice* 2001; **9**: 217–24.

4. Maidment R, Livingston G, Katona C. Just keeping taking the tablets: adherence to antidepressant treatment in older people in primary care *International Journal of Geriatric Psychiatry* 2002; **17**: 752–7.

5. Department of Health. *The NHS Plan* London: HMSO, 2000.

6. Freuhwald S, Loeffler-Stastka H, Eher R, *et al*. Depression and quality of life in multiple sclerosis *Acta Neurologica Scandinavica* 2001; **104**: 257–61.

7. Kupfer DJ, Frank E. Comorbidity in depression *Acta Psychiatrica Scandinavica* 2003; **108(418)**: 57.

8. Harper-Jacques S. Diabetes and depression: addressing the depression can improve glycemic control *American Journal of Nursing* 2004; **104(9)**: 56–9.

9. Sanderson J. *Knowsley Book Prescription Scheme* Knowsley: Knowsley Primary Care Trust, 2006.

10 Williams C. Choosing and using self-help materials *Behavioural and Cognitive Psychotherapy* 2002; **30**: 243–8.

11. Lovell K. *SHADE: a self-help manual for anxiety and depression* Manchester: University of Manchester, 2000.

12. Centre for Clinical and Academic Workforce Innovation (CCAWI). *Primary Care Mental Health: clinical skills for primary care mental health practice* Mansfield: University of Lincoln.

13. Powell T. *The Mental Health Handbook* Bicester: Speechmark, 2003.

14. Mental health link to diet change *BBC News*, http://news.bbc.co.uk/1/hi/health/4610070.stm [accessed November 2007].

15. Mayhew L. The eating cure *Society Guardian*, 4 May 2004.

16. Cornah D. *Feeding Minds: the impact of food on mental health* London: The Mental Health Foundation, 2005.

17. Van der Weyer C. *Changing Diets, Changing Minds: how food affects mental well being and behaviour* London: Sustain in conjunction with the Mental Health Foundation, 2006.

18. Babyak M, Blumenthal JA, Herman S. Exercise treatment for major depression: maintenance of therapeutic benefit at 10 months *Psychosomatic Medicine* 2000; **62**: 633–8.

19. Callaghan P. Exercise: a neglected intervention in mental health care? *Journal of Psychiatric and Mental Health Nursing* 2001; **11**: 476–83.

20. Department of Health. *Exercise Referral Systems: a national quality assurance framework*, 2001, www.dh.gov.uk/en/PublicationsandStatistics/Publications/PublicationsPolicyAndGuidance/DH_4009671 [accessed November 2007].

21. Department of Health. *At Least Five a Week: evidence on the impact of physical activity and its relationship to health* London: HMSO, 2004.

22. Halliwell E. *Up and Running: exercise therapy and the treatment of mild or moderate depression in primary care* London: The Mental Health Foundation, 2005.

14 | Mental health law

Alan Cohen

What this chapter contributes:

how the Mental Health Act (1983) works

the practical application of the act in general practice

sections 2, 3 and 4

how the Mental Health Act (1983) has been used

how the Mental Capacity Act (2005) works

the practical application of the act in general practice.

Background and history

It is possible to trace legislation[1] relating to what were once called imbeciles, mental illness, madhouses and lunacy back as far as 1377, when there are records of the Bethlem Madhouse. However, the more recent history of mental health legislation starts in 1890 with the Lunacy Act, which was replaced in 1959 by the Mental Health Act. This in turn was updated by the 1983 Mental Health Act, which in its turn was due to be replaced by a 2006 act. The proposals were set out in a Mental Health Bill, published in 2004. However, the plans proposed were so completely criticised by a confederation of professional representative groups, the voluntary sector, user groups and civil rights pressure groups that, following a Joint Scrutiny Report, the bill was shelved, and some changes were made to the amended 1983 act. The amended act was promulgated in 2007, and will be known as the Mental Health Act 2007. All of these acts relate to the involuntary confinement of people with a mental health disorder. However, a separate issue that is relevant to primary care is the capacity to make decisions, and the legislation relating to this difficult area was reviewed and a new law promulgated in 2005 – the Mental Capacity Act.

The Mental Health Act (1983)

This, the most current Mental Health Act,[2] was amended in 2007, with an implementation date of October 2008. The aim of the act is to describe the circumstances in which an individual can be detained involuntarily because of a mental health problem; in the terms of the act itself its aim is 'the reception, care and treatment of mentally disordered patients, the management of their property and other related matters'. The act therefore describes what is meant by a 'mental health problem' in legal terms, the circumstances in which an individual can be detained against his or her will, and the review process to ensure that continuing detention is appropriate and in the best interests of the individual and society.

Mental disability

The current definition[3] of mental disability (within the meaning of the 1983 act) is 'mental illness, arrested or incomplete development of mind, psychopathic disorder and any other disorder or disability of mind', which is then split into four subtypes: severe mental impairment, mental impairment, psychopathic disorder, and mental illness.

Severe mental impairment

This is a state of arrested or incomplete development of mind. This includes severe impairment of intelligence and social functioning, and is associated with abnormally aggressive or seriously irresponsible conduct on the part of the person concerned.

Mental impairment

This is a state of arrested or incomplete development of mind (not amounting to severe mental impairment). This includes significant impairment of intelligence and social functioning, and is associated with abnormally aggressive or seriously irresponsible conduct on the part of the person concerned.

Psychopathic disorder

This means a persistent disorder or disability of mind (whether or not including significant impairment of intelligence), which results in abnormally aggressive or seriously irresponsible conduct on the part of the person concerned.

Mental illness

This is *not* defined. This missing definition is especially odd, in that this is the most common form of mental disorder for which people are dealt with under the act.

There are certain exceptions that the act makes clear do not represent a mental disorder, e.g. 'by reason only of promiscuity or other immoral conduct, sexual deviancy or dependence on alcohol or drugs'. These types of exception are clearly important and appropriate; it should be borne in mind that, in previous years, people had been incarcerated for their sexual orientation, or for bearing a child out of wedlock. In today's society neither would be considered as evidence of a mental disorder.

In the 2005 Mental Health Bill, which was eventually shelved, there were a number of areas of contention, in particular the inclusion of People with a Severe and dangerous Personality Disorder (PSPD). It was proposed in the 2005 bill that such a group of people (if they could ever be identified) might be compulsorily admitted to hospital even if they had not committed an offence, if they did not have a specific mental illness, and irrespective of whether or not there was an appropriate treatment in place. Such a recommendation followed a number of high-profile murders by individuals for whom such a diagnosis was eventually made. That the bill was dropped is in part recognition of the wholesale opposition, especially to this section, of the legislation.

Admission to hospital

There are four sections of the Mental Health Act (1983) of which the GP and primary care clinician need to be aware in order to arrange appropriate admission to hospital. There are other sections of the act relating to transfer to hospital from the criminal justice system, but for most GPs specific knowledge of this part of the act is not necessary. For those GPs who work in the prison healthcare system, or who are interested in further reading, contact with the RCGP's special interest group is recommended.

The four sections that relate to admission are:

- section 2: admission for assessment for up to 28 days
- section 3: admission for treatment for up to six months in the first instance
- section 4: admission as an emergency for up to 72 hours in the first instance.

The other section that a GP may encounter is section 136 – the section that police officers can enact to detain a person who they suspect may have a mental health disorder, and who in their opinion is a danger to themselves or others. The section also allows the transfer of that individual to a 'place of safety' for assessment.

One of the criticisms of the 1983 act was that this section 136 seemed to be used far more extensively on people from a black or minority ethnic group than would be expected considering the proportion of this group within the whole population.

Section 2

Section 2 is intended for the admission of a patient with a mental disorder for whom the diagnosis is not known, or for whom a period of assessment is necessary. The period of detention can be up to 28 days.

The criteria for admission are that the patient represents a danger to him or herself (either through self-injury or through self-negligence) or to others.

The process for admission is that an application is made either by an approved social worker (ASW) or by the 'nearest relative'. The application is supported by two medical recommendations. The medical recommendation for admission should precede or be contemporaneous with the application from the ASW to the managers of the Mental Health Trust.

Medical recommendation

Section 2 requires that two doctors sign the medical assessment. At least one doctor should be approved as having special experience of managing mental illness and of the Mental Health Act. The need for such a doctor is described in section 12(2) of the act, and the experience needed for the role is set out in guidance. GPs can be section 12(2) approved if they have at least three years of experience as a principal, and have had experience of managing compulsory admissions, with suitable references from at least one psychiatrist. The CV and references are reviewed by the regional Mental Health Act committee.

The other doctor who signs the medical assessment should have previous knowledge of the patient, and it is usually this role that the GP fulfils. All psychiatric consultants are section 12(2) approved as are most senior registrars.

For most GPs, a compulsory admission is an infrequent occurrence. Indeed it is one of the significant events that can be monitored as part of the Quality and Outcomes Framework.

The process and steps that need to occur to arrange an assessment are usually time consuming and can frequently be confusing. The ideal process is shown in Figure 14.1.

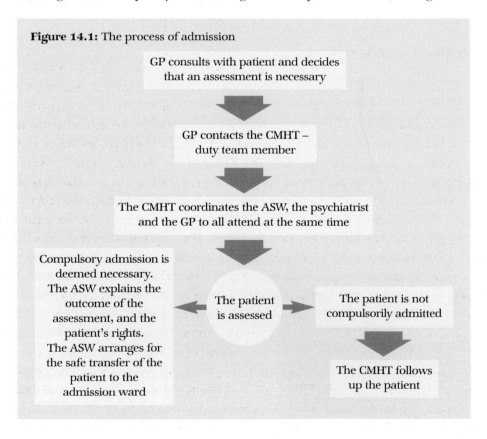

Figure 14.1: The process of admission

GP consults with patient and decides that an assessment is necessary

GP contacts the CMHT – duty team member

The CMHT coordinates the ASW, the psychiatrist and the GP to all attend at the same time

The patient is assessed

Compulsory admission is deemed necessary. The ASW explains the outcome of the assessment, and the patient's rights. The ASW arranges for the safe transfer of the patient to the admission ward

The patient is not compulsorily admitted

The CMHT follows up the patient

Whilst the above diagram is the theoretical process, there are a number of places where there are opportunities for confusion and delay.

Contacting the Community Mental Health Team

If the patient is known to the Community Mental Health Team (CMHT), then this is the most appropriate first port of call. Many trusts in England have crisis intervention teams, which are an alternative place to go following the identification of the need for an assessment. Good practice dictates that whether or not the GP rings the crisis intervention team or the CMHT, only one phone call should be necessary to start the process of arranging an emergency assessment. It is the responsibility of the Mental Health Trust to coordinate the arrangements for a Mental Health Act assessment. It should not be necessary for several phone calls to be made to locate an ASW. In office hours, the CMHT phone number should be answered, as should the number of the crisis intervention team. If these teams are unavailable, and routinely unavailable (there will always be the occasional unforeseen staffing problem – as there is in most practices), then it is helpful to contact the mental health commissioner at the Health Board or Primary Care Trust (PCT) who commissions the service. They will be in a position to ensure that changes are put in place. Out of hours, each Mental Health Trust is required to provide an emergency number that will deal with assessing urgent cases. Again it is their responsibility to ensure that the number is answered, and that they coordinate the ASW, psychiatrist/section 12(2) doctor, and the GP.

Coordinating the assessment

When the GP makes the request for an assessment, the team member will ask for details about the patient, previous history, address, etc. The team will set about trying to coordinate the diary of several busy clinicians and social workers at short notice. The GP should view the assessment visit in the same way that an emergency home visit for a terminally ill patient or a patient having central chest pain is viewed – serious enough to leave patients sitting in the waiting room. Certainly the mental health professionals should also view the visit in the same way. However, if the initial information passed to the team indicates that the risk of harm to others in particular is high, the decision by the ASW may be to ask the police to be present. The police have a sophisticated risk assessment process with varying degrees of response, dependent on the level of perceived risk. Adding in the need to coordinate the attendance of a number of police staff can delay the timing of the assessment. The ASW should have already ensured that a bed is available, and that there is an ambulance on site to transport the patient to the ward should it be necessary. Coordination is therefore quite a complex process, and should be left to the ASW. The assessment visit personnel therefore consists of, at a minimum, an ASW, a psychiatrist or section 12(2)-approved doctor, and the GP. However, the social worker may bring a training ASW, as may the GP or the psychiatrist, and there may be from four to six trained police equipped with stab-proof vests and shields, as well as the ambulance crew. It is not surprising that some assessments can be both difficult to coordinate and stressful for all those who attend – not least a potentially paranoid patient.

Entering the premises

It is the responsibility of the ASW to ensure that, if the premises need to be entered because the patient refuses admission, the correct procedure is followed.

Attending the assessment

The GP has a duty to attend an assessment, in the same way that he or she has a duty to attend any other home visit that has been requested, and is perceived to be appropriate. So if the patient has moved home to an address outside the practice area, refusing an assessment visit may be appropriate. Refusing a request to attend an assessment for a patient who is known to the GP, at a time that is in surgery hours, could be considered inappropriate.

During the assessment

The assessment requires that both doctors agree that compulsory admission is necessary. That is, the patient is a significant risk to him or herself or others. Potentially the two doctors may have a difference of opinion, or they may have a difference of opinion with the ASW who has requested the assessment. Although theoretically possible, in practice this is an unusual occurrence. If it does happen, a pragmatic solution is to repeat the assessment with different staff within 24–48 hours.

After the assessment

If the outcome of the assessment is that compulsory admission is necessary, it is the responsibility of the ASW to arrange transport of the patient to a place of safety – usually the mental health acute admissions ward. It is for that reason that the ASW will have the ambulance crew standing by, rather than waiting for the ambulance to arrive once the decision has been made to compulsorily admit somebody. If the local Mental Health Trust is unable to provide a bed for an assessed patient, it remains the responsibility of the ASW to find a bed elsewhere – in some cases this might be in a private institution. It is not the responsibility of the GP to find the bed. If a person refuses to be admitted despite the assessment and completion of the appropriate forms, the police are empowered to use force to ensure that the patient is transported safely to an appropriate admission ward. In some cases the patient will have pets that need caring for while the owner is compulsorily admitted. Once again this is the responsibility of the ASW, and not the GP, to arrange care for the pets. If the outcome of the assessment is that compulsory admission is not appropriate, it may well be that the CMHT should continue to follow up and support the patient, as there may well be a continuing mental health need that should be addressed.

Claiming a fee for attending an assessment

The attending GP can claim a fee from the PCT or Health Board. This is currently £173.37 (2005 data).

The approved social worker

The ASW is a social worker who has received special training in the assessment of mental health problems and in the administration of the Mental Health Act. They are employed and supported by the Local Authority, and can only work with clients/patients that reside in the jurisdiction of the Local Authority who employs them. The ASW has specific roles within the act, such as being the applicant for admission. It is clear from the previous section that the role of the ASW includes the effective coordination of the assessment process. This coordination role is not the responsibility of the GP, and the only input the GP should have is in requesting the assessment, and then agreeing a mutually convenient time.

The 2005 Mental Health Bill proposed that the role of the ASW be replaced by the approved mental health professional (AMHP). This proposal has been included in the 2007 act. The intention is that the role of the ASW is expanded to allow professionals other than social workers to undertake the role. Whilst there are clearly some technical details to be resolved, to ensure competency etc., the outcome so far as the GP is concerned will be to make access to suitably qualified professionals much easier.

The nearest relative

The nearest relative is a specific term that describes a hierarchical list of relatives who can apply for admission to hospital on behalf of the patient. The list is:

1. husband or wife

2. son or daughter

3. father or mother

4. brother or sister

5. grandparent

6. grandchild

7. uncle or aunt

8. nephew or niece

9. someone, not being a relative, with whom the person concerned normally resides, and has done so for at least five years.

It is an anomaly of the current act that an ASW can apply to the County Court to displace the nearest relative, and that the County Court can appoint an 'acting nearest relative'. Any other relative, or someone with whom the person was living, can also apply to displace the nearest relative. However, patients themselves cannot apply to displace the nearest relative, and it is this part of the act that is in contravention of the European Convention on Human Rights. Changes will be introduced to the amended Mental Health Act on 4 November 2008 to correct this anomaly, so that patients themselves can apply to the County Court for displacement of the nearest relative.

Current good practice encourages every application for admission to be made by the ASW, as this separates the relative from the very difficult decision to be made about whether or not the patient should be admitted against his or her will. It may well be that the relationship between the nearest relative and the patient is strained, especially at the time when the patient may be experiencing a deterioration in his or her mental health symptoms, sufficient to warrant compulsory admission to hospital. To further compound that difficult relationship by putting the onus (legally and) morally on nearest relatives to compulsorily admit their relative is unreasonable. For that reason, it is usually the ASW who makes the formal application for an individual to be admitted.

Section 3

Section 3 is used to admit patients for compulsory treatment. It is used for patients in whom the diagnosis is already known. The section lasts in the first instance for six months, but thereafter can be renewed whilst the patient is still an inpatient for a further 12 months.

The criteria for admission are the same as for section 2 – that the patient is a danger to him or herself or to others.

The application for admission is made by an ASW (to become AMHP), or the nearest relative. Two medical recommendations are necessary, as with section 2.

Supervised Community Treatment

A significant development that was proposed in the amended 1983 act will be the introduction of Supervised Community Treatment (SCT). This replaces the Mental Health Bill proposal of a community treatment order. In summary it applies to patients who have been detained on section 3 of the act (not section 2) or those who have been transferred from the criminal justice system, e.g. sections 37, 48 and 51. There are specific criteria that must be applied for an individual to warrant SCT. The criteria broadly are that the individual must have a mental disorder and that there is appropriate treatment available. The Clinical Supervisor (previously the Responsible Medical Officer [RMO]) must determine if the patient meets the criteria, and then seek agreement from the AMHP. The Mental Health Trust Managers must liaise with the PCT and the Local Authority to ensure that the services required are available prior to the patient leaving hospital. SCT cannot be implemented directly from the community – there must be an admission immediately prior to the community treatment being implemented. The SCT may require that the patients reside at a specific address, or make themselves available for treatment, or desist from specific actions/activities. The SCT provides a power to the clinical supervisor to recall patients to hospital if they become a danger to themselves or others, but there is no power if patients fail to adhere to the other conditions. A patient who has been recalled, if detained for longer than 72 hours, must be referred to the Mental Health Tribunal for review. At the time of writing, the Code of Practice as it relates to the role that primary care and general practice plays in caring for people on supervised community treatment has not been finalised. There are clearly a number of concerns about communication both with the registered GP and the Out-of-Hours service that have not yet been resolved.

Section 4

Section 4 is the emergency admission process, and can only be used when there is no possibility of obtaining a second medical recommendation. A single doctor can make a recommendation to an ASW (to become an AMHP) for compulsory admission for 72 hours. The application has to demonstrate, as it does for section 2 or section 3, that the patient is a risk to him or herself or to others. It also has to demonstrate that the urgency of the admission precludes compliance with the safeguard of obtaining a second medical opinion.

A section 4 can be converted to a section 2 or 3 once the patient is on the ward. Section 4s are relatively unusual, as each Mental Health Trust should be providing an on-call specialist to deal with such eventualities.

Other sections

Although GPs may not need to be involved with other sections of the Mental Health Act, they should be aware of the following.

Sections 5(2) and 5(4)

These allow a current voluntary inpatient to remain on the ward as a compulsory patient. Section 5(2) relates to the doctor on the ward, enforcing admission and assessment for up to 72 hours, and section 5(4) relates to a nurse enforcing admission and assessment for up to six hours.

Section 136

This is the power that police officers have to take an individual, whom they believe to be a danger to him or herself or others as a result of a mental health disorder, from a public place to a place of safety for an assessment. Section 136 cannot be used to admit a patient from his or her own home; they must be in a public place. Section 135 is a warrant issued to an ASW to force admission to a private residence to undertake a Mental Health Act assessment. They are issued by magistrates at the application of the ASW.

Use of the Mental Health Act

The latest report of the Mental Health Act Commission, the *11th Biennial Report, 2003–2005*,[4] provides some interesting statistics on the use of the act. Broadly, during the last six years the number of people admitted under section 2 and section 3 have remained fairly constant at around 25,000 people per year. However, since the act was promulgated, the number of annual admissions have almost doubled. On 31 March 2004, there were 9243 men and 4757 women detained. This is an increase of about 4 per cent on the same date in 2002, and is marginally the highest figure recorded to date – which is significant considering the reducing number of hospital beds.

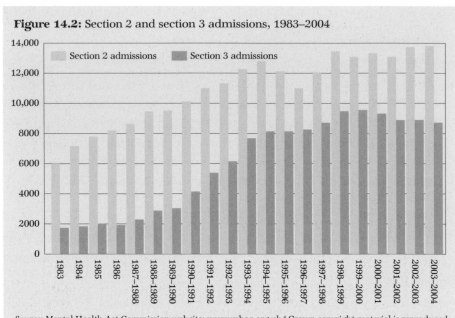

Figure 14.2: Section 2 and section 3 admissions, 1983–2004

Source: Mental Health Act Commission website: www.mhac.org.uk.[4] Crown copyright material is reproduced with the permission of the Controller of OPSI.

Five per cent of those patients sectioned were deemed to be at risk to themselves and to others; of the remaining 95 per cent, 43 per cent were considered a risk to themselves, and 52 per cent were considered a risk to others (see Figure 14.3).

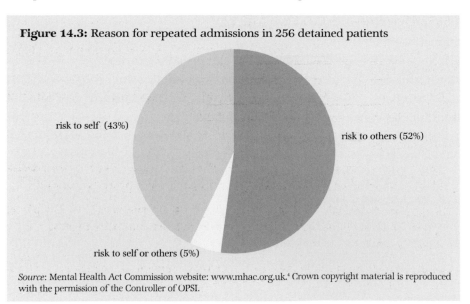

Figure 14.3: Reason for repeated admissions in 256 detained patients

risk to self (43%)

risk to others (52%)

risk to self or others (5%)

Source: Mental Health Act Commission website: www.mhac.org.uk.[4] Crown copyright material is reproduced with the permission of the Controller of OPSI.

The report confirms findings elsewhere that black patients are more likely to suffer a higher than average likelihood of detention under the act (see Table 14.1). Black groups seem to be three to five times more likely to be detained under the act than other groups.

Table 14.1: Ethnic category of patients detained under the Mental Health Act as at 31 March 2005

Ethnic category	Detained patients as of 31 March 2005	
	Number	%
British (white)	9090	69.01
Irish (white)	251	1.91
Any other white background (white)	413	3.14
White and black Caribbean (mixed)	169	1.28
White and black African (mixed)	40	0.30
White and Asian (mixed)	60	0.46
Any other mixed background (mixed)	109	0.83
Indian (Asian or Asian British)	206	1.56
Pakistani (Asian or Asian British)	191	1.45
Bangladeshi (Asian or Asian British)	93	0.71
Other Asian background (Asian or Asian British)	130	0.99
Caribbean (black or black British)	895	6.79
African (black or black British)	425	3.23
Any other black background	405	3.07
Chinese (other ethnic groups)	45	0.34
Any other ethnic group	196	1.49
Not stated/not counted in this table	454	3.45
Total	**13,172**	**100**

Source: Mental Health Act Commission website: www.mhac.org.uk.[4] Crown copyright material is reproduced with the permission of the Controller of OPSI.

Mental Capacity Act 2005

This act is designed to clarify the law relating to those people who are not able to make decisions for themselves.

The Department of Health[5] website and the Mind[6] association both provide a clear summary of the areas that the new legislation covers.

The act is underpinned by five principles:

- a presumption of capacity – every adult has the right to make his or her own decisions and must be assumed to have capacity to do so unless it is proved otherwise

- the right for individuals to be supported to make their own decisions – people must be given all appropriate help before anyone concludes that they cannot make their own decisions

- that individuals must retain the right to make what might be seen as eccentric or unwise decisions

- best interests – anything done for or on behalf of people without capacity must be in their best interests

- least restrictive intervention – anything done for or on behalf of people without capacity should be the least restrictive of their basic rights and freedoms.

The act will set out a[7]

> single clear test for assessing whether a person lacks capacity to take a particular decision at a particular time. It is a 'decision-specific' test. No one can be labelled 'incapable' as a result of a particular medical condition or diagnosis. Section 2 of the Act makes it clear that a lack of capacity cannot be established merely by reference to a person's age, appearance, or any condition or aspect of a person's behaviour which might lead others to make unjustified assumptions about capacity.

Everything done for the person who lacks the capacity to make his or her own decisions should be done with the person's best interest. The act provides a check list for decision makers to consider when assessing what may be in the person's best interest.

Following a European ruling about a man in Bournewood Hospital, it became clear that there is a problem with the current legislation. The European Court of Human Rights found that the UK had acted unlawfully in detaining a man who lacked mental capacity in hospital for psychiatric treatment without the safeguards available to people who are sectioned under the Mental Health Act. This is termed the 'Bournewood Gap'.

Both the Mental Health Act 1983 and the Mental Capacity Act 2005 are in the process of being amended to bring them into line with the ruling from the European Court.

So far as most primary care clinicians are concerned, where a question of an individual's capacity is concerned, specialist advice should be sought from senior psychiatric colleagues.

References

1. Roberts A. *Mental Health History Timeline*, Middlesex University, www.mdx.ac.uk/www/study/mhhtim.htm [accessed November 2007].

2. Her Majesty's Stationery Office. *Mental Health Act 1983* London: HMSO, 1983.

3. www.hyperguide.co.uk/mha/s1.htm [accessed November 2007].

4. Mental Health Act Commission. *In Place of Fear? 11th biennial report 2003–2005* London: The Stationery Office, 2005, www.mhac.org.uk/files/MHAC%2011%20TEXT%20FA.pdf [accessed November 2007].

5. www.dh.gov.uk/en/Policyandguidance/SocialCare/Deliveringadultsocialcare/MentalCapacity/MentalCapacityAct2005/index.htm [accessed November 2007].

6. www.mind.org.uk/News+policy+and+campaigns/Policy/Draft+Mental+Health+Bill+2004.html [accessed November 2007].

7. www.dca.gov.uk/menincap/bill-summary.htm [accessed November 2007].

15 | Risk

John Hague

What this chapter contributes:

the epidemiology of suicide

risk factors

special risk groups

antidepressants and suicide

assessment scales

training

advice on assessing suicide risk

what to do after an episode of self-harm

a discussion on homicide.

On average a GP in the UK can expect one of his or her patients to commit suicide every five years. If a GP spends 30 years in post they will have cared for around six people who have ended their own lives. In contrast to almost every other sphere of medicine the GP will, in many cases, continue to look after the family of the person concerned. Every subsequent consultation with a family member will be a reminder of the event to both parties. This is a considerable burden to bear, even if in every case no errors have been made.

Suicide thus has an enduring effect on those left behind, be they professionals or friends and family of the victim. It is vital that in as many cases as possible everyone feels that every step that could have been taken was taken. Some of the higher-risk groups may present in a 'counter-intuitive' way (for example young drug users), and some high-risk groups may also be counter-intuitive (for example most postnatal suicides occur in comparatively well-off, older, white professional women).

The challenge for primary care is to understand the epidemiology and main drivers for suicide, and then try to minimise the frequency of completed suicide, while at the same time acknowledging the reality that assessing suicidality in the context of a brief primary care consultation is an inexact science.

Box 15.1: Statistics for suicide

- Every GP can expect to have a suicide on his or her list every five years.[1]
- 40 per cent of suicides saw their GP in the month before death.[2]
- Only 25 per cent of these will have been in contact with specialist mental health services in the last year.[1]

Homicide by those suffering with mental illness is comparatively a rarer event,[1] yet remains a devastating event for those involved, with the exacerbating factor that the perpetrator is often a survivor, although a proportion also commits suicide at the time of the homicide.

The epidemiology of suicide

Definition

The convention is to include in mortality statistics every suicide verdict by coroners, and as well every open verdict, unless it is clear that suicide was not considered at the inquest (for example deaths where no clear cause can be found but where death was not self-inflicted).

Statistics

In England the suicide rate has fallen every year since 1998, until 2004, when there was a slight rise in the European Age Standardised Rate from the low of 8.5 per 100,000 in 2003 to 8.6 per 100,000.[3]

Figure 15.1, from the 2005 report on progress in the national suicide strategy, shows how the rates have changed over the years, since 1995.

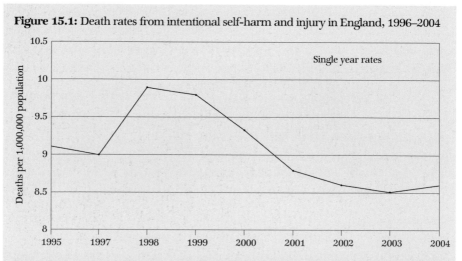

Figure 15.1: Death rates from intentional self-harm and injury in England, 1996–2004

Source: National Suicide Prevention Strategy for England (2006).[3] Reproduced by permission of the National Institute for Mental Health in England.

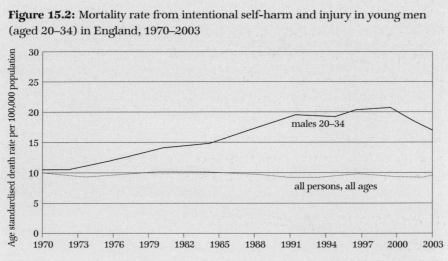

Figure 15.2: Mortality rate from intentional self-harm and injury in young men (aged 20–34) in England, 1970–2003

Source: *National Suicide Prevention Strategy for England* (2006).[3] Reproduced by permission of the National Institute for Mental Health in England.

Over the years since 1970 there has, on average, been a fall in the general rate, along with a fall in the rate for older men and women, but a rise in young men.

There is a significant correlation with the sex of the victim, with most suicides occurring in young males, with on average one woman committing suicide to almost every three men (see Figure 15.3).

The greater number of suicides occurs in those aged under 40.

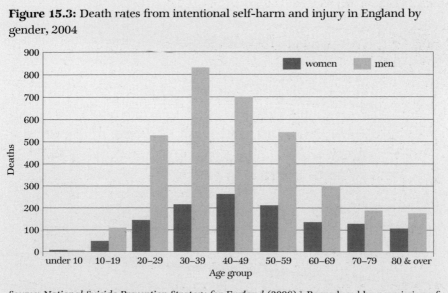

Figure 15.3: Death rates from intentional self-harm and injury in England by gender, 2004

Source: *National Suicide Prevention Strategy for England* (2006).[3] Reproduced by permission of the National Institute for Mental Health in England.

There is a considerable variation geographically (see Figure 15.4).

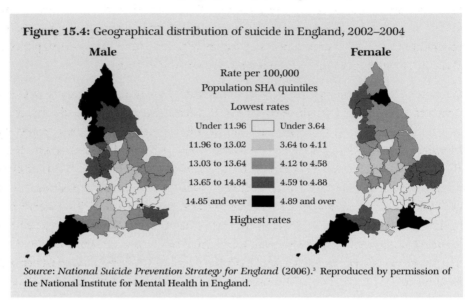

Figure 15.4: Geographical distribution of suicide in England, 2002–2004

Source: *National Suicide Prevention Strategy for England* (2006).[3] Reproduced by permission of the National Institute for Mental Health in England.

There is also variation by day of the week, with most suicides occurring on Mondays; they are also more common after public holidays, and lower before them.[4]

The method of suicide varies by sex, with just under half of men choosing hanging, strangulation or suffocation, compared with 32 per cent of women. In women drug-related poisoning accounts for 42 per cent of deaths (see Figure 15.5). 'Other' methods are discussed in more detail in the 2001 national confidential inquiry into suicide. The main point here is the rarity of use of firearms in suicide in the UK, accounting for only 2.9 per cent of male suicides, and 0.45 per cent of female suicides.[3] This is in stark contrast to the USA, where 60 per cent of suicides involved a firearm.[5]

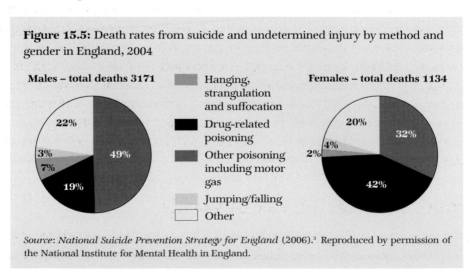

Figure 15.5: Death rates from suicide and undetermined injury by method and gender in England, 2004

Source: *National Suicide Prevention Strategy for England* (2006).[3] Reproduced by permission of the National Institute for Mental Health in England.

Those who commit suicide are often suffering social adversity. Seventy-one per cent were not married, and 41 per cent of those over 65 were widowed. Most were unemployed or on long-term incapacity benefit, and this was most high in the under 25s (64 per cent unemployed; 11 per cent on incapacity benefit long term). Forty-three per cent lived alone. Nineteen per cent were misusing alcohol and/or drugs.[1]

In the inquiry cases (where an inquiry was conducted by the health services, as well as a coroner's court), events in the three months before death were noted. Suicide was commonly preceded by adverse life events with half having suffered adverse events – especially relationship problems. Five per cent of the suicides were preceded by bereavement. Non-fatal self-harm occurred in 25 per cent of the suicides, and suicidal ideas occurred in 29 per cent. Non-compliance with drug treatment, non-attendance, increased alcohol or drug misuse each occurred in about a quarter of cases. Most of the suicides (58 per cent) suffered from affective disorder, 20 per cent from schizophrenia or related disorders, 11 per cent from personality disorders, and 9 per cent from alcohol dependence. Of those who had been in contact with mental health services in the year before they died 64 per cent had a history of ever having harmed themselves, and 19 per cent had a history of violence.[1]

Suicides appear to cluster in the first year after onset of an illness (21 per cent), but this is more common in the over 65s and under 25s. In all only 25 per cent had never had an admission to a psychiatric unit, with this falling to 7 per cent in those with a history of mental illness greater than five years.[1]

Only 24 per cent of patients had been in contact with mental health services in the year before their death.[1] In 1994 'Bandolier' said that 40 per cent of suicides had seen their GP in the month before death.[2] Surprisingly the national confidential inquiry and suicide strategy concentrate mainly on the group in contact with mental health services, despite the fact that this excludes 76 per cent of the suicides.

Of those in contact with mental health services, 19 per cent of suicides were in contact with services in the 24 hours before death, and 48 per cent in the week before death. Seventy per cent of these contacts were routine. In people who committed suicide in the community (84 per cent of the total) 71 per cent had been admitted at some time. Eighty-eight per cent were regarded as being at least moderately recovered at the time of discharge. Eighty-six per cent were regarded as being at low or no immediate risk, with 60 per cent being estimated to be at low or no long-term risk. Twenty-nine per cent were out of contact with services at the time of death. In only 19 per cent of cases was the suicide thought to be preventable.[1]

Groups at increased risk of suicide

In 1994 Gunnell and Frankel showed that various groups had an increased risk of self-harm.[6] These figures have been added to and modified over the years by various authors. The biggest risk is in the four weeks after discharge from a psychiatric hospital, when suicide is between 100 and 200 times more likely. Those with a history of self-harm have an increased risk of between 10 and 30 times. Those who misuse drugs or alcohol have a risk of about 20 times.

In England and Wales suicide rates are six times higher in the prison population than in the general population. In the first month after release ex-prisoners are 35 times more likely to commit suicide; in the first year they are six times more likely to commit suicide.[7]

Various occupational groups are at an increased risk, perhaps because of ease of access to effective means – doctors and farmers share a doubling of suicide risk with the unemployed.[6]

Counter-intuitive risk factors

Two groups are worthy of special mention, those under 25, and mothers in the first year after they have had a baby.

The young often display signs that can worsen their chances of being helped, because their actions can be misinterpreted and cause them to be denied services – a quarter showed clear signs of relapse of their mental illness, with half showing increased use of alcohol or drugs, or increased self-harming behaviour. These 'proxy indicators' can lead to those unfamiliar with these facts failing to help those who appear to be 'disruptive' – when in fact they are in grave danger.[1]

As the confidential inquiry into maternal deaths has shown,[8] suicide is the leading cause of death bar none in mothers in the year after they have given birth. In this group of mothers 87 per cent were white, 83 per cent were aged over 25, and 46 per cent were aged over 30. Fifty-five per cent had previous children, and 54 per cent were seriously mentally ill, with 50 per cent having a previous history of very severe depression or post-partum psychosis. Half of these had been admitted in the past. Fifty per cent were in contact with psychiatric services. Sixty-five per cent died in a violent suicide – double the usual percentage in women, with only 35 per cent dying from overdose.

The inquiry emphasises that pregnancy results in a 50 per cent risk of relapse of a severe and enduring mental illness, and suggests the following 'risk profile':

- white
- older mother
- second or subsequent pregnancy
- 'comfortable life'
- previous mental illness and psychiatric contact
- baby under three months.

Do antidepressants make suicide more likely?

The literature on this subject continues to grow. Despite this growth, uncertainty is the major result in adults, with some studies reporting a link but others failing to find a link. It is hypothesised that the initial agitation or increase in anxiety, seen in a sub-group of people starting taking antidepressants, is responsible for the possible link.

Simon *et al.* looked at records of a group health cooperative covering health care for half a million people in the US states of Idaho and Washington between January 1992 and June 2003.[9] They intended to look at three questions:

1. What is the risk of death or serious suicide attempt during acute-phase antidepressant treatment?

2. Is there an increased risk of death by suicide during the month after starting antidepressant treatment?

3. Are the drugs included in the FDA warning on newer antidepressants of March 2004[10] ('newer antidepressants' – bupropion, citalopram, fluoxetine, fluvoxamine, mirtazapine, nefazodone, paroxetine, sertraline, escitalopram and venlafaxine) associated with a higher risk of death by suicide, or serious suicide attempt, than are older antidepressants?

The findings present a good picture of the epidemiology of suicide. Male and female rates of suicide death were similar, and the rate did not vary significantly in the six months after starting treatment.

The authors then looked month by month at the serious suicide attempts. This showed that the risk was highest in the first month of treatment, and dropped month by month. The surprising finding was that the risk was highest of all in the month before starting medication. Looking more closely at the month before and after starting treatment revealed that the higher rate of suicide attempts during the month before starting treatment was primarily attributable to increased risk in the seven days before the first prescription (65 attempts per 100,000, compared with 10 per 100,000).

Finally the authors looked at the risk of 'newer' antidepressants compared with 'older' antidepressants. The risk of suicide death over the first six months of treatment was 34 per 100,000 for the drugs included in the warning, compared with 51 per 100,000 for 'older' drugs. The risk of suicide attempts leading to hospitalisation was 76 per 100,000 for newer drugs and 129 per 100,000 for older drugs.

The authors conclude that, in answer to their questions, first, the rate of serious suicide attempt is approximately 90 per 100,000, and suicide death during acute-phase antidepressant treatment approximately 40 per 100,000. Second, available data does not indicate an increased risk of suicide or serious suicide attempt after starting anti-depressant medication. Third, the risk was not higher among those treated with newer antidepressants.[11]

In contrast the manufacturers of paroxetine (an SSRI antidepressant) have recently (2006) announced that they had found an increase in suicidal behaviour in those taking paroxetine, compared with placebo, based on an analysis of patients aged 18–64 in clinical trials.[12]

In children the evidence appears more certain, with the MHRA recommending that SSRIs other than fluoxetine should not be used in those under the age of 18, as the balance of risks and benefits is unfavourable.[13]

Gunnell *et al.* looked at the data submitted to the Medicines and Healthcare products Regulatory Agency by pharmaceutical companies in their safety review of antidepressants. They concluded that increased risks of suicide and self-harm caused by SSRIs cannot be ruled out, but larger trials with longer follow-up are required to assess the balance of risks and benefits fully, offsetting any risks with the benefits of the effectiveness of SSRIs in treating depression.[14]

In the elderly, Juurlink *et al.* reported that SSRIs were associated with a five times increased risk of suicide in the first month of treatment, compared with other antidepressants, yet they also said that the risks of undertreatment with other drugs were likely to be worse than the early risks associated with SSRIs.[15]

To summarise, based on available evidence:

- those in primary care should not initiate prescription of antidepressants in children or adolescents

- the benefits of antidepressants, used for licensed indications (not minor depression as a first-line treatment, but in moderate or severe major depression), outweigh the risks

- those being started on antidepressants should be provided with written information

- in particular they should be warned about the possibility of initiation anxiety, and possible worsening of suicidal thoughts, and given clear 'safety net' instructions on what to do if these problems occur – for example being encouraged to phone their primary care team, or out-of-hours service. They could also be given written details of how to contact organisations such as the Samaritans, or other appropriate local organisations

- patients should be monitored as per recommendations in the NICE depression guideline.[16]

Assessing suicidality with scales

In theory the epidemiology of suicide, above, is quite clear, and should make it straightforward to design a simple tool to reliably assess suicide risk. Experience tells a different story in primary care. If about a third of a GP's workload is mental health related, yet delivered in 10 minute consultations, and they can on average expect a suicide once every five years, then the methods used need to be unobtrusive enough as to be applicable in most consultations, yet sensitive enough to spot the one encounter in 20,000–30,000 consultations that represents the chance of preventing the suicide that 'usual practice' has not prevented.

A very comprehensive review of suicide assessment tools was published recently by Brown.[17] Although it was intended to be mainly for use in 'intervention research', the review is directly applicable to primary care as it includes several brief screening measures, and even discusses subscales of common rating scales such as BDI-II, PRIME-MD (part of which forms the PHQ-9) and Hamilton. The review says, however, that 'the predictive value for most suicide measures has not been established', and 'only a few instruments such as the Beck Hopelessness Scale and the Scale for Suicidal Ideation have been found to be significant risk factors for completed suicide'.

The 'Paykel Suicide Items'[18] are examined, with the review saying that there is some preliminary evidence that they may be very useful as a brief screening tool instrument for suicidal ideation, although further study is needed to investigate their concurrent and predictive value. These items present a hierarchical list of questions, with the risk escalating from 'Have you ever felt that life was not worth living?' as the first question, to 'Have you ever made an attempt to take your life?' as the fifth and final question. They can be altered to assess risk over varying time frames.

The review concludes that further research establishing the psychometric properties of suicide assessment instruments as screening or as outcome measures in primary care settings is needed. Thus it is hard to recommend any one scale.

Is training worthwhile?[19]

Nutting *et al.* looked at 21 different US primary care practices, and assessed the effect of one of two different interventions on their ability to detect suicidal ideation.[20] The two interventions were brief training (four conference calls for doctors and nurses, with nurses having an extra eight hours of training on depression management) or 'guided development of quality improvement teams', which consisted of four and a half hours of training, followed by 16 hours in which the participants developed a quality improvement plan, which they then implemented.

The effect of the interventions was to nearly double the detection of depression with suicidal ideation, from 20.5 per cent in usual care practices, to 40.7 per cent in intervention practices. Interestingly there was no effect on starting an antidepressant, referral or suicidal ideation at six months.

Schulberg *et al.* studied suicidal ideation in patients with 'uncomplicated depressive disorder' in 60 practices, screening first with part of the PHQ-9, then using a symptom checklist and an algorithm to gather more information on the level of risk.[21]

The paper shows that 90 per cent of the patients thought to require treatment for depression were at no or low risk of self-harm, with 10 per cent having an intermediate risk. In the low-risk group only 1.1 per cent at three months and 2.6 per cent at six months had suicidal ideation requiring the physician's immediate attention.

These papers mean that there is merit in training health workers in depression and suicide assessment. Once they have learned to perform assessments, then almost all patients with uncomplicated dysthymia, major depression, or both (which is a large proportion of the primary care workload), who are assessed as being at low or no risk, will still be at low or no risk of suicide six months later. This is a simple point of immense practical value in primary care. Another practical point is that it is worthwhile including training in 'the next steps to take' to ensure that action is taken if people are thought to be at risk.

In the UK Green and Gask have developed the STORM (Skills-based Training on Risk Management) package.[22] This focuses on the key skills needed to assess and manage a person at risk of suicide. Three evaluations have shown that it is effective in improving skills, attitudes to suicide prevention and confidence in dealing with suicide risk.

What seems to be worthwhile asking?

First, it is necessary to dispel the myth that asking about suicidal intent will 'plant the idea in someone's head' – this is not felt to be so. Competently asking questions about a person's feelings and intentions is the only way to find out what they are. This needs to be done sensitively in the context of the clinical interview, so that the clinician has the chance to spot possible untruthful answers. The answers also need to be taken in the context of the clinician's knowledge about the patient and his or her condition. Accurate recording of the process is vital, as are consultation skills of a high standard.

Asking the questions in a hierarchy, along the lines of the Paykel items, allows a reasonably rapid judgement to be formed. Another hierarchical tool (the DDRAT) was developed for use as a facilitation tool for training primary care workers,[23] along with some standardised case studies to be discussed during the training. Asking the questions in a hierarchical fashion matches, to some extent, the early stages of Prochaska and Norcross stages of change model of pre-contemplation, contemplation, preparation, action, maintenance, and termination.[24]

So patients need to be directly asked if they have ever thought of harming themselves, whether they have thought about how they might do it, whether they have ever done anything to put the plans into action, what if anything is stopping them from carrying the plans out, and whether they feel that this will continue to stop them in the future (see Table 15.1). This needs to be taken in the context of their illnesses (physical or mental), childbirth, any recent losses (of employment or near ones/relatives) or social isolation, their sex, age, employment status (the unemployed and those in jobs with access to means being more at risk), whether they are in a relationship, whether they abuse drugs or alcohol, and also whether they present any of the indicators specific to the two special risk groups of recent mothers and those displaying 'proxy indicators of risk'.

Table 15.1: Assessing suicide risk – a summary

Examples of questions to ask	Remember
Have you ever thought of harming yourself?	Chronic physical illness
Have you thought how you might do that?	Mental illness
Have you done anything to put your plans into action?	Severe mental illness
What is stopping you from carrying out the plans?	Childbirth
Do you feel that this will continue to stop you in the future?	Any recent losses (of job or near ones)
	Social isolation
	Male sex
	Age
	Employment status (the unemployed and those in jobs with access to means being more at risk)
	In a relationship?
	Abuse of drugs or alcohol?
	Harming oneself by 'violent means' leaves little chance to change one's mind
	Is someone available to supervise the patient?
Risk factors for suicide after childbirth	**Proxy indicators**
White	Clear relapse of illness
Older mother	Increase in drug misuse
Second or subsequent pregnancy	Increase in alcohol misuse
'Comfortable life'	Increase in self-harm
Previous mental illness and psychiatric contact	Non-compliance
Baby under three months	

'Safety netting' is summarised in Box 15.2.

> **Box 15.2:** Safety netting
>
> - Is someone available to supervise the patient if felt to be at risk?
> - Prescribe limited amounts of medication.
> - Ensure the patient knows how to contact the surgery, the out-of-hours service, and also another service such as the Samaritans.
> - Advise the patient and carers on actions to take if they feel more at risk.
> - Arrange follow-up at short intervals until the danger has passed.
> - Always ask for help or advice from specialist mental health services if you are not sure about the level of risk.

The DDRAT is then reproduced as Table 15.2 as an example of how structured questions can lead logically to a proportionate response, according to the degree of risk.

Table 15.2: Pilot primary care mental health risk assessment tool (DDRAT)

In the last 2 weeks have you?	Score	
Thought about killing yourself?	2	
Thought how you would do that?	4	
Done anything to put those plans into action?	6	Add 1 if past history of deliberate self-harm, 1 if recent stable relationship breakdown, 1 if male
If something is stopping you from putting your plans into action, is it likely that the urge to harm yourself will become so strong that you will take action?	8	Add 1 if past history of deliberate self-harm, 1 if recent stable relationship breakdown, 1 if male

Source: Cohen A, Hague J. The DDRAT (Devon and Dorset Risk Assessment Tool), developed in 2003 for use in training, initially in Devon and Dorset.[23]

The score is the number next to the last question that the patient answers 'yes' to, adding the extra points in the last column if applicable. This tool, which was developed for use in training in conjunction with some clinical vignettes, is included as an example of how a hierarchical series of questions can be translated into clinical action (see Table 15.3). It is likely that practitioners will develop their own personal preferred way of handling suicide risk depending on their experience, the local services, and the particular circumstances of the patient and his or her family or friends. The authors of the tool feel that its best use is as a discussion aid in training workshops, with clinical vignettes developed locally to take account of particular local circumstances.

Table 15.3: Suggested actions (DDRAT)

Score	Primary care action	Interface action	Secondary care action
2	Mild/moderate disorder – treat with talking therapy and/or antidepressants	Referral may not be necessary, routine if you think there are other reasons to refer the patient	
4	Moderate disorder – treat with talking therapy and/or antidepressants, and observation in primary care	Referral may not be necessary, routine if you think there are other reasons to refer the patient	
6–7	Moderate to severe disorder – requires treatment and active follow-up with safety netting	Refer routinely	Guarantee to see and assess within no more than 10 working days
8+	Severe disorder – requires urgent action	Refer urgently. Do not leave unsupervised until assessed by specialist	Guarantee to see within that day, consider if MHA assessment needed

Source: Cohen A, Hague J. The DDRAT (Devon and Dorset Risk Assessment Tool), developed in 2003 for use in training, initially in Devon and Dorset.[23]

How reliable is suicide prediction?

The confidential inquiry in 2000 revealed that only 2 per cent of completed suicides were felt to be at high risk at the time of death.[1]

Kapur *et al.* reported on the predictive value of risk assessment after an episode of deliberate self-harm.[25] They found that emergency department staff were more cautious in their risk assessment than specialist staff. This meant that they identified a greater proportion of people who went on to repeat self-harm, but fewer of those assessed as at high risk actually went on to repeat. They found that restricting interventions to those felt to be at high risk of self-harm would prevent fewer than one fifth of repeat episodes.

What to do after an episode of self-harm

- Address all physical issues.

- Assess the risk, as above; arrange urgent specialist assessment if the risk is felt to be high.

- Record the result of the risk assessment.

- Assess the mental health of the person.

- Begin treatment for any conditions (physical or mental) that require treatment.

- Arrange appropriate follow-up for any condition being treated, including referral to specialist services, and safety netting in primary care.

There is evidence that telephone contact at one month may reduce the number of re-attempts at one year. The number of attempts to contact should not be limited; it may be also more effective to contact earlier than one month after the attempt.[26]

Homicide

In England the frequency of homicide has slightly increased since 1997, with the frequency of homicides by females staying static, and that by males rising, and accounting for the rise overall.[1]

The proportion of homicides in which the perpetrator had a history of abnormal mental state is roughly static, and remains at around one third having a lifetime history of mental disorder. The most common disorders were alcohol dependence, drug dependence and personality disorder. Nine per cent of all perpetrators had a history of personality disorder. Five per cent of all perpetrators had a diagnosis of schizophrenia.[1]

At the time of the offence 15 per cent had symptoms of a mental illness. Mentally ill perpetrators were less likely to kill a stranger than those without mental illness.[1]

Only 9 per cent of all perpetrators had been in contact with mental health services in the year before the offence; at least 18 per cent had been in contact with services at some time. The most common diagnoses were personality disorder and schizophrenia, and almost half with any service contact history had a history of alcohol and drug misuse. At the final service contact the immediate and long-term risk of violence was estimated to be low.[1]

Over a quarter of those perpetrators with schizophrenia had no contact with mental health services prior to the homicide. One half of the perpetrators with schizophrenia were out of contact with services by the time of the offence.[1]

Half of the perpetrators with personality disorder had no history of contact with mental health services.[1]

One of the major recommendations from the national confidential inquiry, of relevance to homicide, is that anti-stigma campaigns should be run to emphasise the low risk to strangers posed by people with mental illness.[1]

Taylor and Gunn said: 'the public and politicians believe, or are being encouraged to believe through the mass media, that unless people with a mental disorder are once more segregated, the streets will not be safe'.[27] They analysed homicide figures for England and Wales between 1957 and 1995, and concluded that there was 'little fluctuation in numbers of people with a mental illness committing criminal homicide over the 38 years studied, and a 3 per cent annual decline in their contribution to the official statistics'.

In 2004 Shaw *et al.* reported on an analysis of stranger homicides from 1967 to 1997.[28] They concluded that stranger homicides had increased, but that the increase is not the result of homicides by mentally ill people, and therefore the 'care in the community' policy. Stranger homicides were more likely to be related to alcohol or drug misuse by young men.

In terms of actions to prevent homicide in primary care little can be recommended except that clinicians should strive to deliver high standards of care to all those who present, including those with alcohol and drug problems, and to ensure that specialist help is sought whenever the clinician feels that it is appropriate.

References

1. *'Safety First': five-year report of the National Confidential Inquiry into Suicide and Homicide by People with Mental Illness* London: DH, 2001.

2. Bandolier. *Preventing Suicide*, www.jr2.ox.ac.uk/bandolier/band7/b7-5.html [accessed November 2007].

3. *National Suicide Prevention Strategy for England: annual report on progress 2005* Leeds: National Institute for Mental Health in England, 2006.

4. Johnson H, Brock A, Griffiths C, *et al.* Mortality from suicide and drug-related poisoning by day of the week in England and Wales, 1993–2002 *Health Statistics Quarterly* 2005; **27**: 13–16.

5. Anderson RN, Smith BL. Deaths: leading causes for 2001 *National Vital Statistics Reports*, vol. 52 no. 9, Hyattsville, Maryland: National Center for Health Statistics, 2003.

6. Gunnell D, Frankel S. Prevention of suicide: aspirations and evidence *British Medical Journal* 1994; **308**: 1227–33.

7. Williamson M. *Improving the Health and Social Outcomes of People Recently Released from Prisons in the UK: a perspective from primary care* Sainsbury Centre for Mental Health, 2006, www.scmh.org.uk/80256FBD004F3555/vWeb/flKHAL6L5DLE/$file/health_prison_primarycare.doc [accessed November 2007].

8. *Why Mothers Die 2000–2002: report on confidential enquiries into maternal deaths in the United Kingdom* London: CEMACH, www.cemach.org.uk/getattachment/3e28b22a-7bfb-4287-95a7-dcf2f033f9dc/Why-Mothers-Die-2000-2002-(1).aspx [accessed November 2007].

9. Simon GE, Savarino J, Operskalski B, *et al.* Suicide risk during antidepressant treatment *American Journal of Psychiatry* 2006; **163(1)**: 41–7.

10. US Food and Drug Administration, Center for Drug Evaluation and Research. *FDA Public Health Advisory: worsening depression and suicidality in patients being treated with antidepressant medications* Rockville, MD: FDA, 2004.

11. Hague J. Conversation with a … GP registrar and my iPOD *Primary Care Mental Health* 2006: **4(1)**: 73–4.

12. Lenzer J. Manufacturer admits increase in suicidal behaviour in patients taking paroxetine *British Medical Journal* 2006; **332(7551)**: 1175.

13. *Selective Serotonin Reuptake Inhibitors (SSRIs): overview of regulatory status and CSM advice relating to major depressive disorder (MDD) in children and adolescents including a summary of available safety and efficacy data* London: MHRA, 2003, www.mhra.gov.uk/home/idcplg?IdcService=SS_GET_PAGE&useSecondary=true&ssDocName=CON019494&ssTargetNodeId=221 [accessed November 2007].

14. Gunnell D, Saperia J, Ashby D. Selective serotonin reuptake inhibitors and suicide in adults: meta-analysis of drug company data from placebo controlled, randomised trials submitted to the MHRA's safety review *British Medical Journal* 2005; **330**: 385–8.

15. Juurlink DM, Mamdani MM, Kopp A, *et al.* The risk of suicide with selective serotonin reuptake inhibitors in the elderly *American Journal of Psychiatry* 2006; **163**: 813–21.

16. National Institute for Health and Clinical Excellence. *Depression: management of depression in primary and secondary care* London: NICE, 2004.

17. Brown GK. *A Review of Suicide Assessment Measures for Intervention Research with Adults and Older Adults* University of Pennsylvania, http://sbisrvntweb.uqac.ca/archivage/15290520.pdf [accessed November 2007].

18. Paykel ES, Myers JK, Lindenthal JJ, *et al.* Suicidal feelings in the general population: a prevalence study *British Journal of Psychiatry* 1974; **30**: 771–8.

19. Hague J. Conversation with a … vocational training scheme organiser *Primary Care Mental Health* 2005: **3(4)**: 295.

20. Nutting PA, Dickinson LM, Rubenstein LV, *et al.* Improving detection of suicidal ideation among depressed patients in primary care *Annals of Family Medicine* 2005; **3**: 529–36.

21. Schulberg HC, Lee PW, Bruce ML, *et al.* Suicidal ideation and risk levels among primary care patients with uncomplicated depression *Annals of Family Medicine* 2005; **3**: 523–8.

22. Green C, Gask L. The development, research and implementation of STORM (Skills-based Training on Risk Management) *Primary Care Mental Health* 2005; **3(3)**: 207–13.

23. Cohen A, Hague J. The DDRAT (Devon and Dorset Risk Assessment Tool), developed in 2003 for use in training, initially in Devon and Dorset.

24. Prochaska JO, Norcross JC. Stages of change *Psychotherapy* 2001; **38(4)**: 443–8.

25. Kapur N, Cooper J, Rodway C, *et al.* Predicting the risk of repetition after self harm: cohort study *British Medical Journal* 2005; **330**; 394–5.

26. Vaiva G, Vaiva G, Ducrocq F, *et al.* Effect of telephone contact on further suicide attempts in patients discharged from an emergency department: randomised controlled study *British Medical Journal* 2006; **332**: 1241–5.

27. Taylor PJ, Gunn J. Homicides by people with mental illness: myth and reality *British Journal of Psychiatry* 1999; **174**: 9–14.

28. Shaw J, Amos T, Hunt IM, *et al.* Mental illness in people who kill strangers: longitudinal study and national clinical survey *British Medical Journal* 2004; **328**: 734–7.

16 | The psychological wellbeing of refugees and asylum seekers

Angela Burnett and Liben Gebremikael

What this chapter contributes:

---

presentation and assessment of the mental health of asylum seekers and refugees

practical ways that primary care clinicians can support the care of this group of vulnerable people.

Introduction

Primary healthcare workers in any community will see psychological problems as a significant part of their work. Some refugees and asylum seekers may have mental health problems that precede their experiences of conflict and exile. Others experience stress-related problems related to violence, detention, torture, bereavement, exile or fear of deportation. Exile represents multiple loss – of home, family, friends, familiar places and food, culture, work, as well as of support structures. Eisenbruch describes exile as a form of 'cultural bereavement'.[1]

People may present with psychological difficulties only after they have been in the UK for some time, after other aspects of life are more settled and secure. Some however experience acute problems and may present earlier.

This chapter includes the experiences of an asylum seeker (whose details have been changed to protect his identity), to illustrate the challenges that many people face. We will then discuss psychological issues in further detail and suggest helpful responses. We will use the term 'asylum seeker' for those awaiting a decision on their claim, while 'refugee' refers to those at all stages of the asylum process, including those with a positive decision.

A personal story

Adane is a young Ethiopian man in his early twenties. He had been in the UK for less than a year and soon after arrival he was dispersed to a northern city. He presented to his GP with insomnia, headaches and depression, and was prescribed medication (sleeping tablets, painkillers and antidepressants). However, despite his regular compliance with medication, Adane did not see any improvement.

He was referred to the Ethiopian Health Support Association (EtHSA) by his GP for support and culturally appropriate intervention. During a mental health assessment, three layers of difficulties emerged:

Adane's first concern was the symptoms themselves. Not only were the continuous headache, lack of sleep, low mood and suicidal ideation affecting his daily routine but he was also concerned why this was happening to him and why the medication was not helping.

Second, he was greatly concerned about his current situation. His asylum application was rejected and the long and complex appeal process rendered him fearful and uncertain. As a result of dispersal, he had very little contact with his community and was isolated. His housing arrangement with NASS [the National Asylum Support Service – a Home Office department providing accommodation and subsistence to asylum seekers] terminated when his application failed and he slept on the floor of fellow refugees who had taken him into their home. With no money, he relied on other people's goodwill; as much as he appreciated the help, he felt humiliated and demeaned.

Third, he was weighed down by his past traumatic experiences that led to his exile. He was trying unsuccessfully to avoid thinking and talking about them, hoping that somehow they would disappear. His struggle, however, was defeated by constant reminders through recurrent nightmares and flashbacks, and having to detail his experiences at the immigration tribunal.

In addition he was faced with daily challenges in the form of language and communication barriers, cultural differences, homesickness, unemployment, loss of status, racism and discrimination. Adane revealed in one of his sessions that when his GP suggested a referral to mental health services he immediately refused in fear that he was being deemed an 'ebd', which means 'lunatic' in Amharic (one of the languages spoken in Ethiopia).

Stigma

Many refugees come from countries where mental illness is stigmatised, hidden and never discussed. Recovery is considered impossible and mental health care viewed as unsupportive. Consequently people may be reluctant to seek help, until a situation has advanced so that they cannot cope. Careful explanation of the range of help and treatments available, and that they will not impact negatively on an asylum claim, may be reassuring.

Cultural competence

Health behaviours and expectations of health care are influenced by culture and beliefs. Each culture has its own frameworks for defining psychological health and for seeking help. Behaviour considered as mental illness in Western countries may be interpreted differently in other cultures – viewed perhaps as spirit possession, a sign of divine punishment, genetic weakness or normal behaviour. Additionally, educational, socioeconomic and individual factors are significant influences on personal beliefs and behaviour,[2] so it is important to resist assumptions based on culture and instead to ask for explanation. In addition, we need to be aware of our own social and cultural backgrounds and how they influence our views, interpretations, diagnoses and treatment. However, if a practice is oppressive, it should not just be accepted as 'culture', an example being excessive physical punishment of children, which is common practice within some communities.

Interpreting

The provision of quality interpreting services is essential if access and participation of refugees in health and social care services are to increase. Interpreting is most often considered to be the linguistic translating of the words of the client and the health worker. However, in the context of in-depth personal interviews in a GP consultation or mental health settings, where health issues are discussed and assessments and therapeutic interventions are carried out, the need for an understanding goes far beyond words into cultural, social and belief systems. According to Eisenbruch:

> if western mental health professionals try to identify and treat refugees according to criteria such as those listed in the Diagnostic Statistical Manual (DSM), they run the risk of treating an illness which the refugee does not have and may leave him/her feeling confused. Such misunderstanding of refugees' needs could be avoided if more emphasis were placed on the cultural meanings of the information gathered from the refugees themselves, even if they may at first seem bizarre to the professional.[1]

It is through the availability of well-trained interpreters that appropriate assessment, planning and delivery of care can be facilitated. Their vital role extends beyond linguistic proficiency to the 'knowledge of the way in which both languages are used, which includes idioms, figures of speech, metaphors, similes as well as values, goals and communications styles of those individuals and groups using them',[3] and maintaining confidentiality and professional boundaries.

When working with interpreters, it is important to consider power dynamics. Undoubtedly the clinician holds power in allocating resources, directing assessments and making diagnostic and treatment decisions. The interpreter also holds considerable power 'by virtue of being bilingual and bearing knowledge of both the clinician's and service user's culture. The clinician and the service user are reliant on the interpreter to facilitate communication.'[4] It is therefore important to foster a working relationship where 'the interpreter, clinician and service user feel empowered to play an active and equal role in the therapeutic encounter'.[5]

If you do not share a language with the patient, try to use an interpreter who is not a friend or family member, particularly if issues such as mental health, torture or sexual health may arise, since disclosure of personal information, experiences and feelings may be inhibited. The presence of an interpreter can be reassuring (although fear of a lack of confidentiality may mean that some people feel more relaxed with a telephone interpreter) and interpreters can inform health workers about aspects of culture and language that might otherwise be missed. Check if clients prefer interpreters who are not from their own communities and also be aware that certain languages have different dialects. If possible offer a choice of gender of interpreter, particularly if sexual health, rape or torture may be discussed.

Continuity may help to engender feelings of trust and safety for the client. However, be aware that most interpreters have no specialist training in mental health work and little supervision or support in doing such work (which may cause personal stress by re-stimulating feelings about similar experiences of their own). If possible allow more time for appointments (if feasible, double the time) and include some time before and after the session for briefing and debriefing. This extra time will be a worthwhile investment as you will achieve more with the consultation. Health workers can benefit from training on working with interpreters.

Presentation

Psychological distress is common amongst asylum seekers and refugees. People frequently experience:

- extreme sadness
- anxiety, depression and panic attacks
- problems with memory, concentration and disorientation
- poor sleep patterns (almost universal)
- grief, bereavement reactions, fear of relationships, self-blame
- loss of sense of future
- guilt and shame, self-blame.

These feelings may arise from people's experiences pre-flight, during flight and once they have reached the country of asylum. A recent meta-analysis of the literature on the mental health of refugees has shown that refugee status confers an overall increase in psychological ill-health.[6] The authors found that this is not an inevitable consequence of conflict and trauma but reflects the sociopolitical conditions that they face in host countries, and they conclude that improving these conditions could improve mental health outcomes.

Assessment

Building trust, to enable people to disclose often very traumatic and shameful experiences, can be assisted by continuity, offering people choice of gender of health worker and interpreter, and working at their own pace.

Since expressions of distress and coping strategies differ both between and within cultures, assessment and treatment of psychological health problems of asylum seekers and refugees are complex. Understanding the person's explanatory model (how he or she makes sense of his or her situation), and culturally appropriate responses to distress may be useful, and your interpreter may offer helpful insights to these. Assessments of risk of suicide and child protection may be indicated, although there may be cultural and religious taboos towards talking about self-harm.

It is important to maintain an open mind during a longer period of assessment – cultural differences and communication difficulties may increase the possibility of a misdiagnosis of mental illness. Black and minority ethnic UK residents are known to be disproportionately diagnosed with schizophrenia, sectioned under the Mental Health Act[7] and given high doses of antipsychotic drugs rather than counselling. Therefore be wary of pathologising what may be natural and culturally appropriate expressions of grief and distress following traumatic experiences. Diagnoses such as post-traumatic stress disorder (PTSD) may not reflect the complex way in which historical, political and social factors interact and impact on the experiences of refugee communities.[8] Many behaviour patterns considered to be 'symptoms' could also be regarded as adaptive reactions to conflict, e.g. an exaggerated startle reflex could be an appropriate response to living under gunfire. Although inappropriate in a new environment, it does not necessarily reflect mental illness.[9]

In addition, asylum seekers' and refugees' situation in exile can hardly be described as post-traumatic, as they face ongoing concerns about their safety, racism, poverty and destitution. Using a trauma model can undermine traditional coping strategies, leading to increased helplessness, and a greater dependence on external agencies.[10] Work with asylum seekers and refugees is inherently political in nature – if we focus on individual psychology over the political and social context, our ability to understand people's problems and how they can be relieved most effectively can be reduced.[10]

Torture

Torture has been defined as 'the intentional infliction of severe pain or suffering, whether physical or mental, upon a person in the custody or under the control of the accused' (Article 7.2 (e) (excerpt) of the Rome Statute of the International Criminal Court 1998).

Estimates of the proportion of asylum seekers who have been tortured vary from 5–30 per cent, depending on the definition of torture used and their country of origin. Many people do not initially admit to their experiences of torture, often through shame or embarrassment.

The effects of torture are an accumulation of physical violence, detention (unhygienic cells, inadequate diet) and the psychological consequences of one's own and witnessing others' experiences of torture and of being powerless to prevent it. A survivor of torture may have a preoccupation that his or her body has been irreparably damaged and may experience chronic pain, leading to repeated consultations. The essentials are time, a sympathetic approach and allowing the person to maintain control of the pace of work. A choice of gender for health worker and interpreter may be helpful. The family of a survivor of torture may also need support. Children may feel additional pressures and should be given an opportunity to talk about their feelings.

Rape as a method of torture

Many women, and some men, are survivors of sexual violence including rape. Throughout history rape has been used as a weapon of warfare to degrade and humiliate an enemy. In most cultures, sexual violence and rape are taboo, and survivors may feel very uncomfortable discussing their experiences.

Sexual violence is motivated by a wish to dominate and degrade, and is a very powerful weapon against individuals, families and communities. For both male and female survivors, the resulting dominant emotion is usually that of deep shame. Women may be shunned by their community and family as having been defiled, and are no longer accepted, which has been the experience of many survivors of rape from Kosovo.

Men tend to underreport their experiences of sexual violence. They may have doubts about their sexuality and fear infertility. Both men and women commonly experience sexual difficulties following sexual violence and may need reassurance about sexual function. Persistent unexplained distress and anxiety may be due to a history of sexual violation.

Although some people benefit from talking about their experience of sexual violence, doing so may make others feel very uncomfortable. It may be more effective to help people to develop their own support networks by facilitating the development of meetings and activities, and by addressing the current practical difficulties they face. It is important to address sexual violation in the context of the many traumas and losses experienced.

Insomnia

Insomnia is almost universal amongst refugees and asylum seekers (and is also experienced by 20 per cent of the general adult population and 35 per cent of over-65s). It may be exacerbated by depression, stress, fear, grief, nightmares and inappropriate accommodation. Advice on sleep management should be given such as taking regular exercise, reducing alcohol, caffeine, smoking, avoiding napping during the day, trying to go to bed at the same time each day, allocating a limited time each day to focus specifically on worries/concerns and practising relaxation techniques, meditation or prayer.

If you prescribe a hypnotic, do so only for a limited period (not more than 4 weeks). Some people find mirtazapine 15 mg or trazodone 100–200 mg nocte helpful if insomnia is associated with depression

Physical expressions of distress/'somatisation'

> The mind that has no vent in tears makes other organs weep.
>
> (Henry Vaughan)

People may present with weakness, headaches, abdominal, neck or back pain, or pain throughout the body, with no detectable physical cause. They may be experiencing psychological symptoms but be unable to describe them, due to lack of appropriate language, the stigma of mental health problems, or the belief that health workers are more interested in physical problems.

Take complaints seriously and, after excluding physical pathology, try to find out the meaning and context of the symptoms for the individual. It may be useful to ask patients to record the variability of their symptoms alongside how they are feeling. If symptoms persist (which may be for some time), take a multifactorial approach, trying to address any underlying causes and overcoming social isolation. Consider counselling or complementary therapies such as massage, if available.

Addressing psychological distress

The most valuable inputs for many people are supportive listening and practical assistance to rebuild their lives – restoration of normal activities as far as possible can be the most effective promoter of mental health and can do much to relieve sadness and anxiety. However, some people may be suspicious of health workers, as they may have been identified with the ruling state in their home country, and even been involved in oppression. Trust needs to be earned and may take some time to develop. In addition many people may experience guilt or shame regarding their experiences and may not wish to talk.

Community, religious, spiritual and creative links may be important sources of support. People have survived against huge odds and their resilience can be a strength to utilise.[11]

The factors outlined below have been shown to protect against mental illness for people in exile, and interventions should aim to enhance these:

- contact with family/family reunion
- social support – links to integrated community groups
- strong religious or political ideology
- having a proactive problem-solving approach.[12]

Psychological therapies and counselling

Western models of psychological therapies and counselling are based on the premise that the meeting with 'the client' is to provide a space for exploration of the internal feelings, emotions and ensuing behaviours that appear to be causing distress. Applying these and other prescribed Western models to address the presenting problems of refugees like Adane may possibly render them less effectual.[13] These are models of intervention developed in a Eurocentric framework and need to be attuned to incorporate other dimensions of cross-cultural nature and practical interventions. Discussing emotional difficulties with a professional who is not part of the family or extended community network is unfamiliar – in most cultures professional psychological or counselling services are non-existent. 'Most asylum seekers come from cultures in which the detached introspection of talk therapy is an alien activity.'[14] In some languages there is no word for the term 'counselling'. In Amharic, for instance, the closest translation refers to the idea of giving advice.

Refugee community organisations

What was helpful to Adane (and many other refugees and asylum seekers coming into contact with refugee community organisations (RCOs) and other service providers) was, first and foremost, the fact that someone was taking time to listen and witness the total upheaval of his life. In addition his story was being taken seriously and believed to be true, contrasting with the current pervasive culture of disbelief towards asylum seekers in the UK. The advantage of support being set within the community setting (where this is possible) is not just the absence in communication barrier and cultural difference but the opportunity of establishing closer political alliance.[11,14] (Refugee community organisations may reflect the political divisions in the home country, which may be problematic for some people, if they do not support that particular party.)

Second, the focus of the preliminary intervention took the shape of helping Adane with the practical problems of housing, subsistence and support with his immigration appeals process. The counsellor actively advocated and coordinated support from his GP and other involved agencies to request NASS to provide Adane with accommodation and subsistence on health grounds. This relieved some of Adane's stress and greatly bolstered a trusting relationship and stronger working alliance. 'Practical advice and advocacy is of itself psychologically supportive and recounting of traumatic experience is an option but not a necessity.'[12,14] In our experience of seeing clients in a counselling and consultation setting, we have found that most have learned coping strategies and developed resilience with regard to their past traumatic experiences. However, they find it difficult to comprehend and deal with the post-migration stressors of being labelled as bogus, being left with no support and no employment prospects, which shatter their beliefs and hopes for refuge. It was only after these practical challenges were resolved that Adane was able to find the strength and space to explore the effects of the traumatic experiences in his life.

Group work

Working with refugees in a group setting (whether a therapeutic or social group) has been found to be highly supportive, particularly among young people, in terms of reducing isolation, sharing experiences and inspiring hope and resilience. For many people, hearing that they are not alone in their struggle and stress normalises their feelings and dispels the strong belief that they are going mad.

In summary, psychological intervention and counselling for refugees becomes more effective and beneficial when the act of support and understanding extends beyond the four walls of the counselling room and the traditional 'introspective talk therapy' to include political alliance, advocacy and campaigning, helping with practical problems such as housing and access to other social services. In most instances, it requires contacting, liaising and coordinating services with other agencies; something that is not expected from the traditional counsellor.

Prescribing

Although helpful in some circumstances, medication has limited success in addressing many of the problems that refugees and asylum seekers experience. Antidepressants may help clinical depression, if used in conjunction with practical and social support (mirtazapine and trazodone have been found to be helpful if insomnia is marked). When prescribing, ensure that information about the drug and its possible side effects are clearly understood.

Symptoms causing concern

The following symptoms may cause concern and warrant referral for more specialist help:

- consistent failure to function properly with daily tasks
- active suicidal ideation – the refusal of an asylum claim, detention and threat of deportation pose a heightened risk of suicide and attempted suicide
- social withdrawal and self-neglect
- behaviour or talk that is abnormal within the person's own culture
- aggression.[15]

Domestic violence

Refugee women experiencing domestic violence are especially vulnerable since they lack knowledge of their rights, as well as family and community support. In some cultures, domestic violence is tolerated and women believe they have no recourse to the law. Their claim to accommodation and asylum in the UK may be linked to that of their partner, and they will need independent advice. They may need help to contact specialist agencies and may be extremely reluctant to report domestic violence to the police.

Substance misuse

Limited research is available on the aspect of substance misuse among refugees, with the exception of *khat* (also called *chat*). The general sense, however, is that substance use such as drugs and alcohol is increasing as a coping mechanism. *Khat* is commonly used by people of East African, Middle Eastern and Arab heritage. Currently *khat* is not a controlled substance but there are moves by the Home Office to make it an illegal substance. The effects of *khat* on mental health have been documented predominantly in the Somali community and these include *khat*-induced psychosis. However, the social effects of *khat* are more visible among the refugee community in causing financial hardship and in contributing to a large number of family breakdowns.

Detention of asylum seekers

An increasing number of asylum seekers are detained in detention or removal centres and prisons in the host country. Amnesty estimates that 25,000 were detained in the UK during 2005.[16] Such detention is distressing. For those who have been detained in their own country, the experience of subsequent detention can be devastating. The experience of being locked up will generally evoke powerful memories and these may persist for a long time after release from detention. Of particular concern is the detention of children.

Looking after ourselves

Working with refugees is both rewarding and challenging. It is important not to rescue or raise unrealistic expectations. Avoid making promises that cannot be fulfilled and recognise limitations and vulnerabilities. Encourage independence, although refugees may need assistance to access services. Health workers, including administrative staff, may be exposed to a high degree of distress and need support themselves.

It is easy to feel impotent when faced with such chaos and so many problems. You may feel a huge pressure to meet all needs yourself, while feeling that you do not have the information, skills or time to do so. Where problems do not appear to have any solution, it may help just to listen.

If possible, build networks with others involved in this work, both within and outside your own discipline, and within the statutory and voluntary sectors, so that you are not working in isolation. Some teams have set up monthly facilitated support groups, which give an opportunity for members to discuss difficult issues. Managers need to be aware of the time demands placed on workers caused by people's interpreting needs, multiple and complex difficulties and multi-agency liaison. An email discussion group – the Refugee Network – facilitated by Medact (www.medact.org) offers the opportunity for health workers to discuss issues and share information with colleagues.

Summary

In this chapter we have highlighted some of the issues affecting the psychological wellbeing of asylum seekers and refugees in the UK, and have suggested practical ways in which health workers can help. Practical and psychosocial support has been shown to be more effective in both prevention and care than a more medicalised model, respecting people's individual cultural beliefs, views and practices.

References

1. Eisenbruch M. From post traumatic stress disorder to cultural bereavement: diagnosis of Southeast Asian refugees *Social Science and Medicine* 1991; **33**: 673–80.

2. Helman C. *Culture, Health and Illness* London: Hodder Arnold, 2000.

3. Messent P. From postmen to makers of meaning: a model for collaborative work between clinicians and interpreters. In: R Tribe, H Raval (eds). *Working with Interpreters in Mental Health*, pp. 135–51, Hove: Brunner and Routledge, 2003.

4. Tribe R, Raval H. *Working with Interpreters in Mental Health* Hove: Brunner and Routledge, 2003.

5. Mudarikiri M. Working with interpreters in adult mental health. In: R Tribe, H Raval (eds). *Working with Interpreters in Mental Health*, pp. 182–98, Hove: Brunner and Routledge, 2003.

6. Porter M, Haslam N. Pre-displacement and post-displacement factors associated with the mental health of refugees and internally displaced persons: a meta-analysis *Journal of the American Medical Association* 2005; **294**: 602–12.

7. Minnis H, McMillan A, Gillies M, *et al*. Racial stereotyping: survey of psychiatrists in the United Kingdom *British Medical Journal* 2001; **323**: 905–6.

8. Bracken P. Hidden agendas: deconstructing post traumatic stress disorder. In: P Bracken, C Petty (eds). *Rethinking the Trauma of War*, pp. 38–59, London: Free Association Books, 1998.

9. Burnett A, Thompson K. Enhancing the psychological well-being of asylum seekers and refugees. In: K Barrett and B George (eds). *Race, Culture, Psychology and Law*, pp. 205–24, Thousand Oaks: Sage Publications, 2005.

10. Giller J. Caring for victims of torture in Uganda: some personal reflections. In: P Bracken, C Petty (eds). *Rethinking the Trauma of War*, pp. 128–45, London: Free Association Books, 1998.

11. Jones L. The question of political neutrality when doing psychosocial work with survivors of political violence *International Review of Psychiatry* 1998; **10**: 239–47.

12. Burnett A, Gebremikael L. Expanding the primary mental health team for asylum seekers and refugees *Journal of Primary Care Mental Health* 2005; **3**: 77–81.

13. Watters C. The mental health needs of refugees and asylum seekers: key issues in research and service development. In: F Nicholson (ed.). *Current Issues of Asylum Law and Policy*, pp. 270–85, London: Avebury, 1998.

14. Summerfield D. Asylum seekers, refugees and mental health services in the UK *Psychiatric Bulletin* 2001; **25**: 161–3.

15. Burnett A, Fassil Y. *Meeting the Health Needs of Refugees and Asylum Seekers in the UK: an information and resource pack for health workers* London: Directorate for Health and Social Care/DH, 2002.

16. Amnesty International UK. *Seeking Asylum is Not a Crime: detention of people who have sought asylum* London: Amnesty International, 2005.

17 | Prisoners and offenders
Their primary mental healthcare needs and experience

Mark Williamson

What this chapter contributes:

health characteristics of prisoners

health characteristics of recently released prisoners

a model of care for offenders.

Introduction

Prisoner health and the health of released prisoners and offenders, covering physical health, mental health and primary care and social care issues, is a relatively poorly researched field both in the UK and worldwide. It is therefore important that we use knowledge and information from as wide a scope as possible both geographically and in terms of related population cohorts to try to learn about the key issues affecting prisoner health during incarceration and after release. The author is keen to see the dissemination of the evidence of need, best practice, the development of services that work, the exploration of models of care that will probably work, and a building of interest and attention to this area of health and social care, which, to date, has been relatively neglected by the main bodies of public health, education and research and primary care.

This chapter does not seek to define best practice in primary care mental health – there are other important sources – or to plead for a special approach for offenders in relation to primary care mental health. I am, however, going to describe the characteristics of the offender population, describe the international evidence in relation to the primary care needs of offenders, describe some of the UK health and social care policy context, and propose a model of care for offenders that has at its heart the provision of excellence in primary care mental health services.

In the UK the prison population is increasing and the health problems of prisoners are being increasingly identified as important areas for research and service development. The NHS has recently become responsible for the commissioning of health care of prisoners, taking over this role from the prison service. This significant change, which now more closely aligns the UK with arrangements in the rest of Europe, followed the Reed and Lyne[1] report on the work of Her Majesty's Chief Inspectorate of Prison Team, which identified significant variability in the quality of health care provided for prisoners in UK prisons. There then followed the publication in March 1999 of *The Future Organisation of Prison Health Care*,[2] which outlined the agreement between the Prison Service and the NHS on a formal partnership to secure better health care for prisoners. This important document spelled out a vision for health care in prisons:

> Healthcare in prisons should promote the health of prisoners: identify prisoners with health problems; assess their needs and deliver treatment or refer to other specialist services as appropriate. It should also *continue any care started in the community contributing to a seamless service and facilitating through-care on release* [author's emphasis]. The majority of health care in prisons is therefore of a primary care nature. However, health care delivery in prisons faces a significant number of challenges not experienced by primary care in the wider community.

This paragraph nicely explains the need for continuity of care and the challenges of delivering an effective healthcare solution for prisoners within prison and on release. It states unequivocally the central role of primary care in providing the framework by which the solutions to the various issues can be addressed. Linked to this the prior report by the Health Advisory Committee for the Prison Service (1997) stated that prisons should 'give prisoners access to the same quality and range of health care services as the general public receives from the NHS'.

One of the unspoken realities of prison health is how issues or clinical problem areas overlap significantly, e.g. mental health and substance misuse, substance misuse and communicable disease, primary care, sexual health and public health, and social exclusion issues with all of the above. The co-representation of these issues contributes in the relatively disempowered and marginalised of society to a tendency in care providers to allow them, including prisoners and ex-prisoners, to fall between the stools of the care-providing structures and systems. It must equally be credible that this reality will contribute to the recidivism and ill-health of prisoners after release.

Prisons are designed for punishment, correction and rehabilitation to the community. These goals and the associated prison regimen may conflict with the aims of health care. A literature review[3] showed that the main issues in prison health care are mental health, substance abuse and communicable diseases. Women prisoners and older prisoners were identified as having needs that are distinct from other prisoners and that health promotion and improving the health of the community outside prisons are desirable aims of prison health care. It also found that the delivery of effective health care to prisoners is dependent upon a partnership between health and prison services, and creative methodologies such as telemedicine may be usefully deployed.

Throughout the search to provide the evidence for this chapter it became clear that many of the research papers were simply describing the epidemiology and healthcare needs in the prison setting. Others were descriptions of one-off service approaches that had been shown to be effective in a particular cultural or organisational setting. Very few indeed focused on primary mental health care, the pre-incarceration phase or the post-release period or considered which interventions might be effective.

It is clear to all who work in prisons that every prison has a unique culture, does the same thing uniquely differently from others, and hosts a unique and small subset of the population. These realities confound research findings, preventing them from being easily generalisable. The reverse perspective on the two-way street of this reality is that despite a relative lack of evidence much good work can be effective in each unique setting. Positive results have been shown from a variety of healthcare projects and approaches based as they are on reasoned logical planning and some evidence, even if it has had to be extrapolated from different settings, patient cohorts or prison systems. Hence the very difficulty inherent in trying to generalise should in fact encourage every prison health team to adopt and express a culture of creative solution building for each of the uniquely difficult healthcare problems of the environment. The post-release period can learn from prison-based work and community-based research but again the encouragement to be creative should apply.

The characteristics and outcomes of the prisoner and offender population

The general prisoner population has many important characteristics that, because of the small percentage of prisoners serving life sentences, can be assumed to be retained by the recently released prisoner and offender population. The average GP therefore, though not perhaps considering him or herself as likely to encounter prisoners, will certainly do so and the characteristics of offenders will need to be understood to support a successful consultation.

There are 138 prisons in the UK (127 public, 11 private) housing approximately 80,000 prisoners (in 1992 the figure was 42,000) and the population is slowly rising. Five per cent are female and there are a small number of child prisoners, approximately 100 girls and 3000 boys.

There are about 135,000 prisoners incarcerated per year, and (logically) a slightly smaller number released, of which approximately 50 per cent serve less than six months. These figures mean that there are nearly a million relatives affected by imprisonment annually.

England and Wales has the highest imprisonment rate in Western Europe, though some others are notably increasing their use of this sentence, e.g. the Netherlands. The increasing use of the imprisonment sanction implies a successful approach but in fact it is relatively unsuccessful with an 80 per cent recidivism rate within two years of release. The ex-prisoner population and their families are a significant part of the socially excluded population, and they share similar issues of health, healthcare needs and difficulties in respect of accessing health and social care services.

It is of particular note that there is a dearth of UK-based research in respect of cultural and ethnic diversity, and the outcomes of initiatives focused at addressing these issues. This contrasts with the USA where the contrast between the majority black prisoner population and the largely white prison guards has been troubling for many years. There are now approximately 10,000 foreign nationals in UK prisons so study needs to be done on the effectiveness of health interventions for them, and should link to similar research in respect of the care of refugees in the community and detention centres.

The social exclusion characteristics of prisoners are shown in Table 17.1 (Department of Health figures).

Table 17.1: Social exclusion characteristics

Social exclusion characteristic	Prison population
Have been in local authority care	13 times more likely than the 'non-prison' population
60% are unemployed	13 times more likely than the 'non-prison' population
Regularly played truant	10 times more likely than the 'non-prison' population
Excluded from school	20 times more likely than the 'non-prison' population
Have had a family member convicted of a crime	2.5 times more likely than the 'non-prison' population

Some other characteristics are that:

- 42 per cent of released prisoners have no fixed abode
- 50 per cent on release have no GP
- 50 per cent re-offend within two years
- 50 per cent of prisoners have reading skills < 11-year-olds
- a third of offenders' debt problems worsen in custody
- 125,000 children have a family member in prison.

Of crime (National Offender Management Service figures):

- 70 per cent is drug related

- 40 per cent is alcohol related

- 55 per cent is linked to thinking and behaviour problems

- 50 per cent in the UK is committed by 100,000 offenders

- it is thought a 50 per cent reduction is possible

- the cost of crime by re-offenders is approximately £11 billion per annum

- each prisoner costs the criminal justice system £65,000 per annum

- each prisoner costs £38,000 to incarcerate per year.

On admission to UK prisons 40 per cent of people deny contact with a GP (Department of Health figures), though a more recent regional audit in the North of England (unpublished) suggests this figure is variable and may be as high as 70 per cent. The reliability of offenders as historians must be considered because, as is stated in many studies,[4] they will tend to deceive, or respond in the way they think researchers want them to, when it is perceived to be in their interests to do so.

The fact that the post-release period is a key area for study and for action in terms of service development and improved coordination of care is well illustrated by the findings of Verger et al. in France, reported in 2003.[5] They noted that, while the poor health status of prisoners has been highlighted in Western countries, the surveillance of their mortality has been neglected. They studied the mortality of 1305 prisoners released during 1997 from a French prison. Health status after release was obtained for 86.4 per cent of them. Compared with the general population, ex-prisoners' non-natural mortality rates were significantly increased both in the 15–34 and 35–54 age categories (3.5-fold and 10.6-fold respectively), and the risk of death due to overdose was 124 and 274 times higher in the same categories respectively. Their key finding and opinion was that prevention and care should be reinforced in the pre-release period without waiting for more epidemiological data.

This finding contrasts ironically with, but is also partly explained by, Clavel et al.,[6] who confirmed the benefits of incarceration in prison in relation to mortality. The mortality among a population of male prisoners between 1977 and 1983 was compared with that among the general French population. The overall mortality rate (for all deaths except external causes) was lower among prisoners (standardised mortality rate, SMR = 84; $p < 0.05$). Moreover, the risk of dying from all causes, as well as from malignant neoplasms, diseases of the circulatory system and suicides, fell significantly with increasing duration of imprisonment. These findings suggest that the lifestyle specific to imprisonment might overcome the prejudicial effect of risk factors such as alcohol, tobacco or drug abuse that tend to be common among prisoners after release.

The key message is that, surprisingly and no doubt dependent on setting, to some extent prisons can be a place of relative health and safety for the prisoner population and that therefore prisoners may benefit in healthcare terms from imprisonment and that they are correspondingly extremely vulnerable on release.

In the UK there is a newly established prison health research network that has primary care and public health, mental health and substance misuse subgroups. These are developing planning for research programmes to try to improve our understanding of these issues and to ensure that system-wide learning occurs and is implemented. There is a wide range of NHS initiatives, which will have an effect on the health and social care of this population in the community after release, and which are coincidental with the current transfer of responsibility to the NHS from prisons of commissioning the health services in prisons in the UK.

In the UK we can consider primary care to be that care provided by general practices and their healthcare teams, and the care provided by dentists, pharmacists and opticians. Community care extends this scope to that care provided by community nurses and doctors and social workers. Very little research has been done that looks at how released prisoners have their primary, community and social care and health needs assessed and provided for.

In 1984 Martin[7] compared the medical care of prisoners 'declaring sick', to the medical officer and hospital officers in Bedford Prison, with the medical care given to the medical officer's patients in general practice. The consultation rate of prisoners was higher than that of patients in the practice. It is considered that part of this increase was because household remedies were not available to prisoners except through the prison medical service and part may also have been due to the stresses of life in prison. Few psychoactive drugs were prescribed in prison, primarily to avoid the development of trading in such drugs and the bullying of patients. The problems that prisoners presented reflected the problems of violence and poor hygiene in prison. It was also considered that some problems that more commonly present in prison than in community-based general practice may be related to stress of the circumstances of prisoners and of their environment.

Further findings from Martin et al.[8] showed that these issues persist beyond release, but that willingness of prisoners to access primary care in the community was low. The group of men studied had a high level of illness, neglected their health, and had a high alcohol intake. Many prisoners with active medical problems on discharge from prison were unwilling to take a letter to their own GP. It is apparent that the issues explored were of a primary care mental health nature, which would probably benefit from appropriate intervention.

In 1981 a review[9] of the utilisation of health care showed that the annual consultation rate for men was 48 per prisoner per year, 2.6 times the rate for men studied in a long-term prison, and almost 20 times the rate for men studied in the general population.

The annual consultation rate for female prisoners was three times that of male prisoners. These figures are based on relatively small studies in particular institutions and care must be taken in extrapolating to the prison system as a whole. A great deal can of course be done to manage offender health-seeking behaviour. For all prisoners, the most common problems seen were skin (9.7 per cent), musculoskeletal (8.3 per cent) and psychiatric conditions (8.2 per cent). An examination of practitioners' patterns in providing care demonstrated the primary role of registered nurses, who saw 70 per cent of the patients.

Offender health-seeking behaviour in UK prisons is therefore many times that of the non-prisoner population. This high demand has seen the development of wing-based nurse triage schemes in a number of UK prisons (e.g. HMP Belmarsh), which have been shown to effectively manage demand for doctor appointments. The general trend over recent years has been for an increasingly nurse-led model of care in the prison setting with medical input being programmed in rather than being a first point of call.

A paper from Florida[10] raises the question of the appropriateness of a purely medical model of delivering primary care in the prison setting. In 333 inmates seen on sick call 528 problems were identified. The large number of psychosocial problems (194 out of 528) and the wide diversity of problems (125 in 333 inmates) were documented. The importance of considering alternative models of service delivery and the importance of health education were identified. Subsequent experience in the UK[11] has confirmed the effectiveness of expanding the roles of members of primary healthcare teams, e.g. pharmacists and dentists, and of using the skills, leadership and competences of nurses more appropriately.

An important recent paper from South Carolina[12] nicely explains the benefits of both a supportive nurse–patient relationship in the prison but also the key role of extending the partnership into the community after release. The paper also takes the step of declaring significant benefits on criminal behaviours, particularly those affecting health. They conclude that 'nursing is uniquely positioned to develop prevention, intervention, and treatment strategies for individuals involved in criminal activities before, during, and after incarceration'. This bridging model of services for the prisoner into the community is a theme that appears relatively frequently in the few programmes of care focused on the post-release period.

Wildbore[13] in Manchester has demonstrated that community-sentenced young offenders can benefit from nurse-led health promotion. Forty years ago an increase in 'juvenile delinquency' led to a large prison-building programme for young offenders. Today, the emphasis is on community sentencing and a reduction in prison places. The secondment of nurses into youth offending teams makes it possible to offer primary health services to a group of mainly male, vulnerable people. The ability of health and social care services to provide such input before young people offend is challenging in view of the hard-to-reach nature of this sector of the population. The implication is that services need to be designed to be acceptable to and accepting of these young people.

Mental health

According to Department of Health figures[14] 90 per cent of prisoners have a mental health or substance misuse problem, or both. Seven per cent suffer from severe and enduring mental health problems with approximately 1000 per annum transferred to secure NHS mental health facilities. The delay in such transfers has been a major problem but is rapidly improving. There were 94 UK prison suicides in 2003/04. The prevalence of mental health problems and the subsequent utilisation rates of mental health services by women is approximately twice that seen in male prisoners, and the ratio persists into the post-release period.

With respect to research there is a greater range of studies concerning mental health issues in relation to prison health but again relatively little relating to primary care mental health or to follow-up after release. We know from Reed and Lyne[15] that the quality of services for mentally ill prisoners fell far below the standards in the NHS in 2000. Patients' lives were unacceptably restricted and therapy limited. They called for policy review and improvements in Care Programme Approach, mental healthcare in-reach and improved transfer times into NHS secure hospitals have subsequently resulted.

In 1998 Bisson *et al.*[16] looked at the psychological health of British servicemen and their families who had been held prisoner in Kuwait following the invasion in August 1990. Their study investigated the mental health status of this group of individuals at six and 18 months after the final hostage was released. The Impact of Event Scale scores changed little over time whereas the General Health Questionnaire scores reduced significantly ($p = .001$) over the 12-month period suggesting that, despite ongoing intrusive thoughts and avoidance phenomena, levels of psychological distress did reduce. Those variables most strongly associated with a poor psychological outcome were witnessing physical violence and perceived deterioration in physical and mental health. Poor outcome at six months was strongly correlated with poor outcome at 18 months.

These findings, although related to a different population and circumstance, might help to predict the group of released prisoners from UK prisons who may suffer most psychological harm and require proactive help. Though the serviceman group and their experience are probably relatively unique, the primary mental health nature of their needs is highlighted.

Planning for the post-release period for mentally ill prisoners is believed to be important and is self-evidently something that should occur. Wolff *et al.*[17] found, however, that the quality of planning was variable, often absent and dependent on the presence of well-functioning mental health units in the prison to be effective.

An important US study by McCoy *et al.*,[18] from Chicago, shows the importance of assertive outreach for prisoners with mental health problems who are released. They knew that people with mental illnesses who are released from prison are at high risk of psychiatric decompensation and re-arrest. This paper describes a jail linkage programme for this population that won an American Psychiatric Association Gold Award (2001). Based on interviews with its first 24 participants, they illustrate how the released prisoners experience factors that contribute to recidivism and decompensation. Results suggest that it is possible to identify, engage and retain people in treatment who struggle with many risk factors. They conclude that this programme should be expanded and replicated. The learning from this highlights the risk for the mentally ill after release and the need to retain them in services.

The importance of a case-based targeted support approach is highlighted by a number of other studies in the USA, and in Australia and New Zealand.[19,20]

The risk of the mentally ill moving through a cycle of prisons is a feature of much of the available research. Hartwell[21] in Boston, USA, used data on 247 offenders with mental illness, to identify characteristics that distinguish those who are returned to prison or a psychiatric hospital with those who remain in the community. Sociodemographic, mental health, criminal history and service variables were compared across a range of outcome categories with a focus on those re-institutionalised and those re-incarcerated. Those returning to institutions had somewhat different mental health service and criminal justice histories from the engaged/community group. In particular, the group that is re-incarcerated is more likely released from misdemeanour sentences, and the group being released from felony sentences is more likely to be found in a psychiatric hospital after release from correctional custody. They concluded that these findings have implications regarding the cumulative effects of engagement with the criminal justice system and the process through which persons with mental illness and a criminal history cycle through institutions.

Suicide and self-harm

Suicide rates (standardised) are higher in prisoners than in the general male population by factors that range from 3.5 (Canada) to 6 (England and Wales), and in non-standardised studies by 2 (Poland) to 15 (Australia).

The rates of self-harm in UK prisons, 2005, are as follows:

- 5653 prisoners harmed themselves (7.4 per cent of average prison population), of which:

  - 10 per cent young males
  - 5 per cent adult men
  - 65 per cent young females
  - 28 per cent adult women.

Comparing these last two figures with the relatively small female prisoner population identifies a very significant and excessive morbidity related to the female prisoner population that requires a disproportionate focus of resources.

The 78 suicides and 40 per cent of prisoners who had attempted suicide displayed psychotic symptoms in the week prior to the attempt.

There are significant challenges to the arrangement of treatments; prisoners are often victims of trauma or abuse and often have a range of physical and mental health problems. There are high turnover rates of inmates in any particular prison that affects rapport building and the continuity of care. Importantly, though one can hardly imagine a solution, the Mental Health Act (1983) does not allow for prisoners to be treated without consent until transfer to an NHS bed. The diversity of the prison and offender population means that there should be an appropriately culturally sensitive approach, particularly in relation to primary care mental healthcare needs.

Roth and Presse[22] in the USA investigated parasuicide and the benefits of nursing approaches. Parasuicide refers to the non-fatal, intentional, self-injurious behaviours closely aligned to the UK self-harm concept. These behaviours are frequently exhibited by individuals with features of a borderline personality disorder. In correctional systems, the rate of parasuicidal behaviour among incarcerated female offenders can be high and intertwined with complex behavioural and social issues. Nursing interventions in the management and treatment of parasuicidal behaviours incorporating the principles of dialectical behaviour therapy were developed and implemented at the institution. The treatment approach provided practical, effective nursing interventions including pre-treatment orientation, strategies for use with threats to self-harm and during self-harming episodes, and follow-up treatment. Again, there are no studies that look at parasuicide post-release and which investigate potential treatment modalities. The impact of giving birth to a child who is then after a few months removed from the mother (length of time varies in various countries) at approximately nine months in the UK can only be imagined, and again the research on this small subset of a small subset has not yet been carried out in the UK.

In the UK the new Assessment, Care in Custody and Teamwork (ACCT) documents have been adopted by the prison system and their impact appears favourable. In particular the holistic approach incorporating input from all parts of the prison security and healthcare system, in addition to the increased support and surveillance received by the vulnerable prisoners, seem particularly effective. Definitive assessment of the new system versus the previous F2052SH is awaited though the prison suicide statistics have shown a recent 30 per cent annual fall.

A study by Gunter[23] in the USA found that, although women represent an increasing number of state prison inmates, they are studied less than their male counterparts.

Incarcerated women have higher rates of depression than both community samples and incarcerated men. The diagnosis and treatment of depression in incarcerated women is complicated by the presence of substance abuse, psychosocial stressors, medical problems and personality disorders. The paper showed how a primary care provider based in the community could provide an effective in-reach service to fully meet the primary care mental health needs of the prisoners.

In a study Fogel[24] explored the stressful life event of incarceration for women prisoners and examined its relationship to selected health outcomes. Interviews with 55 women during their first week of incarceration and after six months in prison provided the data for analysis. Specific stresses of incarceration identified by the women included separation from families, worry about their children, and loss of control of their own lives. Psychological stress at time of incarceration was found to be positively related to depression and weight gain after six months of incarceration. Strategies to decrease the stressful nature of incarceration and improve the health status of incarcerated women are recommended by the author. The gender specificity of these findings is likely to be relatively minimal as male prisoners often identify similar psychological stressors [personal observation].

For young people the experience of bereavement seems to complicate the negative mental health effects of imprisonment. A study by Finlay and Jones[25] aimed to pilot a grief awareness programme as a health promotion project for young offenders with complicated grief. Seventeen young offenders in custody at HM Prison Cardiff were opportunistically recruited, interviewed about their bereavement, and offered entry to the programme. Young offenders who reported coping poorly with bereavement were more likely to have used drugs to cope with their emotions, to have had suicidal thoughts, and reported more depression and anxiety. They were also more likely to have been bereaved in late adolescence and to have lost a first-degree relative, with death being sudden, violent or by suicide. Once again it is reasonable to assume that young adult offenders, male or female, might show similar findings.

Such findings highlight the need to consider such aetiologies of behaviour so as to contribute to the use of mitigation and the provision of alternatives to imprisonment in affected young people, and determine and plan effective interventions. The interventions that might be effective in the post-release period appear not to have been studied so a degree of extrapolation is required. The provision in some Primary Care Trusts (PCTs) of a primary care mental health approach for general patients in the community is effective in significantly reducing referrals (by up to 50 per cent) to secondary mental health care [personal communications]. In addition there is evidence from a high-security prison in the UK [personal communications] of an effective primary care mental health approach, again measured by reduced referral to secondary services, and a paper from Brazil[26] promotes the efficiency of the primary care approach, reducing referrals by 36 per cent.

Substance misuse

The key issue for the post-release period that has attracted research interest is drug-related death following release from prison. Bird and Hutchinson,[27] looking at released prisoners from the Scottish jails and young offender institutions, confirmed the theoretical fatal risk to addicts of reduced tolerance following incarceration and the combination of a 'celebratory' fix. It is estimated by the Home Office that that there are approximately 160 ex-prisoners who die from drug overdose in the UK, accidental or intentional, in the first week of release, per year.

Drugs-related mortality in 1996–99 was seven times higher (95 per cent CI [confidence interval]: 3.3–16.3) in the two weeks after release than at other times at liberty and 2.8 times higher than prison suicides (95 per cent CI: 1.5–3.5) by males aged 15–35 years who had been incarcerated for 14+ days. They estimated one drugs-related death in the two weeks after release per 200 adult male injectors released from 14+ days' incarceration. Non-drugs-related deaths in the cohort, in the 12 weeks after release, were 4.9 times (95 per cent CI: 2.8–7.0) the 4.3 deaths expected, which confirmed the findings by Verger[5] on mortality. They concluded that investment in, and evaluation of, prison-based interventions is needed to reduce substantially recently released drugs-related deaths. Seymour et al.[28] also confirmed this finding and the aetiology of the problem. Harding-Pink[29] in 1990 also confirmed the high mortality rate post-release, which is four times the age-adjusted rate for the normal population. Likely risk factors included loss of tolerance to opiates while in prison, and psychological and social stresses following release.

Dual diagnosis, drugs and mental health, is not uncommon in prison. The 1997 Office of National Statistics psychiatric morbidity study[14] identified that histories of abuse, deprivation, homelessness, unemployment and substance misuse are common. Multiple diagnoses of mental health conditions were commonly encountered, especially in remand prisoners; about one quarter of men and one third of women on remand received two or more diagnoses. Services that aim to meet the needs of substance-misusing prisoners will therefore most effectively be delivered in partnership with mental health providers.

The use of benzodiazepines in prison as medication for insomnia has been shown to be a problem that extends into the post-release period and is associated with chronic addiction, mental illness, communicable diseases, criteria of social exclusion and recidivism. Lekka et al.[30] showed that the history of psychiatric hospitalisation, history of illicit drug use, history of unemployment, symptoms of anxiety and hepatitis C virus positivity in their prisoner cohort were independently associated with benzodiazepine use in the prison. Therefore, they concluded, medical and psychiatric interventions focusing on anxiety problems, depression, drug addiction and HCV in this group of benzodiazepine users are warranted.

A paper from Elger[31] in Switzerland advocates the need for better assessment of insomnia and less reliance on benzodiazepines. Her results confirm that insomnia is a frequent complaint among prisoner patients and that at least half of insomnia patients are substance misusers. In non-substance misuse patients, insomnia did not seem to be only a transitory problem of adaptation to incarceration, but a more chronic problem lasting more than three weeks, related to a higher degree of medical and psychological problems before and during incarceration.

It is a feature of the researcher perspective that benzodiazepines are seen as somehow related to a sleep problem; in reality, clinically, they are very problematic drugs of addiction that are commonly used by the offenders as a means to self-medicate their chronic anxiety or depression, or feelings of helplessness. There is no research that currently addresses these issues.

A study in Sheffield[32] confirms the benefits of retention in methadone maintenance programmes on criminal activity (which is the main finding of the larger National Treatment Outcome Research Study – NTORS).[33] *De facto* this small study is looking at many post-release prisoners. A retrospective analysis was made of the criminal records of 57 patients successfully retained in methadone maintenance at two general practices in Sheffield. Their criminal conviction rates and time spent in prison per year were compared for the periods before and after the start of their methadone programme. Overall, patients retained on methadone programmes in the general practices studied had significantly fewer convictions and cautions, and spent significantly less time in prison than they had before the start of treatment.

These findings on drug-related deaths and the importance of the continuity of care principle in methadone maintenance programmes are key factors supporting the establishment of effective handover of care processes and also point to the benefits of bridging services. The national integrated drug treatment strategy, launched in 2006, is now challenging prisons and their local communities to successfully deliver the treatment programmes that have been indicated as likely to be effective by this research. The logistics and the effects on prison regimens are only now becoming evident but the benefits in relation to recidivism and drug-related mortality are clear.

Housing, employment, social care and leisure

There is little evidence from the UK. In a recent paper from San Francisco, Kushel *et al.*[34] describe some of the characteristics and risks associated with homelessness and the links to imprisonment. The USA imprisons approximately ten times the number *pro rata* of the population as in the UK with a significant non-white racial bias, so again the findings may not be particularly generalisable to the UK.

They studied a large sample of homeless and marginally housed adults to examine whether a history of imprisonment was associated with differences in health status, drug use and sexual behaviours among the homeless. Almost one in four participants (23.1 per cent) had a history of imprisonment. Models that examined lifetime substance use showed cocaine use (odds ratio [OR] = 1.67; 95 per cent CI = 1.04, 2.70), heroin use (OR = 1.51; 95 per cent CI = 1.07, 2.12), mental illness (OR = 1.41; 95 per cent CI = 1.01, 1.96), HIV infection (OR = 1.69; 95 per cent CI = 1.07, 2.64), and having had more than 100 sexual partners were associated with a history of imprisonment. Models that examined recent substance use showed past-year heroin use (OR = 1.65; 95 per cent CI = 1.14, 2.38) and methamphetamine use (OR = 1.49; 95 per cent CI = 1.00, 2.21) were associated with lifetime imprisonment. Currently selling drugs also was associated with lifetime imprisonment.

They concluded that, despite high levels of health risks among all homeless and marginally housed people, the levels among homeless former prisoners were even higher and that efforts to eradicate homelessness must also include the unmet needs of inmates who are released from prison. The study also confirms the relative similarities of the homeless or marginally housed population and of prisoners.

Recent national policy initiatives for prison and offender mental health care

Offender Mental Health Care Pathway[35]

This pathway is intended to guide the practice of people who directly deliver services, and support decision making for those who commission them. It contains a large number of templates based on best evidence and good practice. It acknowledges the key issues presented with this paper of the importance of primary care mental health services and the continuity of care between prisons and upon release. This is a key and well-evidenced piece of work that must now be utilised to improve services to prisoners.

Mental health in-reach collaborative launch

The in-reach project is a fundamental component of the prison mental health modernisation agenda and is crucial in the implementation of the strategy set out in the document *Changing the Outlook: a strategy for developing and modernising mental health services in prisons.*[36] The mental health in-reach concept has been delivered through the use of a national collaborative approach first pioneered by Don Berwick in the USA. The focus on delivering best clinical practice makes collaboratives a useful vehicle to potentially take forward the main principles of this paper.

Changing the Outlook[36]

Produced in 2001 this very important document set out a joint Department of Health and Prison Service approach to far-reaching development and modernisation of mental health services in prisons over the next 3–5 years, in line with, and ensuring that prisoners benefit equally from, the National Service Framework for Mental Health and *The NHS Plan*.

The aims of the document are stated as:

- a reduction in the number of prisoners located in prison healthcare centres, with resources re-deployed to provide day care and wing-based support
- a reduction in the average length of time mentally ill prisoners spend in those prison healthcare beds that remain
- a more appropriate skill mix among those providing mental health care, so that prisoners have access to the right range of services to NHS standards
- increased numbers of day care places
- improved wing-based services
- better integration between the Prison Service and NHS staff, to encourage skills transfer among staff, reduce professional isolation, and to facilitate the exchange of information
- quicker and more effective arrangements for transferring the most seriously ill prisoners to appropriate NHS facilities and receiving them back
- increased collaboration by NHS staff in the management of those who are seriously mentally ill, including those vulnerable to suicide or self-harm whilst they are in prison
- improved health and social functioning for patients.

Safer Prisons Report[37]

This is a very important and detailed paper looking primarily at current prisoners rather than the recently released. A brief summary will inevitably miss major issues. The following notes only the recent release period and the key recommendation for post-release:

- in a 4-year study period (1996–2000), 354 people were found to have committed suicide within one year of release from prison, i.e. 88 cases per year
- these deaths clustered immediately after release with 80 (23 per cent) in the first month and 40 in the first week
- this concurs with a recently produced unpublished paper giving a 35 times higher risk of death from suicide than the normal population in the first week following release and a risk of five times in the first year

- the release of prisoners with mental health problems should be coordinated with mental health teams outside prison
- care plans should be jointly reviewed by prison and local staff prior to release
- those 'at risk' of self-harm should be followed up within a week of release.

National strategy for the clinical management of drug dependence in prisons

The drivers behind the new national strategy (2006) for the clinical management of drug dependence in prisons are the high rates of suicide on admission to prison and the concern about drug-related deaths post-release. There has also been legal challenge to the variability of services available in prisons and the lack of equivalence with national and international community-based services. Many prisons have attempted to address these issues but have faced difficulties working with the prison regimen, providing continuity with other health and criminal justice-based services and community teams, and in particular the difficulties arising from the Home Office-originated and restrictive remit of the Counselling, Assessment, Referral, Advice and Throughcare (CARAT) teams. Particular problems remain in respect of dual-diagnosis patients, and those with mostly alcohol problems, which will be the subject of future guidance.

The key elements of the new strategy are:

- opiate substitution therapy for stabilisation of all, and maintenance of some, heroin-addicted prisoners
- approximately £60m of new funding from the Home Office and Department of Health
- a treatment framework for clinical management.

The key treatment options included within the policy are:

- doctor-prescribed management of withdrawal in first-night reception
- stabilisation for five days converting to detoxification, extended detoxification or maintenance therapy
- safe alcohol detoxification
- managed benzodiazepine withdrawal
- clinical monitoring of stimulant withdrawal
- linkage in the prison between CARAT teams and substance misuse teams, and with services before admission and after release
- joint management between substance misuse teams and mental health teams for patients with dual diagnosis
- regular drug testing for prolonged treatment regimens
- psychosocial support.

Reducing Re-offending by Ex-prisoners [38]

There is now considerable evidence of the factors that influence re-offending. Many of the statistics from the Social Exclusion Unit report *Reducing Re-offending by Ex-prisoners* inform this chapter. Building on criminological and social research, the Social Exclusion Unit has identified nine key factors:

- education
- employment
- drug and alcohol misuse
- mental and physical health
- attitudes and self-control
- institutionalisation and life skills
- housing
- financial support and debt
- family networks.

The evidence shows that these factors can have a huge impact on the likelihood of a prisoner re-offending. For example, being in employment reduces the risk of re-offending by between a third and a half; having stable accommodation reduces the risk by a fifth.

That physical health, mental health and drug and alcohol issues are highlighted enhances the importance of the development of services and personal strategies and plans for offenders, in order to better manage these harmful influences. The focus on re-offending helps to strengthen the imperative for better partnership building and joint working between government departments, regional agencies and the health, social and criminal justice systems.

An evidence and principle-based proposal – Integrated Inclusive Care Programmes

The author, in conjunction with Mrs Jackie Prosser and other colleagues from the National Institute for Mental Health in England, took part in the International Trailblazers initiative and developed an approach or vision that seeks to address the current policy gap. The scope of the project is the health and social care services for socially excluded people, including young people, with an emphasis on primary care mental health and continuity of care into, through and on release from the prison system. The approach can be summarised as promoting Integrated Inclusive Care Programmes (IICP) for local health and prison communities. Starting with a list of principles the project promotes the IICP approach and is currently planning how to influence policy, assure the effectiveness legitimacy of the approach, and gain further support.

A brief summary of the concept follows.

Aim

To improve significantly the health of, and the health and social care services available to, socially excluded people, in the community and in prisons, ensuring continuity of care and with a special emphasis on primary mental health.

Key deliverables

- Improve access for mentally ill offenders to the NHS.
- Reduce suicides in and after prison.
- Continuity of primary care for offenders.
- Increasing offender employment.
- Reducing health inequalities parameters.
- Influence partners and Department of Health policy in this area.
- Raising the profile of offender issues in related health and social care programmes delivery.

Principles

We believe that:

- there should be health and social care services designed to be more effective to support the socially excluded
- continuity of care as people pass through, in and out of the prison system is a critical issue, morally and in respect of delivering effective care
- these services should be designed by local stakeholders to be responsive to the needs of the individuals and their families, responding, over time, to a changing population. Access to the services is to be on the basis of choice
- to be effective services will need to be proactive and incorporate such resources as assertive outreach, patient tracking, identified support personnel and advocates
- these services should deliver the same or better quality of care to the socially excluded as is delivered to the population as a whole. This should be measured in relation to patient outcomes thereby reducing health inequalities
- in designing these services it will be important to identify which specific healthcare interventions/service functions are required for a particular local socially excluded population and prison population
- the range of services provided will need to be appropriate, supported by best available evidence and ensure an equivalence of standards of care across the country

- the workforce to deliver these services can be configured in a range of different ways and with a range of different skill mix. Additionally the workforce will need to be well-trained, resourced and supported, working within and between the prison and community

- primary care will be the foundation of these services, delivered by a range of providers, including alternative or Primary Care Trust medical services and incorporating enhanced service and specialist clinician models

- adherence to these principles will prove to be effective and efficient but that the implementation should be as far as possible evidenced based.

The *strategic vision* therefore becomes to make these principles manifest, to improve the health and wellbeing, health care, and social capital of the socially excluded and of prisoners.

Figure 17.1 demonstrates a *horizontal integration over time* and between prison and community services, and a *vertical integration between the range of services* or care pathways required to tailor health and social care to meet the needs of prisoners before and during incarceration, and after release.

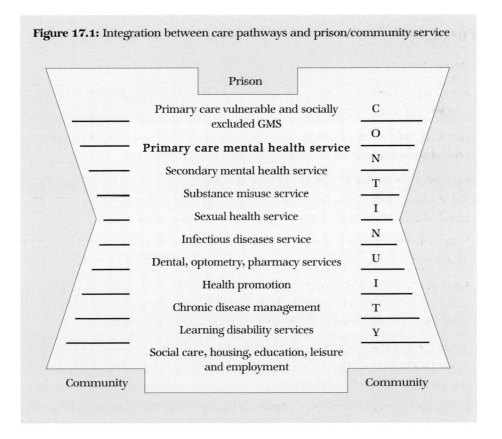

Figure 17.1: Integration between care pathways and prison/community service

Hence the model of care is called an Integrated Inclusive Care Programme (IICP), delivered by a model of service *locally designed for local needs*.

The challenges in taking this forward are seen as:

- need for champions from service users

- engagement of health and social care commissioning structures

- overcoming concerns of the workforce

- lack of workforce

- clinicians' concerns regarding these potential service users

- managing change in the current structures and workforce

- training

- IT systems, records and communication

- making this a priority for local health communities

- delivering creative solutions for the realisation of the principles.

Improving the health, social care and prospects of the socially excluded including prisoners is seen as a significant goal. Are the principles right? In particular is the approach of tailoring services v. providing an equity of services right, morally and in terms of service user acceptability, effectiveness and efficiency? And how and over what timeframe should the pursuit of this vision proceed? The recent Department of Health consultation exercise that resulted in the policy guidance *Our Health, Our Care, Our Say* confirmed a wish for services to be community based wherever possible and to be non-stigmatising.[39] Hence such services should be as normalised as possible whilst retaining a distinctive functionality.

It has been reassuring that this approach has received general support from the Trailblazer International group, at regional and national Care Services Improvement Partnership fora, from a number of local health communities, at executive, public health and health promotion level, and from colleagues at the Department of Health, the NHS Confederation and in the prison health community. The approach resonates with the need for continuity of care, community-based services, and breadth of services, all discussed and affirmed at the recent World Health Organization conference on prison health. Finally the research review that has supported this chapter has revealed the effectiveness of locally designed, multi-agency and multidisciplinary, primary care-based programmes that closely follow prisoners as they move from the prison into the community. The vision presented is therefore seen as a key area for policy development.

Conclusion

The emphasis of the primary care mental health pathway in the IICP model should not be underestimated; it is its most important element. As can be seen from the evidence presented in this chapter, prisoners and offenders suffer from, and are largely under-provided for, significant levels of primary mental health problems. The benefits of the effective provision of care – for anxiety, depression, bereavement, well-controlled psychosis, obsessive-compulsive disorder, post-traumatic stress disorder, personality disorder, mild learning disability, substance misuse, self-harm, eating and body dysmorphic disorders, low self-esteem, all the stuff of primary care mental health – can only currently be theorised because the research evidence is relatively lacking.

Such a development in service provision may well create a step change reduction in recidivism rates, and such service development should be based on coordinated local health and social care investment. In prison settings where these services are provided the care is appreciated by the prisoners and has resulted in reduced referrals to secondary care providers. It is a simple matter of equivalence of access to care that primary care mental health should be better provided in the prison setting, and continued into the community.

Access is everything in health care. The challenges presented and faced by the prisoner and offender population, though significant, can be overcome, and the benefits to them and society, though hard won, will I believe be worthwhile and significant.

References

1. Reed J, Lyne M, HM Inspectorate of Prisons, Home Office, London. The quality of health care in prison: results of a year's programme of semistructured inspections *British Medical Journal* 1997; **315(7120)**: 1420–4.

2. Department of Health. *The Future Organisation of Prison Health Care* London: DH, 1999.

3. Watson R, Stimpson A, Hostick T. Prison health care: a review of the literature *International Journal of Nursing Studies* 2004; **41(2)**: 119–28.

4. Martin RE, Hislop TG, Grams GD, *et al*. Beware of multiple names in database linkage research: prevalence of aliases in female prison population *British Medical Journal* 2005; **331(7512)**: 335–6.

5. Verger P, Rotily M, Prudhomme J, *et al*. Regional Health Observatory-INSERM U-379, Marseille, France. High mortality rates among inmates during the year following their discharge from a French prison *Journal of Forensic Sciences* 2003; **48(3)**: 614–16.

6. Clavel F, Benhamou S, Flamant R. Unite de Recherches en Epidemiologie des Cancers de l'INSERM (U287), Villejuif, France. Decreased mortality among male prisoners *Lancet* 1987; **2(8566)**: 1012–14.

7. Martin E. Comparison of medical care in prison and in general practice *British Medical Journal (Clinical Research Ed.)* 1984; **289(6450)**: 967–9.

8. Martin E, Colebrook M, Gray A. Health of prisoners admitted to and discharged from Bedford Prison *British Medical Journal (Clinical Research Ed.)* 1984; **289(6450)**: 965–7.

9. Demers R, Walsh K. Use of medical services during a 2-month period in the Seattle-King County (Washington) jail *Public Health Reports* 1981; **96(5)**: 452–7.

10. Engebretsen B, Olson JW. Primary care in a penal institution. A study of health care problems encountered *Medical Care* 1975; **13(9)**: 775–81.

11. Signposting to prison health, Sharing Good Practice Conference, May 2005, York.

12. Maeve MK. Nursing care partnerships with women leaving jail. Effects on health and crime *Journal of Psychosocial Nursing & Mental Health Services* 2003; **41(9)**: 30–40.

13. Wildbore A. Opportunities to promote health to vulnerable male teenagers. Trafford Youth Offending Team, Manchester *Nursing Times* 2004; **100(29)**: 36–7.

14. Singleton N, Meltzer H, Gatward R. *Psychiatric Morbidity amongst Prisoners in England and Wales* London: Stationery Office, 1998.

15. Reed JL, Lyne M. Inpatient care of mentally ill people in prison: results of a year's programme of semi structured inspections *British Medical Journal* 2000; **320(7241)**: 1031–4.

16. Bisson JI, Searle MM, Srinivasan M. Follow-up study of British military hostages and their families held in Kuwait during the Gulf War *British Journal of Medical Psychology* 1998; **71(pt 3)**: 247–52.

17. Wolff N, Plemmons D, Veysey B, *et al*. Release planning for inmates with mental illness compared with those who have other chronic illnesses *Psychiatric Services* 2002; **53(11)**: 1469–71.

18. McCoy ML, Roberts DL, Hanrahan P, *et al*. Jail linkage assertive community treatment services for individuals with mental illnesses *Psychiatric Rehabilitation Journal* 2004; **27(3)**: 243–50.

19. Lovell D, Gagliardi GJ, Peterson PD. Recidivism and use of services among persons with mental illness after release from prison *Psychiatric Services* 2002; **53(10)**: 1290–6.

20. Ventura LA, Cassel CA, Jacoby JE, *et al*. Case management and recidivism of mentally ill persons released from jail *Psychiatric Services* 1998; **49(10)**: 1330–7.

21. Hartwell S. Short-term outcomes for offenders with mental illness released from incarceration *International Journal of Offender Therapy and Comparative Criminology* 2003; **47(2)**: 145–58.

22. Roth B, Presse L. Nursing interventions for parasuicidal behaviors in female offenders *Journal of Psychosocial Nursing & Mental Health Services* 2003; **41(9)**: 20–9.

23. Gunter TD. Incarcerated women and depression: a primer for the primary care provider *Journal of the American Medical Women's Association* 2004; **59(2)**: 107–12.

24. Fogel CI. Hard time: the stressful nature of incarceration for women *Issues in Mental Health Nursing* 1993; **14(4)**: 367–77.

25. Finlay IG, Jones NK. Unresolved grief in young offenders in prison *British Journal of General Practice* 2000; **50(456)**: 569–70.

26. Taborda JG, Bertolote JM, Cardoso RG, *et al*. The impact of primary mental health care in a prison system in Brazil. WHO Collaborating Centre for Research and Training in Mental Health, Porto Alegre, Rio Grande do Sul, Brazil *Canadian Journal of Psychiatry – Revue Canadienne de Psychiatrie* 1999; **44(2)**: 180–2.

27. Bird SM, Hutchinson SJ. Male drugs-related deaths in the fortnight after release from prison: Scotland, 1996–99 *Addiction* 2003; **98(2)**: 185–90.

28. Seymour A, Oliver JS, Black M. Drug-related deaths among recently released prisoners in the Strathclyde Region of Scotland *Journal of Forensic Sciences* 2000; **45**: 649–54.

29. Harding-Pink D. Related articles, mortality following release from prison *Medicine, Science and the Law* 1990; **30(1)**: 12–6.

30. Lekka NP, Paschalis C, Papadourakis A, *et al*. Characteristics of inmates receiving prescribed benzodiazepines in a high-security Greek prison *Comprehensive Psychiatry* 2003; **44(5)**: 409–14.

31. Elger BS. Prevalence, types and possible causes of insomnia in a Swiss remand prison. Medecine penitentiaire et Institut universitaire de medecine legale, Geneva, Switzerland *European Journal of Epidemiology* 2004; **19(7)**: 665–77.

32. Keen J, Rowse G, Mathers N, *et al*. Can methadone maintenance for heroin-dependent patients retained in general practice reduce criminal conviction rates and time spent in prison? Institute of General Practice and Primary Care, Northern General Hospital, Sheffield *British Journal of General Practice* 2000; **50(450)**: 48–9.

33. Godfrey C, Stewart D, Gossop M. Economic analysis of cost and consequences of the treatment of drug misuse: 2 year outcome data from the National Treatment Outcome Research Study (NTORS) *Addiction* 2004; **99(6)**: 697–707.

34. Kushel MB, Hahn JA, Evans JL, *et al*. Revolving doors: imprisonment among the homeless and marginally housed population *American Journal of Public Health* 2005; **95(10)**: 1747–52.

35. Department of Health and National Institute for Mental Health in England. *Offender Mental Health Care Pathway* London: DH, 2005.

36. Department of Health. *Changing the Outlook: a strategy for developing and modernising mental health services in prisons* London: DH, 2001.

37. Shaw J, Appleby L, Baker D. *Safer Prisons Report – a national study of prison suicides 1999–2000 by the National Confidential Inquiry into Suicides and Homicides by People with Mental Illness* London: DH.

38. Office of the Deputy Prime Minister. *Reducing Re-offending by Ex-prisoners* London: Stationery Office, 2002.

39 Department of Health. *Our Health, Our Care, Our Say: a new direction for community services* London: DH, 2006, www.dh.gov.uk/en/Publicationsandstatistics/Publications/Publications PolicyAndGuidance/ DH_4127453 [accessed November 2007].

18 | Social inclusion

Brian Fisher

What this chapter contributes:

causes of social exclusion and its relation to health outcomes

how social exclusion presents in primary care

GP role in reducing social exclusion.

Health inequalities, mental health and patient and public involvement – 'unwell some of the time – excluded all of the time'

There's a man I know – well he's been on the go
For years and years and years
And he's a little bit high – and he's a little bit low
And his eyes are thick with tears
Somebody knows him – but nobody shows him
That his life could be his own
Nobody tries – when somebody cries –
'Why must he be alone?' – 'Why must he be alone?'

Insanity man – when will they understand?

When will they shake your hand – and say –
'Hey man – you've been through it'
'Say man – you can do it'?
Insanity man – when will they take the stand?
Well I don't think they can – they say –
'No way man – you can rough it'
'Go 'way man – you can stuff it'

(B. Gladman, song recorded on CD in 2001)[i]

This chapter aims to define social exclusion in the field of mental health and describe how it links with patient and public involvement. It draws heavily on other published work to describe practical approaches that we in primary care can implement to reduce social exclusion and improve the lives of people with long-term severe mental health problems.

Action on inclusion needs to be seen as a moral imperative – a vision of a future where people with mental health problems have the same opportunities to work and participate in their communities as any other citizen.[2]

The effects of social exclusion

Social exclusion means that people with mental health problems do not share in the benefits of society to the same degree as those without. For instance:

- less than a quarter of people with long-term mental health problems are working – the lowest employment rate for any of the main groups of disabled people (see Figure 18.1)

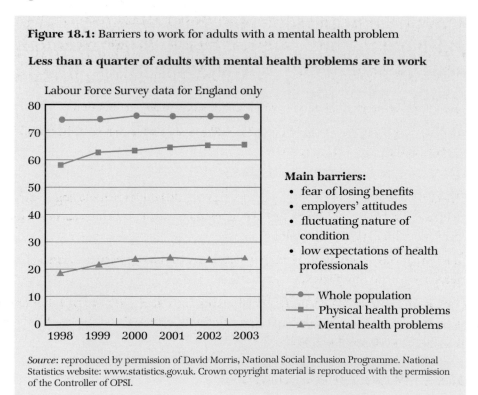

Figure 18.1: Barriers to work for adults with a mental health problem

Less than a quarter of adults with mental health problems are in work

Labour Force Survey data for England only

Main barriers:
- fear of losing benefits
- employers' attitudes
- fluctuating nature of condition
- low expectations of health professionals

— Whole population
— Physical health problems
— Mental health problems

Source: reproduced by permission of David Morris, National Social Inclusion Programme. National Statistics website: www.statistics.gov.uk. Crown copyright material is reproduced with the permission of the Controller of OPSI.

- social isolation is an important risk factor for deteriorating mental health and suicide (see Figure 18.2). Two thirds of men under the age of 35 with mental health problems who die by suicide are unemployed.

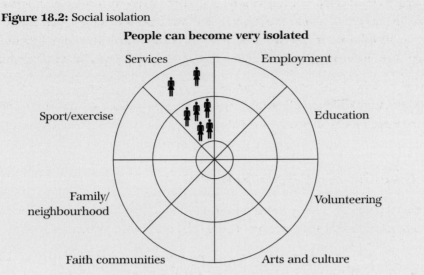

Figure 18.2: Social isolation

People can become very isolated

Sue attends the day centre and the clinic
She has five friends she sees at outpatients or the day centre

Note: the Inclusion Web is introduced at www.ndt.org.uk/projectsN/SI.htm and its use with 150 subjects is reported in Hacking S, Bates P. The Inclusion Web as a tool for person-centred planning and service evaluation *Mental Health Review Journal: research, policy and practice*, 2008 (forthcoming).

Source: reproduced by permission of David Morris, National Social Inclusion Programme, and the National Development Team.

In one survey, 44 per cent of people with mental health problems felt that:

- they had experienced discrimination from GPs, while 18 per cent said they would not disclose their condition to a GP.

Also:

- fewer than four in ten employers say that they would consider employing someone with a history of mental health problems, compared with more than six in ten for someone with a physical disability

- a third of people with mental health problems report having been dismissed or forced to resign from their job.

The statistics are to be found in the Social Exclusion Unit report.[3] On p. 118 it has a graphic representation of the financial results of not tackling the problems. It is clear that this is pressing and important.

Causes of social exclusion

Stigma and discrimination against people with mental health problems is pervasive throughout society. Despite a number of campaigns, there has been no significant change in attitudes.[4] Fewer than four in ten employers say they would recruit someone with a mental health problem.[5] Many people fear disclosing their condition, even to family and friends.

Professionals often have low expectations of what people with mental health problems can achieve. There is limited recognition in the NHS that returning to work and over-coming social isolation is associated with better health outcomes. Employment is not seen as a key objective for people with mental health problems by many health and social care professionals.

There is a lack of clear responsibility for promoting vocational and social outcomes for adults with mental health problems. Services do not always work effectively together to meet individual needs and maximise the impact of available resources.

People can lack ongoing support to enable them to work. £140 million a year is invested by health and social care in vocational and day services for people with mental health problems.[6] But not all of these promote social inclusion as effectively as they could, and links with Jobcentre Plus can be weak. People on benefits often do not believe they will end up financially better off if they try to move into work. Many people lose jobs that they might have kept had they received better support (see Figure 18.3).

People face barriers to engaging in the community. They can struggle to access the basic services they need, in particular decent housing and transport. Education, arts, sports and leisure providers often are not aware how their services could benefit people with mental health problems and how they could make their services more accessible for this group. Many people do not want to participate in activities alone, but feel there is no one they can ask to go with them. People can also face exclusion by law from some community roles such as jury service.

Figure 18.3: Adults with mental health problems claiming incapacity benefit (IB) in England, 1995–2002

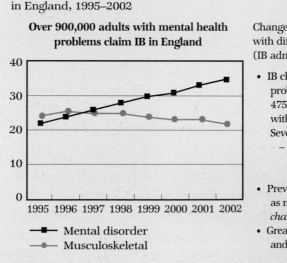

Over 900,000 adults with mental health problems claim IB in England

Mental disorder

Musculoskeletal

Changes in proportions of IB claimants with different diagnoses (IB admin data)

- IB claimants with mental health problems have almost doubled from 475,000 in 1995 to 848,000 in 2002, with a further 58,200 claiming Severe Disablement Allowance
  – doesn't include mental health problems as a secondary condition
- Prevalence of mental health problems as measured by ONS *has not changed over the last decade*
- Greater proportions still on IB after one and three years cf. other claimants

Source: reproduced by permission of David Morris, National Social Inclusion Programme. Department of Work and Pensions website: www.dwp.gov.uk. Crown copyright material is reproduced with the permission of the Controller of OPSI.

Specific groups

Some groups face particular barriers to getting their mental health and social needs addressed:

Ethnic minorities may feel alienated from mainstream (predominantly white) mental health services, and so tend to present late to mental health services. They have often had contact with the criminal justice system, are more likely to disagree with their diagnosis, and can encounter discrimination on grounds of both health status and ethnicity in seeking work.

Young men with mental health problems are at high risk of dropping out of education or work, of becoming involved with crime, and they are a particularly high-risk group for suicide.

Parents with mental health problems – particularly lone parents – have very low employment rates,[7] may not receive sufficient family support and their children may develop emotional problems.[8] Adults with complex needs, such as substance misuse or homelessness in addition to their mental health problems, often struggle to get their needs met by statutory services.[9]

How issues of social exclusion may present to primary care

Presentations may not be obvious and one of the reasons for this is that general practice may be seen as one of the agents of exclusion by our patients. It can be difficult for clinicians to discuss and understand the issues, particularly when patients find them difficult to discuss with people in general and with clinicians in particular.

However, some of the markers that should alert us may include:

- *medically unexplained symptoms*. People presenting with repeated complaints for which we cannot find a physical cause should prompt us to think of psychological factors underlying the presentation. In addition, we should be thinking that social or cultural factors may be relevant

- *depression*. We must always remember that social exclusion in the form of poverty, joblessness and racial discrimination may underlie the symptoms. Unless we ask, we will not understand or be able to help effectively

- *poor compliance with medication*. Again, unless we understand the ways in which culture and information about health affect people's drug taking, we cannot be very useful. Exhortation without understanding is not helpful

- *doctor-dependent behaviours* may also be underpinned by cultural factors. Moving people to independence can be hard, but it will be harder if we don't understand the social forces that drive the behaviour

- *self-harm* may also be a presentation that has social factors at its root. We need to be prepared to explore these difficult areas to support patients in improvement.

In principle, we need to approach mental illness in general and issues of social exclusion in particular through the principle of empowering patients to find their own solutions to their situation. GPs can help analyse and reflect back to patients. We should be working with outside agencies such as community and statutory groups to improve patients' lives. We ourselves are not the solution they need. We can be conductors of an orchestra of people and agencies to support and empower our patients to find their solutions to their problems. This approach is particularly important when issues of social exclusion are centre-field.

What follows is a series of suggestions for how this might be supported in primary care.

Patient and public involvement and community development

The government says, in its discussion paper *A Stronger Local Voice*, that it is committed to:

- developing a health and social care system planned around the needs of individual people and those of the wider community

- creating health and social care services that are, regardless of who provides them, user-centred, responsive, flexible, open to challenge, accountable to communities and constantly open to improvement

- devolving decision making to the local level. Some 80 per cent of the NHS budget is now devolved to Primary Care Trusts (PCTs), meaning that priorities are decided locally.[2]

Patient and Public Involvement (PPI) offers a number of benefits across the NHS[10] both generally and in the field of mental health. One of the exciting consequences of PPI is that the act of involvement itself can be therapeutic for those engaged, quite apart from the improvements to the system that can result. The user movement has made significant improvements to the kind of care that is now offered to users of the service.[11] In the collective process of supporting each other to make change, some individuals have received considerable support. In general, PPI, particularly if it has a community development aspect, can have significant health-protective effects. We see PPI as underpinning an approach to reducing social exclusion in primary care.

I emphasise the importance of community development (CD) in this context. CD can, to some degree, roll back the effects of isolation and can help users back into productive links with others.

CD can be defined as a process that mobilises communities to become participants in both defining problems and developing solutions to health and health service issues. It can involve:

- lay needs assessment, taking a holistic view
- new as well as more appropriate services
- inter-agency work, improving relationships
- builds communities, reduces social exclusion.[12]

There is now good evidence that significant health protection is achieved by bringing people together through encouraging the formation of networks.[13] Confidence increases, transferable skills are learnt, people make friends. A wide range of beneficial effects can be shown.

There is evidence that leg ulcers improve when people become less lonely[14] and child health is better as networks become denser.[15] Longitudinal studies have shown that the impact of social networks on health is especially dramatic in childhood. Studies of children brought up in orphanages have long established that, even with a plentiful diet, children's physical and intellectual growth can be dramatically stunted in the absence of loving relationships.

Survival rates following major surgery or illness in later life are strongly predicted by marital status and the presence of close confiding relationships.[16] People with strong networks recover better from cardiovascular disease (see Figure 18.4).[17]

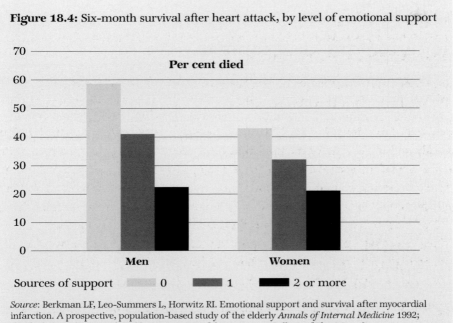

Figure 18.4: Six-month survival after heart attack, by level of emotional support

Per cent died

Men   Women

Sources of support   0   1   2 or more

Source: Berkman LF, Leo-Summers L, Horwitz RI. Emotional support and survival after myocardial infarction. A prospective, population-based study of the elderly *Annals of Internal Medicine* 1992; **117(12)**: 1003–9. Reproduced by permission of the American College of Physicians.[3]

The striking health impact of social networks is seen in Roseto in Pennsylvania. Despite having unhealthy diets, this community had unusually low rates of heart attacks attributable to its close social relationships. When this pattern of community life weakened in the 1970s, death rates rose to the normal rate.[18] Similar causes explain the significantly higher life expectancies of the Finno-Swedish minority in Finland. Putnam found that joining a group halved one's chances of dying within the next year.[19]

The mental health links are important. Bonding social capital provided by family and close friends provides tangible assistance and improves wellbeing and belonging, whereas its absence leads to isolation and depression.[20] Petersen *et al*. conclude that access to and utilisation of social networks are important to success in finding work.[21] Social disorganisation correlates to rates of suicide and crime.[22]

At the national level, a number of studies have found a significant correlation between measures of social capital, especially trust in people, and rates of economic growth (controlling for other factors). Indeed the influence of social capital on economic growth appears to be at least as strong as the influence of human capital.[23]

The implication of this evidence is that supporting PCTs in engaging with their communities will reap significant health and social rewards for individuals, communities and the state, with a positive impact on education, joblessness and crime.

There are a number of examples of CD-supporting developments in mental health. A good example is Lewisham Community Development Partnership (LCDP), based in Southeast London, which has always facilitated the link between PPI and health improvement.[24]

The current political context

In the last quarter of 2006, the omens looked grim for healthcare organisations such as PCTs that focus on the issue of social inclusion and PPI. The incentives offered by Payment by Results and Practice-Based Commissioning (PBC), when applied to mental health, are likely to lead to a focus on organisations finding the cheapest, most efficient approaches to care. Social exclusion may not be seen as important in that context.

In addition, the consolidation of health services as the financial situation bites will lead to a focus on reduction of services and reorganisation into larger units. The process in itself is likely to take people's eyes off social exclusion.

The new arrangements for Local Involvement Networks (LINK – these are the successors to PPI Forums) that are likely to come into force in 2008 are as yet untried. We do not know whether they will enhance PPI in general and what impact they will have on users of mental health services. LINKs will be existing voluntary agencies who will be funded to offer proactive involvement across health and social care organisations, gathering information, and passing it to PCTs and Overview and Scrutiny Committees. There will be a new duty placed on commissioners to respond to patients and the public.[10]

This arrangement attempts to find a balance between a proactive approach building on current energy and experience and a formal approach that can sometimes tie groups down and encourage a defensive attitude by the NHS.

Practice-Based Commissioning and Patient and Public Involvement

From April 2006 each individual practice, or groups of practices, were given a budget with which to buy care for their patients. The budget is based on historical spend on hospital referrals (see Figure 18.5).

If practices generate savings by either doing fewer referrals or by referring patients to cheaper services, often in a community setting, those savings can be used for improved patient care. For instance, if patients with osteoarthritis of the hips are referred to exercise classes rather than operations, the savings could be used to buy more physiotherapists based in the community. This process is underpinned by a nationally agreed tariff for procedures. A tariff is not yet in place for mental health commissioning, but may come into force in 2008 (see Chapter 2). The principle and process as described here will then largely apply.[25]

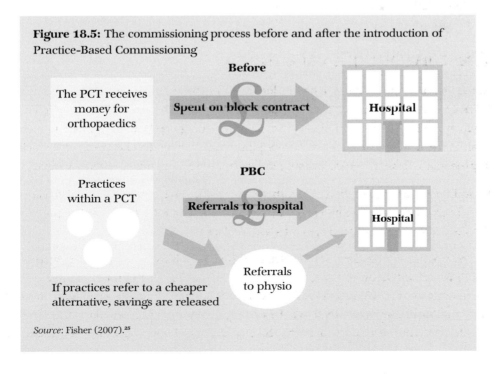

Figure 18.5: The commissioning process before and after the introduction of Practice-Based Commissioning

Before

The PCT receives money for orthopaedics

Spent on block contract

Hospital

PBC

Practices within a PCT

Referrals to hospital

Hospital

Referrals to physio

If practices refer to a cheaper alternative, savings are released

Source: Fisher (2007).[25]

Patient Choice

Patient Choice is a phrase used mainly to describe the ability of individuals to make choices in the NHS system. It is currently exercised mainly at the point of referral, when patients can choose their hospital and are given information to help them make that choice. This includes comparative data such as parking facilities, star ratings, MRSA rates. In reality, there may be few choices in rural areas.

Patients are in theory more likely to choose hospitals with good outcomes and good patient-centred services, thus introducing market forces into the system.

Patient and Public Involvement

There is no formal mechanism for patient or public influence over the general development of services in PBC. For instance, commissioning practices may decide that most diabetics should be cared for outside of hospitals. This may be a sound decision, but there may have been no discussion about this with local people at all. The same is true of non-Foundation Trust hospitals – they can make investment (or dis-investment) decisions with little recourse to local people.

Foundation Hospitals have a mechanism by which patients and staff can influence decisions. The model is based on that developed by trade unions, exemplified by the cooperative movement. There is a large members' group, with a central committee having some powers over decision making. There is debate over its effectiveness, but it is an important and interesting model that could be exported, with improvements, to PCTs.

The difference between PPI and Choice

As currently construed, 'Choice' and PPI are different. Choice is best described as enhancing individuals' ability to get what they want from the system, mainly in referral, but, in future, over management of their care.

In the field of mental health, the individual's ability to influence his or her care is a key issue. The power to discuss with the clinician, for instance, about talking therapies or about prescribed drugs is of great importance. If technology and process could enable a more equal dialogue, this would be seen by many patients as a significant step forward.

PPI should be seen as a more holistic, collective approach, where the local population, as well as individuals – the public as well as patients – offer recommendations for good practice that affects and influences the delivery of care for all. Choice is subsumed within PPI.

What can GPs do to reduce social exclusion and improve PPI?

Social exclusion is a complex issue and many of the solutions lie well outside the purview of general practice, though PCTs have a broader and more relevant set of responsibilities in this regard.

Nonetheless, there are a number of interventions that would make a substantial difference. Key areas on which GPs could focus include:

- developing best practice in issuing certificates to ensure patients stay out of work for as short a time as possible

- encouraging the take-up of benefits

- the promotion of CD and social networks

- promoting the physical health of users of mental health services

- linking with voluntary agencies

- attending Care Programme Approach (CPA) meetings to offer a more holistic view, on occasion

- supporting Patients as Teachers (PAT)

- Patient Participation Group (PPG).

In order to do these things, a practice would need to work closely with other agencies. It would be almost impossible to do all these things in-house. The Royal College of General Practitioners has developed a set of good-practice recommendations.[26] What follows reflects these closely.

Certificates and employment

We are spending time on employment issues in this section because the area is so critical to social exclusion. It is also discussed in Chapter 3 on psychological therapies.

GP advice has been shown to be important in shaping patient and employer beliefs, and influencing patients' return to work. Managing certification is an active part of managing the patient. GPs could consider certification in the same category as writing a prescription. Used appropriately, certification can support recovery and rehabilitation.

People with mental health problems are capable of work. US research[3] found that up to 58 per cent of adults with severe and enduring mental health problems are able to work with the right support.

People with mental health problems do want to work. Thirty-five per cent of people with mental health problems who are economically inactive would like to work, compared with 28 per cent of those with other health conditions. Many successful people have had mental health problems.[3]

As time away from work extends, significant adverse health effects can occur – depression and other psychological problems increase whatever the original diagnosis. The longer a patient is off work the lower the chances of returning. Less than 50 per cent of people with six months' sickness absence ever return to work and few people return to any form of work after 1–2 years' absence irrespective of further treatment. A useful timeline is given at this website of the Department for Work and Pensions.[27]

It is possible to issue a Med 3 certificate without putting the patient off work by offering advice to the employer in the 'remarks' section about workplace adjustments. Also, if the patient is off sick, GPs can suggest work adjustments to enable an early return. These could include graduated work and/or a change in working hours or a workplace assessment by an occupational health professional.

Distinguishing between work problems and other factors is important. If other factors are the main problem, getting back to work may aid recovery. Signing patients off work may risk their job and add to their problems.

Strategies directed towards job retention are of proven value; they are most effective in the first months of sickness absence. These include cognitive behavioural therapy (CBT) and specific work counselling. Returning to work after acute symptoms of depression have eased, but before they have completely resolved, may aid recovery.

Work closely with an employment adviser

A JobcentrePlus Personal Adviser should be helpful to patients. GPs can refer directly to a Disability Employment Adviser by adding a note in the 'remarks' section of the Med 3. See IB204 at www.dwp.gov.uk/medical. Employment advisers hold sessions in some practices and that makes communication and uptake of benefits much easier and more effective. The government is considering making this service more widely available.

The promotion of community development

PCTs and local authorities are increasingly working with Community Development Workers (CDWs). It should not be too difficult to get in touch with a CDW in a GP commissioning cluster or neighbourhood area. In fact, PBC may well stimulate the use of CD in local areas. CDWs can help set up voluntary or non-profit organisations to promote PBC.

CD can help by:

- listening to local people using various methods. These can vary from the conventional questionnaires to qualitative outreach work with communities who can be hard to hear

- helping the practice or commissioning cluster respond to local voices

- working with the developing LINKs organisations.

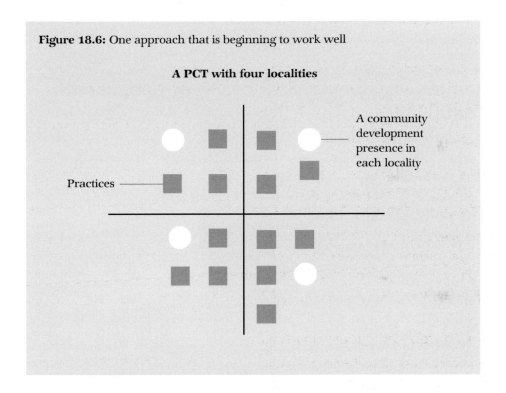

Figure 18.6: One approach that is beginning to work well

A PCT with four localities

A community development presence in each locality

Practices

The LCDP[24] is a leading exponent of this approach. Information is available on its website on the work done with MIND on local needs assessment for mental health.

Another important approach is working with *time banks*.[28] These are community organisations that enable people with time and skills to help others. Time banks provide opportunities for people to perform tasks for others, such as dog walking or giving lifts to the shops. In return, they earn credits to spend on the services of others. All members' time is valued equally. They are based on what people can offer rather than on what services they use. Research has linked participation in a time bank to a reduced reliance on GPs and an overall improvement in health.[29]

Working with national patient groups

Similarly, many national groups have local branches that would, on the whole, be happy to work with practices, clusters and PCTs. To find a list of the biggest mental health charities, see: www.mentalhealth.org.uk/information/organisations-and-websites/key-organisations/.

Another way of linking with local voluntary agencies is through a *social prescribing project*. There are a few of these across the UK – they enable practices to easily and safely refer patients to approved voluntary agencies. A brokering service is useful because there can be so many agencies even in a small locality that practices need help in finding the right one for an individual patient.[30-32]

Maintaining the physical health of people with mental illness

The Disability Rights Commission's study *Equal Treatment: closing the gap*, which promoted the physical health of users of mental health services, showed that people with mental illness have a greater likelihood of major illness, developing health problems at an earlier age than the rest of the population, and dying earlier.[33] Poverty is linked to poorer health, but clinical evidence shows it is not the only factor.

Its investigation focused on primary healthcare services. Many people reported very helpful primary care staff. Others, though, said they had problems with gaining access to services, the attitudes of some staff, and getting the necessary treatment and support. The clinical evidence shows, similarly, that, while many services are equally available to people with mental health problems and/or learning disabilities, this is not universally the case.

In contrast to many clinicians' assumptions, people with mental health problems are interested in their physical health.[34] Indeed, there is evidence that mental health problems make clinicians blind to physical health issues.[35]

The simplest way that practices can respond to these issues is by implementing the Quality and Outcomes Framework process for ensuring that the physical health of patients with mental health problems is maintained and improved. It can be difficult ensuring that there are robust arrangements between the practice and the Community Mental Health Team (CMHT). The practice also needs to include those patients with severe mental illness who are not on the CPA system. One example of a comprehensive approach was spearheaded by the Clinical Governance Resource Group in Lewisham.[36] The key was setting the process up involving local practices and the CMHT. Links between the CMHT and practice nurses have strengthened and make the process fairly seamless for the patient.

Exercise on Prescription is also a useful intervention – most PCTs have such services available.[37] Mild depression responds well to exercise and it has been shown to be helpful in more serious psychiatric conditions.

GPs attending CPAs

This is a simple, though time-consuming, approach to better communication both with the patient and the CMHT. GPs will learn a lot about aspects of their patients' lives they were ignorant of and the CPA team develops a more holistic view of the patients' treatment. It is well worthwhile.

Patients as Teachers

This is a technique for patient involvement that has been used in both hospital and primary care settings. The evidence seems to be[38] that it has a significant effect on clinician behaviour at six months.

The aims of the process are:

- to identify what good practice looks like from the users' points of view

- for users to teach that to clinicians in a supportive environment

- for lay-defined guidelines to be produced

- for mutually agreed outcomes to be monitored against.

PAT is a two-stage process. It is most useful for chronic diseases where users have had a longish contact with services. It can be useful in either primary or secondary care, or across the interface.

Focus groups of clinically relevant patients

For each speciality, the focus groups will be different. The aim is to identify key subgroups. For instance, in ischaemic heart disease (IHD), it might be an Asian group, women, men or the elderly.

Each group is asked the same basic question: 'In your experience, as your illness has been managed over the years, what has worked best for you?' This ensures that the responses will focus more on what works well, rather than just focusing on complaints. In addition, it is sensible to identify a number of subsets of this question. For instance, you might be interested in:

- access

- communication

- information transmission

- quality of care, etc.

The good practice recommendations derived from this process form the agenda for the next stage of the process.

Finally, delegates are identified who are interested in appearing in the educational event.

The educational meeting

Here, the delegates teach clinicians good practice from the patients' points of view. The meeting needs to be advertised as one that will lead to change.

The agenda of the meeting has been defined by the patients in advance. In this meeting, they represent the views of their group. The key change issues need to be identified through the meeting. They will be written up and sent to the participants as a reminder of what the meeting agreed.

Evaluation

This is done at six months to assess from the professional participants whether they feel that their practice has changed in line with the lay recommendations.

The lay guidelines

These can be written up and distributed. They can become an integral part of the clinical governance process.

One particularly relevant example is of a PAT programme focusing on depression.[39] Practices could be working with their PCT in promoting this kind of approach.

Patient Participation Groups and patient panels

Details of setting up and support can be obtained from www.napp.org.uk.

There is some evidence that PPGs can be easy to start but difficult to continue. Also, they end up less offering the practice an alternative view, but become institutionalised and focus on supporting the practice by buying ECG machines.

Another version of the PPG is the *patient panel*. This has been used in Lewisham PCT with support from the LCDP, a community development organisation. Here, the panel is derived from a representative selection of patients from the practice list, say 100. They are written to and asked key questions by the practice and are invited to the practice at least once a year to hold the practice to account.

This version of the panel can also be used for a commissioning cluster – contact LCDP to find out more: lcdp@lcdp4health.demon.co.uk.

Housing

People with mental health problems are one-and-a-half times more likely than the general population to live in rented housing, with higher uncertainty about how long they can remain in their current home.[40]

Clinical staff should work with the person to reduce the risk of losing his or her home, if the accommodation is appropriate. If the person will be homeless he or she should be referred to the local housing authority and work with housing services to identify and address his or her housing and support needs. This can be difficult as local housing departments are notoriously unresponsive. Citizens Advice Bureaux can be very helpful.[41]

It may be helpful to establish referral protocols with local housing advice agencies. It is important to recognise the role that housing staff play in supporting people with mental health problems in the community, and develop collaborative working relationships with them.[42] This can be done, for instance, by offering informal support to housing staff on mental health issues and housing management. Again, community workers have been helpful in facilitating this process.

The Revolving Doors Agency has worked in improving access to care and housing for people with mental health issues who have had contact with the criminal justice system.[43]

Race

This is a highly contentious issue. Some basic facts are agreed, as summarised by the Social Exclusion Unit's report *Mental Health and Social Exclusion*:[40]

- stigma and fear within ethnic minority communities, in combination with a distrust of mental health services, mean that many often seek professional help at a very late stage when their problems can be more serious

- people from ethnic minority groups are six times more likely to be detained under the Mental Health Act than white people

- the prevalence of common mental health problems is fairly similar across different ethnic groups, although rates are higher for Irish men and Pakistani women, and lower for Bangladeshi women

- people from ethnic minority groups are more likely to experience racism, be unemployed, be homeless, have poor physical health and live in deprived neighbourhoods, all of which can contribute to poorer mental health

- there are particular issues for refugees – two thirds have experienced anxiety or depression. They might have faced war, imprisonment, torture or oppression in their home country. In their new country they can also experience social isolation, homelessness, language barriers, hostility and racial discrimination

- adults from ethnic minority groups have higher levels of dissatisfaction with mental health statutory services than white people, and are twice as likely to disagree with their diagnosis.

An important article by Singh and Burns[44] sheds more light than heat on this topic. It suggests that there is little evidence for institutional racism. It suggests that one of the drivers for sectioning patients from African Caribbean backgrounds may be that patients who first present are not referred into mental health services by their own families soon enough and therefore end up in police hands. This may encourage a more violent and institutional response.

It is not easy to offer simple advice to practices in this field. It would make sense to employ staff from a variety of backgrounds. It is essential that clinicians understand the backgrounds of their patients so far as possible. Working with local faith groups can be very helpful. Working with local community development agencies to listen to local people can be very helpful in tailoring services and responses to local need. One agency that has long experience in this field is Social Action on Health.[45]

A simple but comprehensive summary from Mind can be found at: www.mind. org.uk/Information/Factsheets/Diversity/The+African+Caribbean+Community+and+ Mental+Health.htm. Another site of interest is: www.diverseminds.org.uk.

Record Access – patients having access to their full GP record

There is now increasing evidence that enabling patients to see their full GP record has a number of significant benefits.

Evidence of the benefits to patients from Record Access (RA) includes:

- increased trust in/with their clinicians

- an improved relationship with their practice

- improved compliance in medicine-taking

- some evidence that preventative health behaviour is encouraged

- obtaining their own health information without needing to contact the practice (allergies, immunisations)

- empowering patients to care for themselves more effectively

- using consultations with their clinicians more effectively

- saving time for themselves and the practice

- correcting errors in the record.

Most patients want to see their health records. People say that they understand about 60 per cent of what they see without any change of clinician writing style. Although a minority, mainly those with psychiatric difficulties, are upset about what they see, they still feel accessing their record was the right thing to do.[46] RA appears safe, even for patients with serious illnesses such as cancer.

Practices using the EMIS computer system can now obtain kiosks that enable their patients to see their records in the waiting room and a pilot is looking at online access. A good summary of the research in the field can be found by going to www.icmcc.org and clicking on 'record access'.

'People with diagnoses of mental illness often have particular concerns in relation to their records and what better way to ensure their/carer/family engagement than to place them at the heart of the service by driving forward this initiative, enhancing their ability to self-manage and be centrally involved by re-siting the locus of control.'[47]

The RCGP makes the point that we should involve patients, to the extent they prefer, in understanding the cause of their distress, in deciding whether a diagnostic label will be given, and in decision making about management of their mental health problem. RA can assist with this process.

PCTs' responsibilities

PCTs need to both support practices in this work and to ensure wider impact across their area.

In supporting the initiatives outlined above, they should be:

- ensuring that Choosing Health moneys are retained for public health work. Among other things, these should be funding mental health promotion work in schools and workplaces

- supporting job brokers in surgeries and training for practices on the importance of employment of people with mental health problems

- ensuring that every item on a Professional Executive Committee (PEC) or board agenda should include a 'social exclusion impact assessment'

- working with the local authority, local businesses, schools and the media to discuss and reduce stigma

- developing primary care data collection and disease management IT systems that prompt encouragement of self-management, shared decision making and options for health promotion.[48] St Helens PCT has developed its own self-help approach[49]

- supporting their own HR team to develop employment policies friendly to people with mental illness

- ensuring support for practices in their physical health review of patients with mental illness. There is government advice on this[50]

- asking Overview and Scrutiny Committees to do an overview of the area's social exclusion in mental health and then act on the results

- ensuring access to interpreters

- ensuring effective funding and use of primary care mental health workers and gateway workers

- developing a Primary Care Mental Health Strategy that brings together these disparate aspects of skills and care while encouraging PPI at all levels of the system. One excellent example of this has been developed in North Mersey[29]

- ensuring that social inclusion is high on the agenda of the Local Strategic Panel

- bringing psychiatric services closer to drug misuse services, both in the statutory and voluntary sector

- working with the local authority to:
  - develop a community development/PPI programme[51]
  - develop a housing policy sensitive to the needs of patients with mental health problems
  - ensure that practices and others are encouraging and making it easy for patients to take up benefits
  - support education opportunities for people with mental health problems.

The PCT should be commissioning the local mental health service to ensure a wide-ranging approach. The approaches for which evidence is good are detailed most helpfully in the Social Exclusion Unit's set of Action Points.[40] They include:

- an appropriate CPA assessment that includes work assessment

- transforming day services to promote social inclusion. Characteristics should include: access to supported employment; developing referral links with community services; providing advocacy and support; and involving people with mental health problems in the design and operation. There is practical advice from the DH on this[2]

- recognising people's diverse needs around ethnicity, gender and culture, and reflect this in provision, perhaps by commissioning specialist support from local voluntary and community groups

- supporting people to access direct payments

- ensuring training for staff is provided by people with mental problems, perhaps using Patients as Teachers as an approach

- ensuring that mental health services have good PPI in place at all levels

- ensuring access to interpreters

- delivering services in appropriate locations, perhaps in faith organisations.

However, these are simplistic ideas. We still do not really know how to move from needs-based commissioning and medical models to more whole systems/community-based approaches. How do we commission for health and inclusion, rather than commissioning for services that simply deal with the resultant fallout of not doing so?

Conclusion

This chapter has outlined the causes and effects of social exclusion in mental health. It has shown how the impact of social exclusion can be mitigated at a number of levels. We have tried to show that PPI is an essential ingredient of supporting social inclusion and that effective PPI can be therapeutic and health protective.

In addition, we have tried to emphasise the importance of this area to government policy and to local people, wherever they are. This is a moral imperative as well as a practical one. And GPs, their staff and local health organisations must all play their part.

Finally, we acknowledge that we have a long way to go to commission these services effectively.

References

1. www.voicesforum.org.uk/articles.htm [accessed November 2007].

2. Department of Health. *A Stronger Local Voice* London: DH, 2006, www.dh.gov.uk/assetRoot/04/13/70/41/04137041.pdf [accessed November 2007].

3. Social Exclusion Unit, Office of Deputy Prime Minister. *Action on Mental Health: a guide to social inclusion*. Stigma and Discrimination on Mental Health Grounds: Factsheet 1, www.cabinetoffice.gov.uk/upload/assets/www.cabinetoffice.gov.uk/social_exclusion_task_force/publications_1997_to_2006/action_on_mh.pdf [accessed November 2007].

4. Taylor Nelson Sofres. *Attitudes to Mental Illness 2003 Report* London: DH/ONS, 2003.

5. Manning C, White PD. Attitudes of employers to the mentally ill *Psychiatric Bulletin* 1995; **19**: 541–3.

6. Financial mapping returns collated by Mental Health Strategies (2003) (unpublished).

7. Office for National Statistics. *Labour Force Survey: household datasets*, spring quarter 2003, Cardiff: ONS.

8. Morris J. *The Right Support: report of the task force on supporting disabled adults in their parenting role* York: Joseph Rowntree Foundation, 2003.

9. Rankin J, Regan S. *Meeting Complex Needs: the future of social care* London: IPPR/Turning Point, 2004.

10. Department of Health, Farrell C. *Patient and Public Involvement in Health: the evidence for policy implementation. A summary of the results of the Health in Partnership research programme* London: DH, 2004.

11. www.together-uk.org/ [accessed November 2007].

12. Fisher B. Community development in primary care. In: S Gillam, F Brooks (eds). *New Beginnings: towards patient and public involvement in primary health care* London: King's Fund, 2001.

13. Eng PM, Rimm EB, Fitzmaurice G, *et al*. Social ties and change in social ties in relation to subsequent total and cause-specific mortality and coronary heart disease incidence in men *American Journal of Epidemiology* 2002; **155(8)**: 700–9.

14. Ginn J, Arbor SL, Cooper H. Inequalities in older people's health behaviour: effect of structural factors and social relationships *Journal of Contemporary Health* 1998; **7**: 77–82.

15. Runyan DK, Hunter WM, Socolar RS, *et al*. Children who prosper in unfavorable environments: the relationship to social capital *Pediatrics* 1998; **101(1)**: 12–18.

16. Berkman LF, Glass T. Social integration, social networks, social support and health. In: Berkman LF, Kawachi I (eds). *Social Epidemiology* Oxford: Oxford University Press, 2000.

17. Berkman LF, Leo-Summers L, Horwitz RI. Emotional support and survival after myocardial infarction: a prospective, population-based study of the elderly *Annals of Internal Medicine* 1992; **117(12)**: 1003–9.

18. Putnam RD. *Bowling Alone: the collapse and revival of American community* New York: Simon & Schuster, 2000.

19. Putnam R. Social capital: measurement and consequences *ISUMA – Canadian Journal of Policy Research* 2001; **2(1)**: 41–51.

20. Brown G, Harris T. *Social Origins of Depression* London: Tavistock, 1978.

21. Petersen T, Saporta I, Seidel M. Offering a job: meritocracy and social networks *American Journal of Sociology* 2001; **106**: 763–816.

22. Sampson R, Groves W. Community structure and crime: testing social-disorganization theory *American Journal of Sociology* 1989; **94**: 774–802.

23. Whiteley PF. Economic growth and social capital *Political Studies* 2000; **48(3)**: 443–66.

24. www.lcdp.co.uk/index.html [accessed November 2007].

25. Fisher B. Patient and public involvement and Practice Based Commissioning. In: E Andersson, J Tritter, R Wilson (eds). *Healthy Democracy: the future of involvement in health and social care*, Coventry: Involve and the NHS National Centre for Involvement, 2007, www.nhscentrefor involvement.nhs.uk/index.cfm?Content=90 [accessed November 2007; requires registration].

26. www.rcgp.org.uk/PDF/clinspec_printed%20version%20mental%20health.pdf [accessed November 2007].

27. www.dwp.gov.uk/medical/deskaids.asp [accessed November 2007].

28. Garcia I. *Keeping the GP Away: community time banks and health* London: New Economics Foundation, 2002.

29. *Creating Mentally Healthy Communities: a proposed model for Commissioning for Health and not just for Illness*, adapted from the North Mersey Mental Health Improvement Programme Primary Mental Health Care Think Tank, July 2005.

30. www.wlct.org/gmahn/socpres.pdf [accessed November 2007].

31. www.natpact.nhs.uk/uploads/LSPPSum.doc [accessed November 2007].

32. www.imaginementalhealth.org.uk [accessed November 2007].

33. http://83.137.212.42/sitearchive/DRC/library/health_investigation.html [accessed November 2007].

34. Meddings S, Perkins R. What 'getting better' means to staff and users of a rehabilitation service: an exploratory study *Journal of Mental Health* 2002; **11(3)**: 319–25.

35. Dean J, Todd G, Morrow H, *et al*. Mum, I used to be good looking. … Look at me now: the physical health needs of adults with mental health problems: the perspectives of users, carers and front-line staff *International Journal of Mental Health Promotion* 2001; **3(4)**: 16–24.

36. Allen D, Harvey S, Marstin P, *et al*. Enduring mental illness and physical health care *Practice Nursing* 2004; **15(7)**: 356–60.

37. www.rethink.org/living_with_mental_illness/treatment_and_therapy/other_treatments/exercise. html [accessed November 2007]

38. Fisher B, Gilbert D. Patient involvement and clinical effectiveness. In: S Gillam, F Brooks (eds) *New Beginnings: towards patient and public involvement in primary health care* London: King's Fund, 2001.

39. Fisher B, Gibbon M, Benson A, *et al*. Patients as teachers: is there shared decision making in the treatment of depression? *Clinical Governance Bulletin* 2005; **6(1)**: 7–9, www.rsmpress.co.uk/cgbsept05.pdf [accessed November 2007].

40. www.socialexclusion.gov.uk/downloaddoc.asp?id–300, Factsheet 6.

41. www.adviceguide.org.uk [accessed November 2007].

42. Office of the Deputy Prime Minister. *Achieving Positive Shared Outcomes in Health and Homelessness* London: ODPM, 2004.

43. www.revolving-doors.co.uk [accessed November 2007].

44. Singh SP, Burns T. Race and mental health: there is more to race than racism *British Medical Journal* 2006; **333**: 648–51.

45. www.safh.org.uk/ [accessed November 2007].

46. Baldry M, Cheal C, Fisher B, *et al*. Giving patients their own records in general practice: experience of patients and staff *British Medical Journal* 1986; **292**; 596–8.

47. Dr Chris Manning, personal communication.

48. *Lewisham Depression Programme: supporting practices to deliver improved care* London: Lewisham PCT, 2003.

49. www.ohwhatarelief.com/ultrasis/reliefGateSh/ [accessed November 2007].

50. www.dh.gov.uk/assetRoot/04/13/82/90/04138290.pdf [accessed November 2007].

51. www.lewishamstrategicpartnership.org.uk [accessed November 2007].

52. www.dh.gov.uk/assetRoot/04/13/10/68/04131068.pdf [accessed November 2007].

19 | Mental health policy and primary mental health care
Present and future

Andrew McCulloch and Alan Cohen

What this chapter contributes:

it reviews current mental health policy and current policy on primary mental health care

the impact of current policy

it sets out some policy issues that need to be addressed if primary mental health care in England is to be improved.

Introduction

Before embarking on our review of mental health policy it is worth making explicit a few assumptions about what policy is and why we have it. Koontz and Weihrich define policy or policies as 'General statements or understandings which guide thinking on decision making.' This definition bears further thought.[1] Key issues arising include:

1. policy may be written or spoken publicly, through documents, broadcasts and speeches, but it may not be. History is littered with implicit, secret and even illegal policy making. Whilst there is no direct equivalent of Suez or the Iran–Contra scandal in mental health it is likely that private messages about health priorities are disseminated from the Department of Health via Strategic Health Authorities (SHAs) and Primary Care Trust (PCT) Chief Executives, for example, and that these may sometimes run counter to stated policy priorities

2. policy may exist at a national, regional, local or organisational level. This chapter is concerned with national (English) policy. However, mental health is strongly impacted also by UK policy as welfare benefits are a reserve power

3. whilst policy guides developments and actions it does not and cannot mechanically determine the outcomes – clinical behaviour is notoriously difficult to change using policy statements unless they are supported by evidence-based change models, which may include incentives, product champions, education and peer pressure.

Having said all that it may be stating the obvious to point out why governments generate mental health policy. After all, mental ill health costs some £100bn to the exchequer each year[2] and good mental health is associated with all kinds of improved social outcomes in areas such as education, employment and productivity, criminal justice and child rearing. What is perhaps interesting is how government's overall philosophy on social intervention manifests itself in specific mental health policies. Arguably, in the case of the 'New Labour' government we see a clear impact from thinking around active and responsible citizenship, as expressed by Etzioni and others,[3] balanced with the state's clear commitment to provide services for mentally ill people, which goes back for centuries. We have also recently seen statements from government which suggest that it wishes to promote happiness and equates happiness with mental health – a simplistic and perhaps dangerous conflation.[4]

Mental health policy prior to New Labour

The Conservative administration that existed up until the 1996 election had a range of mental health policies, strands of which are still relevant today. In terms of services the fundamental plank of policy was to shift specialist services towards working with people with severe and enduring mental illness, the implication being that the vast majority of people with common mental disorders would be treated in primary care. However, the implications of this for primary care were not worked through in policy terms.

In the early 1990s the Department of Health, particularly under the leadership of talented then-junior ministers such as Stephen Dorrell, Tim Yeo and John Bowis, produced some wide-ranging policy documents that encapsulated both the spectrum of services required across primary, secondary and tertiary care (e.g. *The Spectrum of Care* in 1996)[5] and the public health interventions required to tackle mental health at a social level (e.g. *Key Area Handbook* in 1993).[6] Whilst these documents contain many flaws, such as a focus on mental illness rather than mental health and a lack of clear plans to develop comprehensive services, equally they set the foundation for the development of more comprehensive mental healthcare policy.

Mental health policy under New Labour

Mental health policy showed very strong development in the first term of the New Labour government, but appears to have tailed off more recently. When the National Service Framework (NSF) for Mental Health was published in 1999,[7] the Sainsbury Centre for Mental Health commented: 'For the first time, Government has set out a comprehensive agenda for mental health which acknowledges that the whole system of mental health care must be made to work if we are to succeed in modernising care.'[8]

The core aims of the NSF appeared and appear to be:

1. improving public mental health (albeit the document does not adopt a public health approach)

2. reducing suicide

3. modernising mental health care at all levels

4. addressing the public safety agenda

5. improving the quality of care for service users and support for carers (see McCulloch et al.).[9]

The NSF is interesting because whilst it is very comprehensive in many ways it can be seen as a logical extension of the previous government's policy[10] and it shares its fundamental failure to reconcile safety and containment issues with care and public mental health.

However, the year after the NSF came *The NHS Plan*.[11] For many this was seen as signalling the government priority on mental health – to develop comprehensive community care for people with severe mental health problems. The *Plan* set the three critical targets of developing:

- 50 early intervention teams by 2004

- 335 crisis resolution teams by 2004

- 220 assertive outreach teams by 2003.

The rush to develop these teams, and the failure to achieve the first two targets, directed much management activity in specialist services in the first years of the new century. However, the steam now seems to have gone out of this activity and we are even seeing some of these teams threatened with closure as the financial consequences of Agenda for Change and Payment by Results impact directly and indirectly on mental health services.

Primary mental healthcare policy

The cynic might reasonably observe that policy on primary mental health care is the same as it has always been. Primary care must soak up the vast majority of people with common mental disorders and in addition must address the physical health of people with severe mental disorders. In addition, one third of people with a diagnosis of a severe mental health problem are only managed in primary care. There remains little focus on developing a resourced and systematic policy for primary mental health care. However, there have been important developments.

The NSF set two standards around tackling common mental disorders:

Standard Two

Any service user who contacts his or her primary mental healthcare team with a common mental health problem should:

- have his or her mental health needs identified and assessed

- be offered effective treatments, including referral to specialist services for further assessment, treatment and care if he or she requires it.

Standard Three

Any individual with a common mental health problem should:

- be able to make contact round the clock with the local services necessary to meet his or her needs and receive adequate care

- be able to use NHS Direct as it develops, for first-level advice and referral on to specialist helplines or to local services.

However, it does not set out a strategy for delivering this given the evidence that it did not happen in 1999, and does not happen now:

1. diagnosis rates for common mental health problems in primary care are low – perhaps 60 per cent or less[12,13]

2. many people are treated with suboptimal or ineffective treatments such as unfocused counselling

3. many others are treated only with medication when combination therapies may be more effective

4. access to primary care services for people with mental health problems, both during office hours and as emergencies 'out of hours', is difficult. The Disability Rights Commission report into access identified many of the problems.[14] The change in the way that out-of-hours services are funded and managed has also reduced the accessibility of the service to people with mental health problems. Helplines such as NHS Direct and SANELINE have been heavily hit by cuts in funding and capacity has been reduced.

Whilst there is no over-arching policy framework for primary mental health care in England that contains key elements such as delivery systems, funding, targets and monitoring, there have been some modest and relevant policy initiatives. Specifically *The NHS Plan* announced the intention to develop new primary care and community mental health workers.[11] Funding was made available from 2003/04 for 1000 such workers.[15] It was planned that these graduate workers would fulfil, *inter alia*, some of the following tasks:

- support delivery of brief focused interventions and self-help tools for common problems

- strengthen information delivery to patients

- support practice-based information systems, audit and outcome measurement.

Implementation of this initiative has so far had patchy results and only 600 workers have been appointed, arguably a drop in the ocean. Generally it would seem that where graduate workers are properly supervised and form part of the overall clinical team in a planned way, they can make a useful contribution. Where this is not the case, or where the role or lines of support and accountability are unclear, they are less effective. To put it another way, it could be argued that the introduction of 1000 graduate workers – a small number relative to the need and even the number of GPs – is a classic 'orphan' initiative that was not thought through in terms of a comprehensive plan for primary mental health care. It has been left to PCTs, practices and mental health trusts to join it up for government – a high-risk approach.

The other most important recent initiative was the announcement of two cognitive behavioural therapy (CBT) pilots in Newham and Doncaster, as part of the Improving Access to Psychological Therapies Programme (IAPT). These pilots may herald a much more systematic roll-out of CBT within primary care, which would give primary care another major string to its bow in the treatment of common mental disorders.

There have been few other significant initiatives on primary care from a mental health policy perspective; other initiatives have come from within generic primary care policy development. The impact of these on mental health and a possible forward agenda have been summarised in the recent consensus statement published by the Mental Health Foundation on behalf of a number of organisations including the Pharmaceutical Schizophrenia Initiative.[16] There is also a useful paper from the National Institute for Mental Health called *Cases for Change: primary care* but it is merely a discussion paper.[17]

At the time of writing a detailed response is awaited from the government on the criticisms contained in a recent report from the Disability Rights Commission that shows, once again, that people with mental health problems have poorer access to primary care and worse physical health outcomes than the general population.[14] This would be an opportunity for the government to set out a more strategic approach to improving primary mental health care.

Primary care policy and its effect on mental health services

It is not appropriate to summarise here all the changes in policy that have an influence on primary care – that would require at least one book in its own right, rather than just a section of a chapter!

The two most recent changes in policy that are having the greatest influence on primary care are the changes that follow from the new General Medical Services (nGMS) contract, and the impact of Practice-Based Commissioning. Both of these are dealt with elsewhere in this book (see Chapters 1 and 2).

However, the current policy that has the greatest potential benefit to change the way that primary care can provide effective mental health services is the IAPT programme.

In December 2004, Lord Layard, a health economist, presented data to a Downing Street seminar, on the association between mental illness and worklessness. His premise drew on a number of well-known and evidenced statements:

- there are 1 million people receiving incapacity benefit who have a mental health problem – which is more than the total number of people unemployed

- 90 per cent of those are not in contact with specialist mental health services, and suffer from depression and/or anxiety

- effective interventions exist for depression and anxiety, including medication and CBT

- a number of programmes run by the Department of Work and Pensions (DWP) have shown that CBT, and programmes related to CBT such as condition management programmes, can support people to return to work

- the CBT service is best delivered through a treatment team or treatment centre approach, which can ensure high-quality psychological assessments and interventions.

Lord Layard proposed that new treatment centres were created to provide CBT and employment advice to people whose long-term employment was at risk because of mental health problems. Treatment centres would serve a population of about 250,000 people, and, across England, some 10,000 new therapists would be needed to staff these centres or teams.

Funding for these teams would come from the savings generated by people returning to work early. Savings would be generated from reduced healthcare costs (both physical and mental health costs), reduced payments on benefits and increased taxation revenue (as people return to work earlier), reduced social costs through improved outputs, and improved quality of life.

The pilots in Doncaster and Newham are designed to test not only the applicability of the CBT treatment centre approach, but to understand and quantify the economic gains that could fund this programme nationally.

Analysis

Despite some good work that has been done in defining a policy agenda for specialist services, although this appears to have run out of steam of late, there is little in the way of a policy framework for primary mental health in England. Yet we know that primary care is the fundamental plank for a successful mental health service because:

- the vast majority of common mental disorders and 30 per cent of severe disorders are treated there

- mental disorders account for at least one third of the disease burden in primary care

- many disorders remain ineffectively treated with enormous costs for the NHS, individuals and society

- primary care manages the biggest entry gate to secondary care – secondary care is compromised without good primary care

- primary care looks after the physical health of the vast majority of people with mental health problems and they suffer severe inequalities in physical health.[14,18]

In some ways the policy framework on primary mental health care is strategically more important than that for secondary care.

It seems to the authors that there are seven key issues that need to be tackled in order to develop a strategy for primary mental health care.

The organisation and location of primary mental health care

First, the current organisation of primary mental health care in England, with a very few exceptions, is irrational due to its historically received nature. Whilst our primary care services overall are excellent by international standards, our primary mental health care falls short on a range of indicators. Particular failings relative to international or theoretical best practice include:

- almost all patients see a fully trained doctor for a brief interview on presentation – this is expensive and the skills, competences and knowledge of the GP do not match the task, and neither does the length of the consultation

- almost all care is delivered in a healthcare setting but much of the need presents elsewhere (e.g. education, workplace, youth settings, the street)

- intermediate care is not well developed – so the step up to secondary care is too 'steep' (see *The Neglected Majority* for a useful discussion)[19]

- somatisation, which is mental health related, is often dealt with via referrals to acute services – a disaster both in financial terms and reinforcing the patient's dysfunctional beliefs about his or her health.

There are many policy options that have merit in terms of developing more efficient structures for the delivery of primary mental health care, including:

- training a variety of workers including community psychiatric nurses, psychologists and practice nurses to undertake mental health assessments in primary care

- using IT-based assessment tools that patients could complete prior to a consultation

- providing primary mental healthcare workers in settings other than GP surgeries such as schools, workplaces, sexually transmitted infection (STI) clinics and homelessness facilities

- developing mental health intermediate care teams outstationed in primary care and delivering interventions such as assessment, psychological therapies, medication management and lifestyle interventions

- delivering psychoeducational interventions and complementary therapies to tackle somatisation.

The training and development of staff

Second, policy and practice development in primary care will not be delivered without a step change in the quality and quantity of staff training and development. Fewer than 40 per cent of GPs have any postgraduate training in mental health, and where this occurs it relates to a secondary care population of patients rather than a primary care population.[20] Fewer than 2 per cent of practice nurses are trained in mental health.[21]

Clinical governance

Third, the quality of primary care practitioners' response to mental health issues seems to vary across individuals and practices from the world class to the desultory. To some extent we would expect performance to be variable, but we need a clear strategy for dealing with the 'tail' of poor performance. Continuing personal development, outcome measurement and information systems all have an important role, as does peer pressure.

Access to evidence-based treatments

Fourth, there is no doubt that GPs are severely hampered in their ability to access evidence-based treatments. There can be long waiting lists for the range of evidence-based forms of psychotherapy including CBT. Other treatments such as exercise therapy[22] are often not readily available. Unless there is a strategy to deliver a full range of evidence-based treatments in primary care GPs will continue to rely on the prescription pad.

Information systems and information management

Fifth, the *Mental Health Information Strategy* sets out a vision embracing a single electronic patient record with potential for information sharing, outcome tracking and assisted decision making.[23] Implementation of this strategy or any similar approach could have an enormous positive impact on the quality and efficiency of primary mental health care, but the authors are not aware of any PCT that has implemented it.

Addressing the whole person

Sixth, GPs are, of course, experts in delivering primary physical health care. Yet often the physical health of people with mental health problems is neglected.[14] There is also an even bigger issue about the interaction between physical and mental health such as the interactions between cardiovascular disease, diabetes, depression and schizophrenia for example. Thus it is important that GPs address both the physical concomitants of presenting mental ill health and the mental concomitants of presenting physical ill health. In order to achieve this, fundamental changes may be required such as:

- inclusion of this issue in basic training and CPD

- development of simple lifestyle assessment tools covering issues such as relationships, alcohol, diet, exercise and cognitive style that patients can self-complete

- development of much better integrated mental and physical health promotion.

Services for younger people, older people and people from ethnic minorities

Seventh, there is much evidence that these groups experience a number of problems accessing primary mental health care including:

- higher thresholds for diagnosis

- discrimination

- not seeing the service as youth or culturally friendly

- problems with the setting or style of the service.

Many of these problems might be solved by a combination of providing innovative delivery systems for primary care in varied settings and the development of link workers, advocacy and culturally sensitive services.

Conclusion

If we develop competent primary mental healthcare services in this country the potential prize is enormous in terms of economics, human health, wellbeing and happiness, parenting and education. Almost all the domains of life could potentially benefit. Importantly healthcare resources could also be used more effectively through better use of GPs and other staff, more rational care pathways and reductions in frequent attenders. Given the enormity of the prize, we have to ask 'How much longer will it be before government develops a systematic policy on primary mental health care?'

References

1. Koontz H and Weihrich H. *Management* New York: McGraw-Hill, 1988.

2. Mental Health Foundation. *The Fundamental Facts: 2007 edition* London: MHF, 2007.

3. Etzioni A. *The Active Society* New York: Collier-Macmillan, 1968.

4. McCulloch A. Understanding mental health and mental illness. In: C Jackson, K Hill (eds). *Mental Health Today Handbook*, pp. 3–10, Brighton: Pavilion, 2006.

5. Department of Health. *The Spectrum of Care: local services for people with mental health problems* London: DH, 1996.

6. Department of Health. *Key Area Handbook: mental illness* London: HMSO, 1993.

7. Department of Health. *National Service Framework for Mental Health: modern standards and service models for mental health* London: DH, 1999.

8. The Sainsbury Centre for Mental Health. *The National Service Framework for Mental Health: an executive briefing* London: The Sainsbury Centre for Mental Health, 1999.

9. McCulloch A, Glover G, St John T. The National Service Framework for Mental Health: past, present and future *Mental Health Review* 2003; **8(4)**: 7–17.

10. McCulloch A, Parker C. Mental health inquiries, assertive outreach and compliance: is there a relationship? In: N Stanley, J Manthorpe (eds). *The Age of the Inquiry*, pp. 133–50, London: Routledge, 2004.

11. Department of Health. *The NHS Plan: a plan for investment, a plan for reform*. Cm 4818-1. London: The Stationery Office, 2000.

12. The Sainsbury Centre for Mental Health. *Primary Solutions* London: The Sainsbury Centre for Mental Health, 2003.

13. The Royal College of Psychiatrists. *GPs and Hospitals Often Fail to Spot Mental Health Problems* [press release] London: The Royal College of Psychiatrists.

14. Disability Rights Commission. *Equal Treatment: closing the gap* London: DRC, 2006.

15. Department of Health. *The Mental Health Policy Implementation Guide* London: DH, 2001.

16. The Mental Health Foundation and the Pharmaceutical Schizophrenia Initiative. *Primary Concerns* London: MHF, 2007.

17. National Institute for Mental Health. *Cases for Change: primary care* Leeds: NIMHE, 2002.

18. Jenkins R, McCulloch A, Friedli L, *et al. Developing a National Mental Health Policy*. Maudsley Monograph. Hove: The Psychology Press, 2002.

19. The Sainsbury Centre for Mental Health. *The Neglected Majority* London: The Sainsbury Centre for Mental Health, 2005.

20. Kerwick S, Jones R, Mann A, *et al*. Mental health care training priorities in general practice *British Journal of General Practice* 1997; **47**: 225–7.

21. Crosland A, Kai J. They think they can talk to nurses: practice nurses' views of their roles in caring for mental health problems *British Journal of General Practice* 1998; **48(432)**: 1383–6.

22. Mental Health Foundation. *Up and Running* London: MHF, 2005.

23. Department of Health. *Mental Health Information Strategy* London: DH, 2001.

20 | NICE guidelines, algorithms and guideline implementation
The challenges of implementing NICE mental health guidelines in primary care

Stephen Pilling, Katy Price, Nicola Bent and Gillian Leng

What this chapter contributes:

an overview of NICE guidelines for mental health problems

principles of implementation.

Introduction

Over 90 per cent of mental health problems in the UK are managed in primary care[1] and it is estimated over 30 per cent of primary care consultations have a mental health component to them.[2] For the majority of patients treatment in primary care is a positive and appropriate choice, although problems of access to some services, in particular psychological interventions,[3] remain in both primary and secondary care. As the evidence base for mental health interventions has grown, so have the demands on clinicians to make appropriate decisions on care and treatment. The provision of mental health services in primary care now includes not only anxiolytic or antidepressant medication or counselling but also an increasing range of psychosocial interventions such as guided self-help,[4] computerised cognitive behavioural therapy (cCBT)[5] and different types of complex psychological intervention as well as increasing evidence base on the differential effects of drugs.[6] To add to the complexity of the challenge facing primary care mental health services the evidence base is increasingly driving the incentive (Quality and Outcomes Framework [QOF])[7] and monitoring schemes (e.g. the Healthcare Commission's annual health check, www.healthcarecommission.org.uk) used in primary care.

Clinical practice guidelines provide one important method that will enable primary care services to meet these challenges. The clinical practice guidelines developed by the National Institute for Health and Clinical Excellence (NICE) set the national standards for good practice in England and Wales. In Scotland the Scottish Intercollegiate Guideline Network (SIGN) has a similar function. NICE guidance is increasingly being used in Northern Ireland, following a recent formalisation of the relationship between NICE and the Northern Ireland Executive. The development and implementation of these guidelines in primary care presents a number of challenges for guideline developers and clinicians alike, and include: the limited evidence base for a number of interventions in primary care as opposed to secondary care settings; the limited utility of heterogeneous diagnostic entities such as depression; the structural changes that may be required to existing resources to fully support a stepped-care framework; and the resource implications of some of the NICE recommendations, for example the increased emphasis on psychological therapies. Whilst the challenges presented by the first two of these problems will be acknowledged, the focus of this chapter will be on issues of the kind exemplified by the latter two. The chapter will also make reference to the evidence base for implementation that has been well summarised elsewhere by Grimshaw *et al.*[8] and Grol and Jones[9] in relation to guidelines generally and specifically in relation to NICE mental health guidance by Pilling and Price.[10] In brief this evidence can be summarised by saying that implementation programmes can bring benefit (albeit usually modest) if they are underpinned by a good evidence base and adopt a multifaceted, organisationally sophisticated approach to implementation that includes such things as behavioural specificity in the wording of recommendations, educational outreach and patient-specific reminders. Factors such as these have influenced the NICE implementation programme that is described below. The presentation of guidance in accessible forms is also of considerable importance; current NICE guidelines are provided in summary form for professionals, known as quick reference guides, giving health professionals an easy overview of all the recommendations in an easy-to-use format. NICE also produces a version of the guidance for patients and their carers. For primary care professionals in particular, key headlines about NICE guidance are available through the Update for Primary Care (see www.nice.org.uk for more information).

Some of the challenges specific to NICE guidance are listed below and include:

- the organisational changes that are required if NICE guidelines are to be fully implemented including the development of a stepped-care framework (see Whitty and Gilbody[11] – but see below for a fuller discussion), the restructuring of services to move away from less effective interventions (for example the use of trauma-focused forms of treatment as opposed to more general forms of treatment for post-traumatic stress disorder [PTSD]) and the retraining of staff in evidence base interventions

- volume of guidance: NICE publishes two to three clinical practice guidelines on mental health and an average of ten clinical guidelines covering all topics per year. This is in addition to other NICE guidance including the Technology Appraisals. The past five years have seen considerable expansion of new guidance in mental health. It is not anticipated that this will continue at the same rate as the major disorders are covered and the primary focus switches to an update and revision of existing guidance. Mental health guidance also varies in the degree with which it applies to primary care. Some guidance, for example that on depression, is focused largely on primary care whereas other guidance, for example schizophrenia, has a focus largely on secondary care. Nevertheless all mental health guidelines have some important implications for primary care

- the increased demand for psychological treatments from a policy perspective (for example the Department of Health Improving Access to Psychological Therapies programme [IAPT], www.dh.gov.uk). There is the patient perspective – where increasing demands for psychological therapies emerge from the public and their representatives. There is also the commissioning perspective, particularly where the resource base is not increased sufficiently to meet the demand and therefore requires a restructuring of existing resource.

NICE guidelines in mental health

Table 20.1 sets out the completed and current programme of work that demonstrates not only the volume but also the comprehensive nature of the programme. A few areas require new development, most notably alcohol (although this is addressed in NICE's public health programme) and some disorders of childhood, but the current programme covers most of the common and severe mental disorders.

Table 20.1: NICE guidelines in mental health

Guideline	Date of launch
Schizophrenia	December 2002
Eating disorders	January 2004
Self-harm	July 2004
Depression	December 2004
Anxiety (generalised anxiety disorder and panic disorder)	December 2004
Management of violence	February 2005
Post-traumatic stress disorder	March 2005
Depression in children	September 2005
Obsessive-compulsive disorder	November 2005
Bipolar disorder	July 2006
Dementia	November 2006
Antenatal and postnatal mental health	February 2007
Drug misuse – psychosocial interventions	July 2007
Drug misuse – detoxification	July 2007
Attention deficit hyperactivity disorder	July 2008
Personality disorder – borderline	December 2008
Personality disorder – antisocial	December 2008

Key priorities for NICE mental health guidelines in primary care

All NICE guidelines now include key priorities for implementation; the priority is determined by the likelihood that the recommendations will contribute most to either a reduction in the variation of practice or an improvement in outcomes, or better still a combination of the two. The key recommendations from existing published NICE guidelines that relate directly to primary care mental health are summarised in Table 20.2. Where an existing QOF target exists these are highlighted in the table. As can be seen from Table 20.2 a number of themes emerge, principal amongst which are: recognition and detection of disorders; the development of stepped-care models; the use of registers particularly for severe mental illness (and the associated management of physical health problems); and a shift in focus away from the use of medication to psychosocial interventions particularly in mild to moderate disorders. The following section contains a more detailed discussion of these four priority areas.

Recognition and detection

The recognition and detection of mental disorders present a number of challenges in primary care that are briefly discussed below and which may account in part for the under-detection of common mental health problems in primary care. Different disorders will present different challenges, for example an individual with anorexia nervosa may not perceive him or herself to have a problem despite beliefs to the contrary of family, friends or doctor. In contrast a rape victim suffering from PTSD may simply feel too ashamed to seek help. Some of the general problems faced in recognition and detection can be obtained from a consideration of the case of depression, the most common mental health problem encountered in primary care.

First, many people with depression simply do not seek help. The reasons for this include: not believing that any help could be provided (28 per cent); that one should be able to cope with the problem oneself (28 per cent); that it was not necessary to contact a doctor (17 per cent); that the problem would get better by itself (15 per cent); too embarrassed to discuss it with anyone (13 per cent); and afraid of the consequences of the treatment, for example hospitalisation (10 per cent).[12] Second, even when a person presents with depression in a primary care setting the problem is not recognised. For example, although the annual rate of depression in primary care may exceed 10 per cent, studies indicate that the annual rate recognised in primary care is only about 3 per cent.[2] A major reason behind this is that many people with depression may consult for physical complaints and not consider themselves to have any psychological problems, despite the presence of depressive symptoms. Third, there may be limited treatment options available, or which are judged to be acceptable (for example, the difficulty in accessing psychological treatments), for those patients who are identified. For instance, although many patients may be offered antidepressant medication,

Table 20.2: Key mental health recommendations

Guideline	Key recommendations
Schizophrenia	• Registers for people with schizophrenia (QOF) • Physical health checks/monitoring (QOF) • Early identification of the disorder • Joint management plans with secondary care
Eating disorders	• Recognition and detection in primary care • Management of bulimia nervosa (for example guided self-help, access to specialised CBT) • Management of chronic anorexia nervosa including physical health care
Self-harm	• Respect and dignity for service users • Risk and mental state assessment • Referral advice • Prescribing for people who self-harm through poisoning
Depression	• Appropriate diagnosis of mild/moderate/severe depression (QOF) • Reduced prescribing of antidepressants for mild depression • Two-week review to follow up with all patients who have been newly prescribed antidepressants • Development of alternative interventions such as exercise, guided self-help and cCBT for mild/moderate depression
Anxiety	• Recognition and diagnostic process to include personal history, any self-medication, and cultural or other individual characteristics • Providing the patient with written information and information about self-help and support groups • For panic disorder or generalised anxiety disorder, use CBT, selective serotonin reuptake inhibitors (SSRIs) or guided self-help (in order of descending effectiveness)
Post-traumatic stress disorder	• Recognition and detection in primary care • Watchful waiting • Limitations on use of medication, focus on symptom management (e.g. sleep)
Depression in children	• No drugs to be initiated in primary care • Stepped-care model • Provision of psychological interventions
Obsessive-compulsive disorder	• Recognition and detection in primary care • Psychological therapies • SSRIs as first-line treatment
Bipolar disorder	• Recognition and detection in primary care • Registers (QOF) • Physical health checks and monitoring (QOF)

a significant proportion decline the offer, fail to obtain the antidepressants from the pharmacist or do not complete the treatment as prescribed.[13] Finally, the stigma associated with mental health problems generally,[14] and the public view that people with depression are neurotic or irritating,[15] may account for the reluctance of depressed people to seek help. One solution to this problem would be to develop a set of routine screening questions for mental health problems but there are significant technical and practical problems which suggest that this is unlikely to be a feasible approach. The National Screening Committee (NSC) (www.nsc.nhs.uk/) sets out the key criteria by which any screening tool or programme should be judged. A brief review of these criteria quickly establishes that the sensitivity, specificity and positive predictive value of most current screening measures in mental health fail to meet the criteria. (For an example of these criteria at work see the report on screening in postnatal depression.)[16] NICE mental health guidelines now follow the NSC approach and have not recommended the use of population-based screening tools but rather have focused on the use of specific questions for groups felt to be likely to have a high incidence of a disorder, significantly above the base rate for the population as a whole.

A number of examples of this approach are given below and which build on the GPs' own concerns about patients or draw on the evidence of the known risks of certain subgroups, for example the increased rate of depression in patients following a myocardial infarction or who have a history of past episodes of depression. Such an approach also allows for electronic supports to clinical decision making, for example EMIS-delivered prompts to ask a question to a person known to belong to a vulnerable group. This approach is also further reinforced in the QOF where asking specific questions about depression is rewarded for patients on the diabetes or CHD registers. In encouraging the recognition and detection of depression, the NICE depression guideline[6] recommends that those patients with a past history of depression, significant physical illnesses causing disability or other mental health problems such as dementia be asked two questions (often referred to as the 'Whooley questions'):[17]

- 'During the last month, have you often been bothered by feeling down, depressed or hopeless?' and

- 'During the last month, have you often been bothered by having little interest or pleasure in doing things?'

As described above this also links into the QOF indicator that people on the diabetes and CHD register should be screened for depression using two standard screening questions. The QOF also recommends that positive answers to these questions are followed with an assessment of severity using an assessment tool that should lead to a classification of depression into mild, moderate and severe. This would further support the implementation of NICE guidance on the treatment of depression. Use of a decision support tool (such as that shown in Box 20.1) may also assist GPs in acting on a diagnosis.

Box 20.1: Assessing the severity of depression in primary care

Key symptoms:

- persistent sadness or low mood, and/or
- loss of interests or pleasure
- fatigue or low energy.

At least one of these, most days, most of the time for at least two weeks.

If any of above present, ask about associated symptoms:

- disturbed sleep
- poor concentration or indecisiveness
- low self-confidence
- poor or increased appetite
- suicidal thoughts or acts
- agitation or slowing of movements
- guilt or self-blame.

Then ask about past, family history, associated disability and availability of social support.

1. Factors that favour general advice and watchful waiting:

- four or fewer of the above symptoms
- no past or family history
- social support available
- symptoms intermittent, or less than two weeks' duration
- not actively suicidal
- little associated disability.

2. Factors that favour more active treatment in primary care:

- five or more symptoms
- past history or family history of depression
- low social support
- suicidal thoughts
- associated social disability.

3. Factors that favour referral to mental health professionals:

- poor or incomplete response to two interventions
- recurrent episode within one year of last one
- patient or relatives request referral
- self-neglect.

4. Factors that favour urgent referral to a psychiatrist:

- actively suicidal ideas or plans
- psychotic symptoms
- severe agitation accompanying severe (more than ten) symptoms
- severe self-neglect.

ICD-10 definitions:

- mild depression: four symptoms
- moderate depression: five or six symptoms
- severe depression: seven or more symptoms, with or without psychotic features.

In addition algorithms such as that shown in Figure 20.1 from the NICE anxiety guideline can support GPs to decide on the best treatment approach when both anxiety and depression are present, or it is difficult to distinguish between the two.

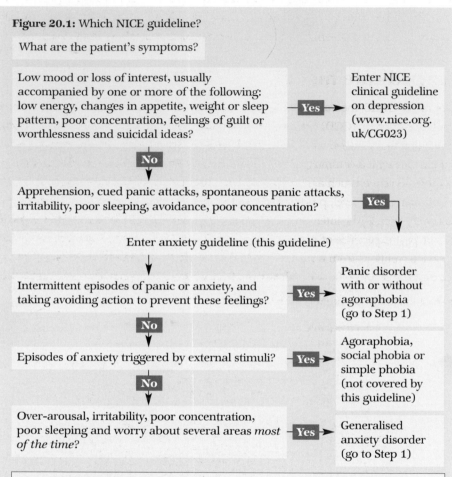

Figure 20.1: Which NICE guideline?

What are the patient's symptoms?

Low mood or loss of interest, usually accompanied by one or more of the following: low energy, changes in appetite, weight or sleep pattern, poor concentration, feelings of guilt or worthlessness and suicidal ideas? — **Yes** → Enter NICE clinical guideline on depression (www.nice.org.uk/CG023)

No ↓

Apprehension, cued panic attacks, spontaneous panic attacks, irritability, poor sleeping, avoidance, poor concentration? — **Yes**

Enter anxiety guideline (this guideline)

Intermittent episodes of panic or anxiety, and taking avoiding action to prevent these feelings? — **Yes** → Panic disorder with or without agoraphobia (go to Step 1)

No ↓

Episodes of anxiety triggered by external stimuli? — **Yes** → Agoraphobia, social phobia or simple phobia (not covered by this guideline)

No ↓

Over-arousal, irritability, poor concentration, poor sleeping and worry about several areas *most of the time*? — **Yes** → Generalised anxiety disorder (go to Step 1)

Stepped approaches to care

This guideline provides recommendations for care at different stages of the patient journey, represented as different steps:

	Panic disorder See page:	Generalised anxiety disorder See page:
Step 1: Recognition and diagnosis	5	5
Step 2: Treatment in primary care	6–7	8–9
Step 3: Review and consideration of alternative treatments	6–7	8–9
Step 4: Review and referral to specialist mental health services	6–7	8–9
Step 5: Care in specialist mental health services	10	10

Source: NICE (2004).[16] Reproduced by permission of NICE.

In a similar vein, the NICE guideline on eating disorders[19] recommends that young women with low body mass index (BMI), patients consulting with weight concerns who are not overweight, women with menstrual disturbances or amenorrhoea, patients with gastrointestinal symptoms, patients with physical signs of starvation or repeated vomiting, and children with poor growth are asked specific questions such as 'Do you think you have an eating problem?' and 'Do you worry excessively about your weight?'

Stepped-care models

Many of the NICE mental health guidelines such as depression, anxiety and obsessive-compulsive disorder (OCD) are structured around a stepped-care model. This is based on the idea that the patient should be offered the most effective, least intrusive intervention first. Most patients with a common mental health problem for which there is evidence for a low-intensity intervention such as guided self-help or exercise would be expected to start at this level of intervention level, progressing only to more complex interventions if they have not had benefit from lower-intensity interventions. Of course some individuals with a severe disorder or past experience of not benefiting from lower-level interventions may immediately receive interventions from a higher level in the system. Some idea of the range of interventions can be seen from the stepped-care model developed for depression (see Figure 20.2).

Figure 20.2: Stepped-care model for depression

Who is responsible for care?	What is the focus?	What do they do?
Step 5: Inpatient care, crisis teams	Risk to life, severe self-neglect	Medication, combined treatment, ECT
Step 4: Mental health specialists, including crisis teams	Treatment resistant, recurrent, atypical and psychotic depression, and those at significant risk	Medication, complex psychological interventions, combined treatments
Step 3: Primary care team, primary care mental health worker	Moderate or severe depression	Medication, psychological interventions, social support
Step 2: Primary care team, primary care mental health worker	Mild depression	Watchful waiting, guided self-help, cCBT, exercise, brief psychological interventions
Step 1: GP, practice nurse	Recognition	Assessment

Source: NICE (2004).[6] Reproduced by permission of NICE.

Stepped care has been proposed as a method for organising the services for disorders like depression because its phased structure represents a more efficient way of organising services that may help to address the gap which currently exists between the demand and supply of psychological therapies. Gilbody and Bower describe a way to overcome this problem by 'increasing efficiency of provision through the adoption of briefer "minimal interventions" within stepped care models'.[20] Indeed, for Gilbody and Bower without the adoption of a stepped-care framework they are pessimistic that it will be possible to effectively implement the depression guideline in primary care. One element present in many NICE guidelines for common mental disorders (for example depression in adults and children, and PTSD) and an important first step in many stepped-care models is *watchful waiting*. This is defined in the guidelines as 'an intervention in which no active treatment is offered to the person with [*the disorder*] if in the opinion of the health professional the person may recover without a specific intervention. All such patients should be offered a follow up appointment.' This is often accompanied with basic advice on anxiety management, sleep hygiene and diet and exercise. This is not a new idea; it is an approach that GPs have used for many years. Inclusion of this approach in the NICE guidelines, however, indicates that the evidence base supports the use of this approach, which can be helpful to professionals in giving strength to the argument that this is an active intervention. The guidelines also provide clarity on the nature of the intervention, and recommendations on the length of time to follow up. The depression guideline for adults[6] includes watchful waiting as a key priority for implementation. 'For patients with mild depression who do not want an intervention or who, in the opinion of the healthcare professional, may recover with no intervention, a further assessment should be arranged, normally within 2 weeks ('watchful waiting').' This is based on the knowledge that many – but not all – cases of mild depression will remit without intervention. Therefore unnecessary intervention may bring little benefit, and, depending on the nature of the intervention, potentially do harm.[21]

The increased emphasis on psychological treatments

Out of the 14 currently published mental health guidelines from NICE, 11 have as key recommendations for implementation psychological therapies as either a first-line treatment or one to be used concurrently with medication. Whilst the majority of primary care professionals are in favour of these approaches for their patients, many have experienced frustration in terms of access to psychological therapies, particularly in relation to referral criteria, waiting lists and locality of treatment.[3,22] Whilst resource limitations are undoubtedly a significant issue it is important to point out that the NICE guidelines see the development of psychological interventions not just as the provision of six to eight sessions of counselling or 16 to 20 sessions of CBT. There is increasing evidence that a wide range of psychological interventions can be effective including guided self-help for depression and anxiety,[23] cCBT for depression and anxiety, and exercise for depression. Many of these interventions can be delivered in primary care by a range of staff including graduate mental health workers (GMHWs). Indeed, emerging evidence[24,25] Richards *et al.* suggest that by working within a stepped-care framework GMHWs and others with similar levels of experience can make a significant contribution to the coordination and delivery of a wide range of psychosocial interventions for people with moderate to severe depressive disorders.[25] This approach is commonly referred to as collaborative or enhanced care[26] and has a strong evidence base for effectiveness.[6]

Some examples of these brief interventions and how they may be provided are given below. Guided self-help, for example, is recommended for use in the guidelines on depression in children and adults, anxiety, eating disorders and OCD. Guided self-help is a brief intervention, generally based on a CBT approach, in which the patient is supported to use self-help materials (such as a booklet or chapters from a book), usually over two to three sessions, with the follow-up sessions often delivered by telephone. The intervention can be delivered by graduate primary care mental health workers, assistant psychologists or practice nurses. Self-help materials can also be beneficial on their own, and a number of trusts in the UK have established a 'Books on Prescription' scheme. Here professionals in primary care can prescribe a self-help book for a problem such as depression or anxiety. The patient then goes to a local library to 'cash in' the prescription, and can borrow the book for a period of time. In February 2006, NICE published a technology appraisal that recommended the use of cCBT. This technology delivers CBT by computer (using software on a CD-ROM or website), which patients can use either on their own or with some level of facilitation from a graduate worker or possibly a suitably trained receptionist. It normally involves approximately eight weekly sessions of CBT.

Implicit in the increased emphasis on psychological treatments is a decreasing emphasis on the use of medication for the treatment of some but not all common mental disorders. We will not rehearse the details of the evidence base here but it may be helpful to highlight a few key findings from the evidence reviewed by the NICE guidelines. For example, the NICE depression guideline group concludes that for mild depression the risk–benefit ratio of antidepressants did not warrant their routine use in primary care (see the Medicines and Healthcare products Regulatory Agency report on the use of SSRIs from the Committee on Safety of Medicines, www.mhra.gov.uk), preferring to recommend a number of psychosocial interventions of the kind described above as preferred treatment options.[6,18,19] For moderate and severe depression the guideline group did not find any clear evidence of a differential benefit of antidepressants over CBT but did find for moderate depression that it was more cost-effective to offer antidepressants as the first-line treatment.[27] However, for severe depression health economic modelling suggests that starting with combination treatment of antidepressants and CBT is not only more clinically efficacious but also more cost-effective.[27]

Another example is the use of medication in the treatment of PTSD where it was not possible to find convincing evidence of clear clinical benefit from any form of psychotropic medication for the treatment of PTSD symptoms[28] as opposed to other commonly co-morbid problems such as depression or sleep disturbance. Unfortunately this is at odds with the data, which shows that some 60 per cent or more of patients with PTSD treated in secondary services are on medication. In contrast the evidence is strong for the efficacy of some psychological treatments (both for trauma-focused CBT and eye movement desensitisation and reprocessing [EMDR]) but not for others. These others include debriefing, which appears to be harmful, and counselling, which is considerably less effective.[29] This highlights two key issues: the need to switch away from medication and the need to provide the right kind of psychological treatment.

Registers and the primary care role in physical health care for severe mental illness

People with severe mental illness (SMI) – including schizophrenia and bipolar disorder – have significantly higher rates of physical morbidity and mortality than that of the general population. SMI is associated with: raised ten-year coronary heart disease (CHD) risk scores (people with SMI are twice as likely to die of CHD than the general population); lower high-density lipoprotein (HDL) cholesterol levels; raised cholesterol/HDL cholesterol ratios; diabetes mellitus; and smoking.[30] It is CHD and not suicide that is the biggest killer in this group of patients. Although antipsychotic medications and increased socioeconomic deprivation are factors in the increased risk, excess risk factors for CHD are not wholly accounted for by these. Osborn et al. concluded that there is an urgent need for CHD screening and relevant interventions for smoking cessation and diabetes, as well as advice on diet and exercise in patients with SMI.[30]

The NICE guidelines on schizophrenia[31] and bipolar disorder[32] both contain prominent recommendations on physical health, in particular the bipolar disorder guideline. The recommendations on physical health in the bipolar guideline include having a physical health check, normally in primary care, as soon as practicable after the initial presentation, annual physical health checks, and monitoring of specific medications. Physical health checks should include assessment of:

- lipid levels, including cholesterol in all patients over 40 even if there is no other indication of risk
- plasma glucose levels
- weight
- smoking status and alcohol use
- blood pressure.

Physical health checks for SMI are also included in the QOF 2006. Currently indicators MH8 and MH9 state that practices should be able to produce a register of people with schizophrenia, bipolar disorder and other psychoses (4 points), and that these patients should have an annual review including routine health promotion and prevention advice relevant to their age, gender and health status (23 points).

Putting NICE guidance into practice

The above section has set out the key aspects for implementation from NICE guidelines, but how can the uptake of guidance be improved? Successful implementation is critical to the success of the NICE work programme. Much has been learned in recent years about the effectiveness and efficiency of guideline dissemination and implementation strategies. NICE and the National Collaborating Centres are involved in dissemination of the guidelines and support implementation through professional organisations, patient groups and by working with organisations involved with NICE guidance both within and outside the NHS.

NICE supports the implementation of its guidelines via an implementation strategy that can be seen on the NICE website (www.nice.org.uk/usingguidance). The strategy aims to support organisations to meet the set of core and developmental standards for NHS organisations relating to NICE guidance, set by the Department of Health in *Standards for Better Health* (July 2004)[33] and national standards, local action, health and social care standards, and planning framework, 2005–2008. The Healthcare Commission assesses how NHS organisations perform against the standards.

As discussed above there is no ideal strategy or intervention that will guarantee successful implementation. The NICE implementation support strategy has been developed with this in mind and includes the following key themes:

- effective dissemination
- developing a supportive environment by working with key partners
- developing implementation tools
- spreading shared learning
- evaluating success.

It is known that guidelines will only be used in practice if they are owned and implemented locally. This means that structures and processes for implementation have to be established locally. NICE has developed a *How to Put NICE Guidance into Practice* guide[34] for organisations that provides an implementation model to help NHS organisations comply with the Departments of Health's *Standards for Better Health*.[33] The guide is based on experience in the NHS and work described in published literature. The guide refers to the following implementation tools that are produced as part of the strategy and are available via the NICE website:

- *forward planner* summarises published and forthcoming NICE guidance. It explains which sectors are likely to be affected, and whether it will impact on work commissioned by the NHS under Payment by Results

- *slide sets* support early awareness-raising activities. They highlight messages from the guidance and make a number of suggestions for its implementation. They can be edited to suit local need

- *audit criteria* help organisations to plan clinical audit projects based on the key priorities of the guidance. Data collection tools are provided that can be used for the data collection part of the audit cycle either in the NICE format (produced in Word) or cut and pasted into local clinical audit templates. The use of the provided audit tools will enable services within a trust, and whole trusts, to benchmark implementation through the collection of comparable data

- *costing tools* help assess the financial impact of implementing NICE guidance. They comprise a national costing report and a flexible Excel costing template. The latter can be used to identify costs and savings or the need to shift resources

- *implementation advice* points people to national support available and highlight relevant resources, tools or examples of good practice

- *commissioning guides* provide support for local commissioning, including needs assessment and opportunities for disinvestment.

Additional resources developed by NICE to support implementation in primary care include a range of joint *Pulse/NICE publications* called 'Guidelines in action'. These are published for selected clinical guidelines and contain a 10-point plan for GPs to use to help put the NICE advice into practice, key practice points, case studies and question and answers on how to overcome obstacles.

The *Evaluation and Review of NICE Implementation Evidence (ERNIE)* database gives details on how NICE guidance has been used and is available on the NICE website. It provides bibliographical references to external literature around implementation and examples of evaluation reports produced by the Institute.

The *Shared Learning* database helps to share practice and provides real-life examples of what works, including generic processes and guidance-specific examples from primary care.

The Institute also develops *online educational tools* to raise awareness of the recommendations in some of the NICE guidelines and these are targeted at general practitioners and healthcare professionals in primary care.

Effective implementation at a local level

Evidence suggests that to maximise the probability of clinical practice guidelines being implemented, consideration of local circumstances is required. PCTs should encourage implementation, promote local ownership and have a crucial role in overseeing audit, monitoring, performance management and clinical governance. They have a role in identifying local variations in care provision but also address the greater challenge of encouraging professional change once variability has been identified.

Mental health care operates within a complex multi-agency and multi-sectoral environment. Successful implementation depends on effective collaboration between primary and secondary care services. This coordination of implementation across sectors is a challenge, but it is clear that, given that so many mental health conditions present in both primary and secondary care, and that their management is often shared, joint working is needed.

Guidelines implementation requires clear leadership, wide stakeholder engagement, a project management approach and a planned programme of activities with appropriate time scales. Involvement of service users and carers is critical for the implementation of national guidance, in the planning, delivery and evaluation of care. Key local priorities should be identified and a baseline assessment against these priorities should be carried out. The challenges to implementation should be considered (such as financial resources, service changes, training and capacity issues), a phased implementation plan should be developed, and monitoring and evaluation activities around implementation should be considered and actioned.

In terms of facilitating organisational changes required to implement guidelines successfully, the role of commissioning presents a substantial lever. Financial incentives within the GMS contract relating to NICE guidelines around mental health encourage implementation, as mentioned earlier.

Practice-Based Commissioning (PBC) is where practices or localities commissioning as a group agree to directly commission or manage the delivery of services for their patients. An indicative budget for this is agreed with the PCT, although the PCT would continue to hold the actual budget and would remain responsible for the service-level agreements with service providers, including monitoring and invoicing functions. However, the practice or localities would make the commissioning decisions and be able to reallocate resources freed up through cost-effective commissioning to new patient services. Mental health services are within the remit of PBC.

The aim of Payment by Results (PbR) is to provide a transparent, rules-based system for paying trusts. Currently payment is linked to activity and adjusted for case mix for some acute care services. NICE works with the Department of Health team that sets the tariff to ensure that the cost of implementation is adequately reflected in the tariff.

At present PbR does not apply to mental health services. A project is underway to develop proposals on how it may be applied to inpatient, outpatient and community-based health care provided to adults of working age and older people. One suggestion is that one-off mental health problems, which can be overcome through a course of psychological treatment over a discrete period of time, may be suitable for inclusion in a mental health tariff.

The future challenge for the implementation of NICE guidance is around developing the organisational structures, professional and personal cultures within which evidence-based, best-practice care can be provided. The use of NICE guidelines will help to achieve a service in which patients and their carers can expect the same high standard of high-quality care irrespective of where they can seek help.

Conclusion

In the seven years it has been established NICE has achieved its initial goal of providing the NHS in England and Wales with national evidence-based, best-practice guidance. Its programme of guidance has made evidence-based medicine accessible to both professionals and patients and their carers. However, the challenge of effective implementation of this guidance still remains. This chapter has set out what NICE has produced in terms of products and what it intends to do in supporting implementation. Primary care has to be the major focus for the implementation of NICE mental health clinical guidelines; further development of the links between NICE guidance, its implementation programme, the QOF and the Healthcare Commission's assessment is crucial to support this. Such a programme also needs to engage with patient groups and their representatives because in the end what they get out of the guidance is what really matters.

References

1.   Goldberg D, Huxley P. *Common Mental Disorders: a bio-social model* London: Routledge, 1992.

2.   Goldberg DP, Jenkins L, Millar T, *et al.* The ability of trainee general practitioners to identify psychological distress among their patients *Psychological Medicine* 1993; **23(1)**: 185–93.

3.   Layard R. *The Case for Psychological Treatment Centres*, 2006, cep.lse.ac.uk/layard/psych_treatment_centres.pdf [accessed November 2007].

4.   Bower P, Richards D, Lovell K. The clinical and cost-effectiveness of self-help treatments for anxiety and depressive disorders in primary care: a systematic review *British Journal of General Practice* 2001; **51(471)**: 838–45.

5.   National Institute for Health and Clinical Excellence. *Information about NICE Technology Appraisal 97, Computerised Cognitive Behaviour Therapy for Depression and Anxiety: understanding NICE guidance – information for people with depression and anxiety, their families and carers, and the public* London: NICE, 2006, www.nice.org.uk/nicemedia/pdf/TA097publicinfo.pdf [accessed November 2007].

6. National Institute for Health and Clinical Excellence. *Clinical Guideline 23, Depression: management of depression in primary and secondary care* London: NICE, 2004, www.nice.org.uk/CG023NICEguideline [accessed November 2007].

7. NHS Employers. *Revisions to the GMS Contract 2006/07: delivering investment in general practice*, 2006, www.nhsemployers.org/primary/primary-902.cfm [accessed November 2007].

8. Grimshaw JM, Thomas RE, MacLennan G, *et al.* Effectiveness and efficiency of guideline dissemination and implementation strategies *Health Technology Assessment* 2006; **8(6)**: iii–iv, 1–72.

9. Grol R, Jones R. Twenty years of implementation research *Family Practice* 2000; **17(suppl. 1)**: S32–5.

10. Pilling S, Price K. Developing and implementing clinical guidelines: lessons from the NICE schizophrenia guideline *Epidemiologia e psichiatria sociale* 2006; **15(2)**: 109–16.

11. Whitty P, Gilbody S. NICE, but will they help people with depression? The new National Institute for Clinical Excellence depression guidelines *British Journal of Psychiatry* 2005; **186**: 177–8.

12. Meltzer H, Bebbington P, Brugha T, *et al.* The reluctance to seek treatment for neurotic disorders *Journal of Mental Health* 2000; **9(3)**: 319–27.

13. Hansen DG, Vach W, Rosholm J-U, *et al.* Early discontinuation of antidepressants in general practice: association with patient and prescriber characteristics *Family Practice* 2004; **21(6)**: 623–9. Epub 2004 Nov 1.

14. Sartorius N. Iatrogenic stigma of mental illness *British Medical Journal* 2002; **324(7352)**: 1470–1.

15. Priest RG, Vize C, Roberts A, *et al.* Lay people's attitudes to treatment of depression: results of opinion poll for Defeat Depression Campaign just before its launch *British Medical Journal* 1996; **313(7061)**: 858–9.

16. Shakespeare J. *Evaluation of Screening for Postnatal Depression against the NSC Handbook Criteria* London: National Screening Committee, 2001.

17. Whooley MA, Avins AL, Miranda J, *et al.* Case-finding instruments for depression: two questions are as good as many *Journal of General Internal Medicine* 1997; **12(7)**: 439–45.

18. National Institute for Health and Clinical Guidance. *Clinical Guideline 22, Anxiety: management of anxiety (panic disorder, with or without agoraphobia, and generalised anxiety disorder) in adults in primary, secondary and community care* London: NICE, 2004, www.nice.org.uk/nicemedia/pdf/CG022 NICEguidelineamended.pdf [accessed November 2007].

19. National Institute for Health and Clinical Guidance. *Clinical Guideline 9, Eating Disorders: core interventions in the treatment and management of anorexia nervosa, bulimia nervosa and related eating disorders* London: National Institute for Clinical Excellence, 2004, www.nice.org.uk/nicemedia/pdf/cg009niceguidance.pdf [accessed November 2007].

20. Gilbody S, Bower P. Stepped care in psychological therapies: access, effectiveness and efficiency. Narrative literature review *British Journal of Psychiatry* 2005; **186**: 11–17.

21. Coyne JC, Palmer SC, Thompson R. Questionnaires for depression and anxiety: routine screening entails additional pitfalls *British Medical Journal* 2001; **323(7305)**: 168.

22. Richards DA, Lovell K, McEvoy P. Access and effectiveness in psychological therapies: self-help as a routine health technology *Health and Social Care in the Community* 2003; **11(2)**: 175–82.

23. Mead N, MacDonald W, Bower P, *et al.* The clinical effectiveness of guided self-help versus waiting-list control in the management of anxiety and depression: a randomized controlled trial *Psychological Medicine* 2005; **35(11)**: 1633–43.

24. Pilling S, Leibowitz J, Cape J, *et al*. Developing an enhanced care model for depression using primary care mental health workers: implications for the care and management of young men with depression. In: P Fonagy, G Baruch, D Robins (eds). *Reaching the Hard to Reach: evidence-based funding priorities for intervention and research* London: Wiley, 2006.

25. Richards D, Lankshear A, Fletcher J, *et al*. Developing a UK protocol for collaborative care: a qualitative study *General Hospital Psychiatry* 2006; **28(4)**: 296–305.

26. Simon G. Collaborative care for depression *British Medical Journal* 2006; **332**: 249–50.

27. Simon J, Pilling S, Burbeck R, *et al*. Treating moderate and severe depression with antidepressant therapy or combination of antidepressants and psychological therapy: a decision analysis supporting a clinical guideline *British Journal of Psychiatry* 2006; **189**: 494–501.

28. National Institute for Health and Clinical Guidance. *Clinical Guideline 26, Post-Traumatic Stress Disorder (PTSD): the management of PTSD in adults and children in primary and secondary care* London: NICE, 2005, www.nice.org.uk/nicemedia/pdf/cg026niceguideline.pdf [accessed November 2007].

29. Bisson JI, Ehlers A, Matthews R, *et al*. Systematic review and meta-analysis of psychological treatments for chronic post traumatic stress disorder *British Journal of Psychiatry* 2007; **190**: 97–104.

30. Osborn DPJ, Nazareth I, King MB. Risk of coronary heart disease in people with severe mental illness: cross-sectional comparative study in primary care *British Journal of Psychiatry* 2006; **188**: 271–7.

31. National Institute for Health and Clinical Excellence. *Clinical Guideline 1, Schizophrenia: core interventions in the treatment and management of schizophrenia in primary and secondary care* London: NICE, 2002, www.nice.org.uk/nicemedia/pdf/CG1NICEguideline.pdf [accessed November 2007].

32. National Institute for Health and Clinical Excellence. *Clinical Guideline 38, Bipolar Disorder: the management of bipolar disorder in adults, children and adolescents, in primary and secondary care* London: NICE, 2006, www.nice.org.uk/nicemedia/pdf/CG38niceguideline.pdf [accessed November 2007].

33. Department of Health. *Standards for Better Health* London: DH, 2004

34. National Institute for Clinical Excellence. *How to Put NICE Guidance into Practice* London: NICE, 2005, www.nice.org.uk/media/848/D0/HowtoputNICEguidanceintopracticeFINAL.pdf [accessed November 2007].

Further reading

Fixsen DL, Naoom SF, Blase KA, *et al*. *Implementation Research: a synthesis of the literature* Tampa, FL: University of South Florida, Louis de la Parte Florida Mental Health Institute, the National Implementation Research Network (FMHI Publication #231), 2005, http://nirn.fmhi.usf.edu/resources/publications/Monograph/ [accessed November 2007].

Greenhalgh T, Robert G, Bate P, *et al*. *Diffusion of Innovations in Health Service Organisations: a systematic literature review* Oxford: Blackwell BMJ Books, 2005.

Grol R, Wensing M, Eccles M (eds). *Improving Patient Care: the implementation of change in clinical practice* Oxford: Elsevier, 2004.

Layard R. *Mental Health: Britain's biggest social problem?* 2004, www.strategy.gov.uk/downloads/files/mh_layard.pdf [accessed November 2007].

Layard R. *Sainsbury Centre Lecture: therapy for all on the NHS*, 2005, www.scmh.org.uk/80256FBD004F3555/vWeb/flKHAL6H3D4F/$File/Layard%20Lecture%20SCMII%20120905.doc [accessed November 2007].

21 | **The workforce in general practice**
Staff numbers and categories

Alan Cohen

What this chapter contributes:

a review of the different professionals working in primary care

a review of their numbers and roles.

Any discussion of workforce numbers in relation to a single aspect of primary care is problematic. Tasks and roles in primary care are fluid. People with significant mental health problems may present with ostensibly physical symptoms and/or may also have physical health problems. Physical health problems, such as neurological disorders, terminal illness, or life-threatening events like heart attacks, can also have substantial mental health components.

The communities that primary care serves will be home to people with the full range of mental health problems. Inner cities in particular will have a high percentage of service users with a dual diagnosis of mental health problems and drink/drug misuse. Social circumstances of decaying housing, poverty, low income and blighted hopes reap a large crop of people with mental health problems. It is in these communities that acute services are often most stretched – all of which compounds the pressures on primary care.

Primary care staff provide health care to all age groups, so the well-known specialist distinctions between child and adolescent services, adult services, substance misuse, and care of elderly people have less relevance in primary care.

The same staff also support people who have received the full range of healthcare services: medical and surgical, paediatric and geriatric, obstetric and gynaecological, cardiac and diabetic. Many of these have their own National Service Frameworks (NSFs) and guidelines, which compete for attention with those for mental health.

General practice in the UK is very much about the delivery of multidisciplinary care. Since so much of the work of general practice has such a significant mental health component, it is appropriate that every member of that multidisciplinary team has some experience and knowledge of the care of people with mental health problems. Members of the primary care multidisciplinary team include both traditional members such as general practitioners, practice nurses and receptionists, as well as new posts specifically targeted at people with mental health problems, such as graduate mental health workers and gateway workers.

General practitioners

There are currently around 33,000 GPs in the UK. The Royal College of General Practitioners (RCGP) and the British Medical Association (BMA) published a workforce survey in 2001 which suggested that there was a shortfall of approximately 10,000 GPs in current workforce planning.[1]

To a large extent this figure arises from changing career patterns. More GPs take mid-career breaks for family reasons. Many more are retiring early. Sabbatical breaks are becoming the norm rather than the exception. GPs are embarking on a range of other health service roles such as education, research and providing advice to primary care organisations. All of these areas further erode time spent in delivering care to service users.

To this must be added the as yet unclear effects of changing patterns of health care, such as the shift of clinical care from long-stay hospitals to the community. Quality-assured care adds further pressures to the workforce, as does the implementation of new policies and practices, and having to provide evidence that this has been done effectively.

The educational needs of new GPs in mental health have been defined, and are constantly reviewed, by the Joint Committee for Postgraduate Training in General Practice (JCPTGP). They are also reflected in the curriculum for examination for membership of the RCGP. For more details see Chapter 22 on training.

The way that GPs work

The RCGP produces a number of Fact Sheets that summarise the overall workload and characteristics of general practice in the UK. The following information is taken from those Fact Sheets.

Seventy-seven per cent of the 33,000 GPs in the UK work full time; this has fallen from just over 80 per cent in 2001. It is said that over 98 per cent of the population are registered with a GP, but finding an accurate reference that demonstrates this level of coverage was not possible.

The average list size, the number of people registered with an individual GP, has fallen over the years. Table 21.1 demonstrates the changes.

Table 21.1: Average list sizes of unrestricted principals, 1985–2003, UK

1985	1988	1990	1992	1994	1997	1999	2001	2002	2003	% change
2011	1938	1893	1875	1847	1818	1788	1785	1776	1745	-13.2

Although the list size has fallen over time, the details are more complex, as the pattern of GP working has changed, with an increasing number of doctors electing to move from full-time commitments to part-time working.

The average consultation rate has increased over the last ten years. In 2001 there were 106 million consultations by men, and 155 million consultations by women, a total of 261 million consultations, or over 700,000 consultations daily. The average consultation rate is just over five consultations per person per year. As later evidence will show about a third of these 261 million consultations have a significant mental health component, which is around 230,000 consultations daily. If there are 33,000 GPs in the UK, this means that at a minimum each GP has at least seven patients per day with a consultation that has a significant mental health component.

The duration of the consultation has increased slowly over the decades: in the 1970s the average consultation rate was about seven minutes; by the 1990s it was about nine minutes; and into the twenty-first century the average length has increased to just over ten minutes. However, it should be noted that there is frequently a difference between the booked appointment time, which for many practices is ten minutes, and the time actually spent with the patient, which according to the Audit Commission report was 13.3 minutes. The same report identified that the average consultation time for a practice nurse was 19.6 minutes.

Although the duration of the consultation is increasing, it may still not be long enough for people with special needs. The Disability Rights Commission formal inquiry (see Chapter 19) makes recommendations about the consultation duration for people with learning disabilities and with mental health problems.

The reason why people attend their GP is a complex subject, and is discussed in more detail in Chapter 4. However, the Office of Health Economics has calculated the number of people who attend their GP for specific conditions (see Table 21.2).

Some 5 million people are considered to have consulted their GP for a mental health condition, yet, as discussed later, a third of consultations have a significant mental health component, and there are some 261 million consultations annually. So 5 million people are responsible for some 80 million consultations annually. The implications for managing this group effectively, using high-quality evidence-based interventions, are clear.

Table 21.2: Number of people who attend their GP for specific conditions

Disease/condition	Patients (000s)
Respiratory system	13,876
Musculoskeletal system and connective tissue	9937
Skin and subcutaneous tissue	9775
Circulatory system	8047
Genitourinary system	6738
Digestive system	6476
Injury and poisoning	5832
Infectious and parasitic diseases	5496
Mental and behavioural disorders	5270
Eye and adnexa	4025
Ear and mastoid process	4007
Endocrine, nutritional and metabolic diseases	3986
Nervous system	3012
Neoplasms	1500
Blood and blood-forming organs	651
Pregnancy, child birth and the puerperium	348
Congenital anomalies	309
Conditions of the perinatal period	59

Source: Office of Health Economics (2004).[2]

GPs with a special interest

The NHS Plan[3] proposed the development of 'specialised' GPs who would take on particular clinical interests in their local communities. Guidance jointly published by the Department of Health and the RCGP set out the role and capabilities of general practitioners with a special interest (GPwSIs) in mental health.

The GPwSI service may provide some or all of the following.

Clinical

This involves providing assessment, advice, information and treatment on behalf of primary care colleagues for patients with common mental health problems. Different models will dictate where or to whom this service is provided. In most cases, the GPwSI would be working alongside other mental health providers, either as part of an integrated Community Mental Health Team (CMHT), alongside a specialist Mental Health Provider in a Mental Health Trust or as part of a Specialist-Liaison Primary Care Mental Health Service.

Education and liaison

This usually involves dissemination of good practice across the primary care organisation, training and education in the identification, prevention and management of common mental health problems, supporting practices to develop audit and monitoring systems for patients with enduring mental health problems, and developing and implementing clinical guidance and protocols for the assessment and treatment of common mental health problems.

Leadership/service development

Supporting the development of care pathways across the primary–secondary community interface to improve the capacity of GPs and others in primary care to deliver effective mental health services. This role is encompassed in the current role of mental health leads for Primary Care Trusts (PCTs).

Beyond this, the activities of the GPwSI service depend on the needs of the primary care organisation and can include provision of the following. The additional provisions depending on the needs of the PCT and the skills of the GPwSI are:

- leadership across the commissioning and service development domains of primary care mental health services

- assessment under Section 12 of the Mental Health Act

- specific psychological services, such as cognitive behavioural therapy, family therapy, group therapy, psychodynamic psychotherapy

- GPwSI service to specific patient populations, for example eating disorder, chronic fatigue syndrome, fears and phobias, depression.

nGMS contract

As described elsewhere there are significant elements of the nGMS contract that relate to mental health. The GPwSI can play a useful role in advising the PCT, and primary care colleagues, on interpretation and implementation of these indicators.

Competences recommended to meet the service needs

These are based on the Department of Health/RCGP guidance. These will depend on the core activities of the service provided, although a GPwSI should be able to demonstrate elements of those listed below.

Generalist

The competences to deliver a GPwSI service should be seen as a development of generalist skills including good communication skills, competence in teaching and training healthcare professionals, and a commitment to cascading knowledge and skills. Further, it would be expected that all GPwSIs in mental health have a good knowledge and understanding of the common mental health problems that present in primary care and of the range of pharmacological, social and psychological interventions available (though not necessarily the skills or expertise to use them). They should be capable of adapting to the changing requirements of any post, to learn and reflect accordingly.

The competences in Table 21.3 have been defined following stakeholder (professionals and users of the service) consultation.

Evidence of training for competences

Generalist skills

Primary care organisations will need to ensure that the GP is a competent and experienced generalist, as well as having the specific competences and experience for the special interest area. This can be assessed in a number of ways but is readily demonstrated by GPs who have passed the MRCGP examination and who are current members of the College.

Special interest skills

Also required is a six-month full-time or equivalent experience providing community mental health services. Alternatively, evidence is needed of working under direct supervision with a specialist clinician in relevant clinical areas, with at least monthly contact with a specialist provider. The number of sessions should be sufficient to ensure that the GPwSI is able to meet the competences of the service requirements, the skill being assessed and the level of expertise required. For clinicians with little or no experience in providing mental health services this should be in the order of 40–50 sessions. *At least some of this experience should be in a community or primary care setting.*

Otherwise, it is necessary to have a personal development portfolio showing evidence of advanced clinical skills and knowledge. Also, there must be evidence of attendance at relevant courses or self-directed learning to meet educational requirements identified through the personal development plan. An example would be motivational interviewing skills, Section 12 Approval Training. Also, evidence of annual appraisal and revalidation in his or her special interest area must be presented.

Translating these requirements for competences, and an ability to demonstrate the acquisition of competences, can be undertaken in a number of ways. To be attractive to the largest number of clinicians it will need to be flexible to meet the needs of the young, aspiring GP, the more mature, experienced GP, and the nurse practitioner.

There is no national register of GPwSIs in mental health, so that, although the above detailed description of the role and competences associated with such a post is available, there is no evidence that GPwSIs are being recruited, or that they are fulfilling their desired role. That there are significant numbers of GPwSI in other clinical areas demonstrates that the post itself is fundamentally sound, but, for other reasons, it appears that there is less attraction in appointing specialist GPs to this clinical area.

Table 21.3: Stakeholder-defined competences

Competences	Clinical	Education/facilitation	Leadership
Knowledge	Local epidemiology, presentation, natural history, complications, investigation, treatment of the common mental health problems and how they may present in primary care Mental Health Promotion Good knowledge of serious mental health problems, including assessment, treatment and significance of care pathway approach Knowledge of basic psychological/psychosocial skills, such as problem solving, brief intervention, motivational interviewing, basic CBT skills, working with families, behavioural therapy	Understanding of local primary care educational structures and opportunities Good understanding of local mental health service provision Working knowledge of the Misuse of Drugs Act, Children Act and Mental Health Act Good understanding of roles, responsibility and structure of primary care organisations and how to influence them to bring about improvement in delivery of mental health services	National, local and professional strategies and guidelines, and how these may relate to service configuration within the primary care organisation Understanding of primary care structures and how these may affect delivery of services within the primary care organisation Understanding of service redesign and care pathways
Skills	Excellent communication skills Skilled at brief and minimal intervention	Able to keep up to date with national and local priorities, treatment changes and services Able to liaise with educational providers delivering training etc. to primary care practitioners, e.g. deanery structures, primary care organisation-protected learning events	Able to work across clinical networks Able to work effectively in a multidisciplinary team Good change management and clinical skills
Attitudes	Able to engage with patient group in a manner that facilitates good history taking and treatment of mental health problems Able to provide patient-centred care	Able to work in a multidisciplinary team and use other members of the team, and to understand their roles, e.g. social services, educational services, voluntary sector Able to take an evidence-based approach to service delivery	Able to take a whole-system approach to patient care, recognising that effective health care involves taking a multiprofessional approach to service planning

Nurses

There are approximately 25,000 practice nurses in the UK, many of whom work part time. District nurses and health visitors work closely with general practice surgeries to deliver high-quality multidisciplinary care, but differ from practice nurses in that they are not employed by the GP.

Many practice nurses believe they would provide better care if they were better skilled in identifying mental health problems.[4] They say that knowing when and to whom to refer people with mental health problems would be beneficial both to service users and to the practice.

In 2003 the Department of Health published guidance on the development of practitioners with a special interest, to mirror the development of GPwSIs. Although theoretically there is no reason why there should not be a practice or district nurse with a special interest in mental health, the author is unaware of such a post. Such practitioners could have a significant role in the implementation of the recently introduced Quality and Outcomes Framework (QOF) targets for depression, mental health, dementia and learning disability.

Nurses in primary care have an increasingly sophisticated role in providing care, and this is reflected in the career pathway available for practice nurses. Four levels of practice-employed nurse are recognised:

- healthcare assistants
- practice nurse
- specialist nurse
- nurse practitioner.

Table 21.4 describes the broad areas of responsibility and roles for each type of nursing grade. These are intended to be indicative of the difference in roles and responsibilities, rather than an absolute 'definition'.

Certainly the opportunities offered by increasing expertise in practice nursing staff to deliver on the structured approach for people with mental health problems as outlined by NICE guidelines, and implemented through the QOF, are significant. All roles of practice nursing staff could have a part in improving the management and follow-up of people with mental health problems.

Practice receptionists and administrators

Practice receptionists have a vital role to play in primary care and are responsible for managing access between service users and doctors. They are the first people with whom users communicate with when contacting practices by phone or in person.

Table 21.4: Roles and responsibilities for each nursing grade

Healthcare assistant	Practice nurse	Specialist practice nurse	Nurse practitioner
Prepares consulting rooms and maintains stocks of examination instruments and specimen collection materials	Delivers nursing care Runs clinics Provides health promotion advice Carries out immunisations and smear tests	Delivers nursing care, including running specialist clinics Educates patients Carries out immunisations and smear tests Inducts new staff	Assesses patients Plans and implements care Provides specialist advice and maintains records Is a lead specialist in a defined area of nursing care, also providing specialist education and training to other staff and students, and undertaking research and lead clinical audits in own specialist area
Maintains vaccine stock levels and stock rotation as agreed with the practice nurses	Inducts new staff Has knowledge of chronic disease management, general health care, family planning and well-woman care		
Maintains and orders drugs, instruments and clinical supplies			
Cleans, autoclaves and correctly stores instruments			
Takes and records blood pressures using templates			
Performs ECGs, venepuncture and testing of urine specimens			
Performs other clinical tasks as trained and agreed to meet the needs of the practice			

Receptionists may have difficulties in communicating with people with more severe mental health problems. They might perceive the behaviour of some service users as threatening. And, while some service users may be unable to cope with pre-booked appointment systems, the volatility of their mental health might also mean they suddenly need an urgent appointment.

There is little research into how receptionists perceive people with mental health problems. The Marylebone Health Centre in London did some work that involved input from the reception staff. Their perceptions were found to be accurate and useful, but this was an isolated, innovative approach. Training that heightens awareness for non-medical staff would be of great benefit.

The Primary Care Programme of the Care Services Improvement Partnership (CSIP) has recently published a document called *Key Skills for Key Staff* that sets out the knowledge, skills and competences needed by the primary healthcare team.[5] It makes clear that it is not possible to describe what each member of the team needs to know, but accepts that there should be some local negotiation and debate, in relation to local circumstances, as to what knowledge, skills and competences should be held by each individual. This reflects the reality of primary care, in that a large practice in rural Shropshire will work in a different way from a small single-handed practice behind King's Cross Station. Ultimately the same knowledge, skills and competences need to be present, but who does what, and how, will vary due to local circumstances.

Key Skills for Key Staff also sets out a pragmatic developmental agenda for practices to acquire the capabilities needed by use of a simple mnemonic 'HEALTH':

H = Health promotion

E = Evidence

A = Assessment

L = Lifestyle

T = Treatments

H = Holistic approach.

There is also a useful table that describes the key skills needed by a primary healthcare team. For each 'key skill' there are identified:

- *What* knowledge, skills and competences are recommended to adequately meet the mental health needs of individuals and families in everyday primary practice?
- *Why* are such knowledge, skills and capabilities required?
- *How* can attainment of key capabilities be demonstrated?
- *When* does this apply to the new General Medical Services (nGMS) contract?
- *Where* can you find out more information to enhance your competences?
- *Which* nationally recognised learning outcomes – Essential Shared Capabilities (ESC) and National Occupational Standards (NOS) – are you able to demonstrate?

This development is clearly extremely valuable.

Counsellors

The emergence of practice counsellors has been one of the outstanding developments in primary care in recent years.

This development has been influenced by a number of factors, including the shift in emphasis of the work of CMHTs, the added flexibility given to practices by practice fund-holding, and a genuine concern among GPs to provide more effective care for service users whose problems result from chaotic life experiences.

The work of primary care counsellors is often concerned with listening and talking to people with mental health problems. Their work contrasts with that of CMHTs and clinical psychologists who tend to deliver interventions to people in response to a defined clinical diagnosis.

Counsellors have the support of a strong professional organisation, the Association of Counsellors and Psychotherapists in Primary Care (CPC). However, not all practice counsellors belong to this or other professional bodies, and lack of professional standards can result in poor or even dangerous treatment for service users.

More information on the types of way that counsellors work is included in Chapter 11, 'Talking therapies'.

The effectiveness of counsellors has been addressed by a number of studies.[6-11] One of the most quoted studies was undertaken by the National Primary Care Research and Development Centre, under the direction of Professor Bower and colleagues.[12] The study, based in Manchester and London, looked at the effectiveness of usual GP care, non-directive counselling, and cognitive behavioural therapy (CBT). The study followed patients for up for 12 months, and looked at mental health outcomes, and in a subsequent paper[13] compared the cost-effectiveness of the three interventions. They found that, at four months, people who received either non-directive counselling or CBT improved faster than those who received usual GP care. However, at 12 months there was no difference in outcome for the three groups. The cost-effectiveness study, limited by the relatively small size of the study populations, concluded that at four months psychological intervention was cost-effective, but that at 12 months there was no difference between the three interventions.

In 2001, Chilvers and colleagues[14] compared the use of antidepressants and non-directive counselling for people with mild and moderate depression. Their conclusion was that both interventions were equally effective although those taking antidepressants improved more quickly at eight weeks, compared with those receiving non-directive counselling. They recommended that patients be given the choice of which intervention they would prefer.

Graduate primary care mental health workers

The NHS Plan[3] proposed the creation of a new paraprofessional called a 'graduate mental health worker'. The original intention of this new post was to appoint 'One thousand new graduate primary care mental health workers, trained in brief therapy techniques of proven effectiveness, [which] will be employed to help GPs manage and treat common mental health problems in all age groups, including children.' It went on to estimate that, by 2004, more than 300,000 people would have received extra help from these new workers.

The type of work that these graduate workers would undertake was summarised in guidance published by the Department of Health as:[15]

- supporting the delivery of brief, evidence-based, effective interventions and self-help for people with common mental disorders of all ages

- strengthening the information available for patients

- supporting the development of practice-based information systems, audit and outcome measurement

- improving service users' satisfaction with care

- improving knowledge within the practice about the network of community resources for people with mental health problems.

Following extensive consultation, in 2003 the National Institute for Mental Health in England (NIMHE) published best-practice guidance, *Primary Care Graduate Mental Health Workers*.[16] This reviewed the role of graduate workers, and summarised their potential work areas as:

- client work

- practice teamwork

- work in the wider community.

These three broad descriptions of their potential contribution have remained in place since 2003.

That general practitioners were recognised as needing support to deliver evidence-based interventions was a major advance – this was the first time that there was a specific allocation for primary care mental health. Even though it was not ring-fenced, and there was no specific 'must do' target, it still represented a major potential advance for treating 90 per cent of people with mental health problems who are managed entirely in primary care.

The financial allocation, added to the PCTs' baseline budget, was, for all of England, £25m. From this allocation, resources would be top sliced to fund the training programmes that needed to be set up to recruit and train these new workers. The salary that most graduate workers would be likely to earn was between £15K and £17K per annum. Each PCT was allocated resources to employ two or three new workers, depending on its size. With a little over 300 PCTs at that time, together the allocation represented 1000 new workers.

Whilst the principle of developing a role in primary care that supported GPs to deliver evidence-based interventions for people with common mental health problems was warmly welcomed, some of the practical issues raised questions as to the usefulness of these new workers. Some of these included developing a career pathway; some feared that people would use these posts as a 'stepping stone' to clinical psychology, and that therefore job retention for these posts would be poor. Other concerns related to: the degree of integration into general practice; the graduate worker's ability to manage patients whom the experienced GP could not satisfactorily manage; and the graduate worker not being trained to assess a patient, but just trained to deliver evidence-based interventions.

NIMHE's *Primary Care Graduate Mental Health Workers*[16] is an extremely useful guide. It covers not only the background to the post, but also extensive practical experience from the Northwest of England in recruiting, training and working with these new staff. The guide includes help in defining what role is needed for these new staff, and how they would fit into a redesigned primary care mental health service. It describes good employment practice including job descriptions, and experience of training, recruiting and retaining individuals to these posts.

Graduate mental health workers have now been in place for between three and four years, and questions are now being asked about their effectiveness. *Primary Care Graduate Mental Health Workers*[16] offers extensive practical guidance and advice – but has that advice been translated into better outcomes for patients, or, even, more patients being treated than previously?

The National Primary Care Research and Development Centre in Manchester, commissioned by the Department of Health,[17] has recently published an evaluation of the policy, which provides some interesting data on the success of this new workforce.

The evaluation found that fewer than the potential 1000 new workers were actually employed. The figure from the Department of Health, in its five-year review of the National Service Framework Implementation,[18] was that 600 graduate workers were in place in 2004/05. Whilst the study did not describe the regional variation in take-up of places, there is some anecdotal evidence that the Northwest and Northeast regions were effective at recruiting and training graduate workers, whilst London was particularly poor. The evaluation paper attempted to survey all graduate mental health workers, by approaching them through their training programmes. They achieved a creditable 82 per cent success, but this was 82 per cent of 358 individuals, not quite the 600 claimed by the Department of Health in its five-year review.

The evaluation paper looked at their clinical workload and found that only two thirds of the surveyed graduate workers saw patients. Further, for those graduate workers who did see patients, they saw, on average, 5.4 new patients per month. The authors of the study usefully point out that, if the 1000 graduate workers were all to see patients (and in fact only 60 per cent do see patients), then 65,000 patients would have been treated, instead of the 300,000 expected. Interestingly, 60 per cent of the people attending graduate workers attended for three or fewer sessions, although each session on average lasted 50 minutes. Ninety-three per cent of patients seen by the graduates suffered from anxiety, depression or psychosocial life events. The most frequent interventions offered by the graduates were guided self-help (60 per cent) and support and non-directive counselling (52 per cent), in line with NICE guidelines.

The paper was able to show that those graduate workers fully integrated into general practice were more likely to see patients, and more likely to stay in post – 50 per cent of those who were not integrated stated that they wished to apply for clinical psychology posts.

The evaluation points out that the data are drawn relatively early in the development of these posts, and that there are a number of confounding features that make absolute interpretation of the results difficult. Its conclusion is that the implementation of the policy should be considered a 'partial success'.

The fact that there has not been universal take-up of these posts, and that several years after their introduction there are still significant shortfalls in the number recruited, may be a reflection of the success of the policy.

A more cynical observer, reviewing the evidence related to counselling, and the evidence about people with mild common mental health problems, might however have made the point that perhaps these people would have improved without the intervention of the graduate worker. Clearly further research is needed to determine the way this valuable resource can best be used, and to understand more clearly the natural history of people with mild disorders.

References

1. British Medical Association and Royal College of General Practitioners. *General Practice Workload* (Information Sheet No. 3) London: RCGP, 2004.

2. Office of Health Economics. *Compendium of Health Statistics, 15th Edition 2003/04* London: OHE, 2004.

3. Department of Health. *The NHS Plan. A plan for investment. A plan for reform*, 2000, www.dh.gov.uk/en/Publicationsandstatistics/Publications/PublicationsPolicyAndGuidance/DH_4002960 [accessed November 2007].

4. L Young RCN, personal communication, 2002.

5. Primary Care Programme of the Care Services Improvement Partnership *Key Skills for Key Staff* Cheshire: CSIP, 2006.

6. Hazzard A. Measuring outcome in counselling: a brief exploration of the issues *British Journal of General Practice* 1995; **45**: 118–19.

7. Bower P, King M. Randomised controlled trials and the evaluation of psychological therapy. In: N Rowland, S Goss (eds). *Evidence-Based Counselling and Psychological Therapies*, pp. 79–110, London: Routledge, 2000.

8. Chambless D, Hollon S. Defining empirically supported therapies *Journal of Consulting and Clinical Psychology* 1998; **66**: 7–18.

9. Jacobson N, Christensen A. Studying the effectiveness of psychotherapy: how well can clinical trials do the job? *American Psychologist* 1996; **51**: 1031–9.

10. Roth A, Fonagy P. *What Works for Whom? A critical review of psychotherapy research* London: Guildford, 1996.

11. Rowland N, Bower P, Mellor-Clark J, *et al*. Counselling for depression in primary care (Cochrane Review). The Cochrane Library, Issue 2, Oxford: Update Software, 2001.

12. Ward E, King M, Lloyd M, *et al*. Randomised controlled trial of non-directive counselling, cognitive-behaviour therapy and usual GP care for patients with depression. I: Clinical effectiveness *British Medical Journal* 2000; **321**: 1383–8.

13. Bower P, Byford S, Sibbald B, *et al*. Randomised controlled trial of non-directive counselling, cognitive-behaviour therapy and usual GP care for patients with depression. II: Cost effectiveness *British Medical Journal* 2000; **321**: 1389–92.

14. Chilvers C, Dewey M, Fielding K, *et al*. Antidepressant drugs and generic counselling for treatment of major depression in primary care: randomised trial with patient preference arms *British Medical Journal* 2001; **322**: 775.

15. Department of Health. *Fast Forwarding Primary Care Mental Health: graduate mental health workers*, 2003, www.dh.gov.uk/en/Publicationsandstatistics/Publications/PublicationsPolicyAnd Guidance/DH_4005784 [accessed November 2007].

16. National Institute of Mental Health in England and the North West Development Centre. *Primary Care Graduate Mental Health Workers: a practical guide* Manchester: NIMHE North West, 2005.

17. Harkness EF, Bower P, Gask L, *et al*. Improving primary care mental health: survey evaluation of an innovative workforce development in England *Primary Care Mental Health* 2005; **3(4)**: 253–60.

18. Department of Health. *The National Service Framework for Mental Health: five years on*, 2004, www.dh.gov.uk/en/Publicationsandstatistics/Publications/PublicationsPolicyAndGuidance/ DH_4099120 [accessed November 2007].

Further reading

Andrews G. Should depression be managed as a chronic disease *British Medical Journal* 2001; **322(7283)**: 419–21, www.bmj.com/cgi/content/extract/322/7283/419 [accessed November 2007].

Andrews G, Henderson S (eds). *Unmet Need in Psychiatry: problems, resources, responses* Cambridge: Cambridge University Press, 2000.

Bebbington PE, Dunn G, Jenkins R, *et al*. The influence of age and sex on the prevalence of depressive conditions: report from the national survey of psychiatric morbidity *Psychological Medicine* 1998; **28**: 9–19.

Bedi N, Chilvers C, Churchill R, *et al*. Assessing effectiveness of treatment of depression in primary care: partially randomised preference trial *British Journal of Psychiatry* 2000; **177**: 312–18.

Boot D, Gillies P, Fenelon J, *et al*. Evaluation of the short-term impact of counselling in general practice *Patient Education and Counselling* 1994; **24**: 79–89.

Bower P. Factors that predict patient outcome in primary care psychological therapies: current evidence and methodological issues *Primary Care Psychiatry* 2000; **6**: 15–21.

Bower P. Primary care mental health workers: models of working and evidence of effectiveness *British Journal of General Practice* 2002; **52**: 926–33.

Bower P. Primary care mental health workers: a qualitative study of a developing role in five sites in the North West, unpublished report, NPCRDC, University of Manchester, 2003.

Bower P, Foster J, Mellor-Clarke J. *Quality in Counselling in Primary Care: a guide for effective commissioning and clinical governance*, NPCRDC, University of Manchester, 2001, www.npcrdc.man.ac.uk/PublicationDetail.cfm?ID=37 [accessed November 2007].

Bower P, Richards D, Lovell K. The clinical and cost-effectiveness of self-help treatments for anxiety and depressive disorders in primary care: a systematic review *British Journal of General Practice* 2001; **51**: 838–45.

Briggs A. Economic evaluation and clinical trials: size matters *British Medical Journal* 2000; **321**: 1362–3.

British Association for Counselling. *Code of Ethics and Practice for Counsellors* Rugby: BAC, 1992.

British Association for Counselling. *Guidelines for the Employment of Counsellors in General Practice* Rugby: BAC, 1995.

British Association for Counselling. *Counsellor Accreditation* Rugby: BAC, 1998.

Broadhurst A. Clinical psychology and the general practitioner *British Medical Journal* 1972; **1(2002)**: 739–45.

Clark A, Hook J, Stein K. Counsellors in primary care in Southampton: a questionnaire survey of their qualifications, working arrangements and casemix *British Journal of General Practice* 1997; **47**: 613–17.

Cooper H, Lester H, Freemantle N, *et al*. A cluster randomised controlled trial of the effect of primary care mental health workers on satisfaction, mental health symptoms and use of services: background and methodology *Primary Care Psychiatry* 2003; **9**: 1–7.

The Counselling versus Antidepressants in Primary Care Study Group. How disabling is depression? Evidence from a primary care sample *British Journal of General Practice* 1999; **49**: 95–8.

Crosland A, Tomson D, Freer M. *Primary Care Mental Health Graduate Workers: issues of content, delivery and implementation of a programme of training* Newcastle upon Tyne: Centre for Primary and Community Care Learning, Northumbria University, 2002.

Department of Health. *Mental Health Policy Implementation Guide*, 2001, www.dh.gov.uk/en/Publicationsandstatistics/Publications/PublicationsPolicyAndGuidance/DH_4009350 [accessed November 2007].

Department of Health. *Treatment Choice in Psychological Therapies and Counselling: evidence based clinical practice guideline*, 2001, www.dh.gov.uk/assetRoot/04/05/82/45/04058245.pdf [accessed November 2007].

Dowrick C, Dunn G, Ayuso-Mateos J-L, *et al*. Problem solving treatment and group psychoeducation for depression: multicentre randomised controlled trial *British Medical Journal* 2000; **321**: 1–6.

Eastman C, McPherson I. As others see us: general practitioners' perceptions of psychological problems and the relevance of clinical psychology *British Journal of Clinical Psychology* 1982; **21**: 85–92.

Friedli K, King M, Lloyd M. The economics of employing a counsellor in general practice: analysis of data from a randomised controlled trial *British Journal of General Practice* 2000; **50**: 276–83.

Friedli K, King M, Lloyd M, *et al*. Randomised controlled assessment of non-directive psychotherapy versus routine general-practitioner care *Lancet* 1997; **350**: 1662–5.

Gask L, Rogers A, Roland M, *et al*. *Improving Quality in Primary Care: a practical guide to the National Service Framework for Mental Health* Manchester: National Primary Care Research and Development Centre, University of Manchester, 2000, www.npcrdc.man.ac.uk/PublicationDetail.cfm?ID=36 [accessed November 2007].

Gilbody S, Whitty P, Grimshaw J, *et al*. Educational and organisational interventions to improve the management of depression in primary care: a systematic review *Journal of the American Medical Association* 2003; **289**: 3145–51.

Goldberg D, Huxley P. *Common Mental Disorders* London: Routledge, 1992.

Grant C, Goodenough T, Harvey I, *et al*. A randomised controlled trial and economic evaluation of a referrals facilitator between primary care and the voluntary sector *British Medical Journal* 2000; **320**: 419–23.

Harvey I, Nelson S, Lyons R, *et al*. Randomized controlled trial and economic evaluation of counselling in primary care *British Journal of General Practice* 1998; **48**: 1043–8.

Hemmings A. Counselling in primary care: a randomised controlled trial *Patient Education and Counselling* 1997; **32**: 219–30.

Hemmings A. Counselling in primary care: a review of the practice evidence *British Journal of Guidance and Counselling* 2000; **28**: 233–52.

Katon W, Von Korff M, Lin E, *et al*. Population based care of depression: effective disease management strategies to decrease prevalence *General Hospital Psychiatry* 1997; **19**; 169–78.

Kendrick T. Depression management clinics in general practice? *British Medical Journal* 2000; **320**: 527–8.

Kendrick T, Burns T, Freeling P, *et al*. Provision of care to general practice patients with a disabling long term mental illness; a survey in 16 practices *British Journal of General Practice* 1994; **44**: 301–9.

King M, Broster G, Lloyd M, *et al*. Controlled trials in the evaluation of counselling in general practice *British Journal of General Practice* 1994; **44**: 229–32.

Lai P, Hubbling D, Persaud R. Non-directive counselling versus routine general practitioner care [letter] *Lancet* 1998; **351**: 750.

Lovell K, Richards D. Multiple access points and levels of entry (MAPLE): ensuring choice, accessibility and equity for CBT services *Behavioural and Cognitive Psychotherapy* 2000; **28**: 379–91.

Lovell K, Richards DA, Bower P. Improving access to primary care mental health: uncontrolled evaluation of a pilot self-help clinic *British Journal of General Practice* 2003; **53**: 133–5.

Mellor-Clark J, Connel J, Barkham M. Counselling outcomes in primary health care: a CORE system profile *European Journal of Psychotherapy, Counselling and Health* 2001; **4**: 1–22.

Mellor-Clark J, Simms-Ellis R, Burton M. *National Survey of Counsellors in Primary Care: evidence for growing professionalisation* London: RCGP, 2001.

Meltzer H, Gill B, Petticrew M, *et al*. *OCPS Surveys of Psychiatric Morbidity in Great Britain, Report 1: the prevalence of psychiatric morbidity among adults living in private households* London: Her Majesty's Stationery Office, 1995.

National Institute for Health and Clinical Guidance. *Clinical Guideline 22, Anxiety: management of anxiety (panic disorder, with or without agoraphobia, and generalised anxiety disorder) in adults in primary, secondary and community care* London: NICE, 2004, www.nice.org.uk/nicemedia/pdf/CG022NICE guidelineamended.pdf [accessed November 2007].

National Institute for Health and Clinical Excellence. *Clinical Guideline 23, Depression: management of depression in primary and secondary care* London: NICE, 2004, www.nice.org.uk/CG023NICEguideline [accessed November 2007].

NHS Centre for Reviews and Dissemination. Improving the recognition and management of depression in primary care *Effective Health Care Bulletin* 2002; **7(5)**, www.york.ac.uk/inst/crd/ehc75.pdf [accessed November 2007].

Otto MW, Pollack M, Maki KM. Empirically supported treatments for panic disorder: costs, benefits, and stepped care *Journal of Consulting and Clinical Psychology* 2000; **68**: 556–63.

Priest R, Vize C, Roberts M, *et al*. Lay people's attitudes to the treatment of depression: results of opinion poll for Defeat Depression Campaign just before its launch *British Medical Journal* 1996; **313**: 858–9.

Proudfoot J, Goldberg D, Mann A, *et al*. Computerized, interactive, multimedia cognitive-behavioural program for anxiety and depression in general practice *Psychological Medicine* 2003; **33**: 217–27.

Rain L. *Counselling in Primary Care: a guide to good practice* Leeds: MIND, 1996.

Richards D, Lovell K, McEvoy P. Access and effectiveness in psychological therapies: self-help as a routine health technology *Health and Social Care in the Community* 2003; **11**: 175–82.

Richards D, Richards A, Barkham M, *et al*. PHASE: a 'health technology' approach to psychological treatment in primary mental health care *Primary Health Care Research and Development* 2002; **3**: 159–68.

Scogin FR, Hanson A, Welsh D. Self-administered treatment in stepped-care models of depression treatment *Journal of Clinical Psychology* 2003; **59**: 341–9.

Seligman M. The effectiveness of psychotherapy: the consumer reports study *American Psychologist* 1995; **50**: 965–74.

Sibbald B, Addington-Hall J, Brenneman D, *et al*. *The Role of Counsellors in General Practice* London: RCGP, 1996.

Sibbald B, Ward E, King M. Randomised controlled trial of non-directive counselling, cognitive-behaviour therapy and usual general practitioner care in the management of depression as well as mixed anxiety and depression in primary care *Health Technology Assessment* 2000; **4(19)**.

Simon G, Von Korff M, Rutter C, *et al*. Randomised trial of monitoring, feedback and management of care by telephone to improve treatment of depression in primary care *British Medical Journal* 2000; **320**: 550–4.

Simpson S, Corney R, Fitzgerald P, *et al*. A randomised controlled trial to evaluate the effectiveness and cost-effectiveness of counselling patients with chronic depression *Health Technology Assessment* 2000; **4(36)**.

Speirs R, Jewell J. One counsellor, two practices: report of a pilot scheme in Cambridgeshire *British Journal of General Practice* 1995; **45**: 31–3.

Von Korff M, Goldberg D. Improving outcomes in depression *British Medical Journal* 2001; **323**: 948–9.

22 | Meeting the challenges of educating and training a primary care mental health workforce

Les Ashton and Mike Scanlan

What this chapter contributes:

some of the challenges that the education agenda faces in delivering the above

some of the recent key factors that have influenced the mental health education and learning agenda

some examples of educational practice that may meet these challenges.

Good mental health is important to everybody's daily functioning and relevant to patients' ability to be involved in the care provided by general practitioners (GPs). It is hard to define, but is more than the absence of mental illness and includes concepts such as self-efficacy, self-worth and empowerment.[1]

A practitioner is expected to treat a wide variety of different mental health problems. Yet there are some underlying principles of knowledge, skills and attitudes that any practitioner should be aware of, for each of those conditions.

The challenges facing primary care mental health education and learning agenda

The ideal aims and objectives underpinning any mental health training aimed at GPs or other primary care practitioners, primary healthcare workers (PHCWs) including nurses, other clinicians and administrative staff should be as follows.

Aim

To improve the mental health care offered by practitioners in primary care with resultant improved outcomes for patient care.

Objectives

- To enhance and improve the knowledge base of primary care practitioners, GPs and PHCWs.

- To provide practitioners, GPs and PHCWs with increased mental health skills.

- To increase the psychological mindfulness of practitioners. This will enable primary care staff to routinely explore whether a wide range of presenting issues have psychological causal and maintaining factors.

- To enable practitioners, GPs and PHCWs to feel more secure about their mental health role. This entails having a raised awareness of what can be achieved in a primary care consultation and also when specialist or other interventions are required.

How are these aims and objectives to be achieved within a working environment where the only constant is change? New policy emerges at a pace that exceeds the rate of learning and there has been an emphasis on new ways of working in order to enable service redesign. Expert or evidence-based approaches, such as National Institute for Health and Clinical Excellence (NICE) guidance, and quality measures, such as the new GP contract Quality and Outcomes Framework (QOF), have not only influenced how practitioners practice but also service redesign. These initiatives and policies have often been introduced with little regard to the educational needs or resources necessary for their implementation.

Educational programmes have in some cases supported new roles, e.g. the graduate mental health worker initiative, but in other areas, such as refashioning of existing roles and services, they have not always been an integral part of their development. With limited resources and funding, how does an organisation balance addressing the educational needs of its existing workforce with that of the needs of new roles emerging out of service redesign?

With revalidation a high priority for everyone, continuing professional development has to be managed. A high number of appraisals may have been performed across primary care organisations. but if the educational needs arising from such activities have not been addressed (for whatever reason) their worth and value could be questioned.

There has been a much welcomed drive in moving away from Cartesian thinking around the mind–body split towards a more holistic approach to mental health issues. This equally has given greater prominence to concepts such as *wellbeing* and *happiness*, which have brought their own educational requirements.[2,3]

Competence frameworks now define roles and job specifications. Yet, investment in multi-professional and inter-professional education is essential if our workforce is going to be *fit for purpose* in meeting these competence requirements. In an environment of ever-decreasing budgets and limited financial resources, how will education ever receive the financial backing it deserves in order to effect efficient change? For too long, education provision has been given little or minimal priority weighting and has often been seen as an add-on or someone else's responsibility.

The message needs to be that mental health is everybody's core business and so is the education agenda!

The biggest challenge facing the need to educate and train the primary care workforce around mental health issues is establishing this agenda as central and integrated within an individual's and organisations' everyday core business.

Educational provision has also undergone major changes with a shift to workplace and work-based learning approaches. With an incremental rise in e-learning resources and the move to portfolio learning this has meant that, from an educational provision perspective, there is now a huge variety of approaches and resources to suit all types of learners and learning styles. However, as the sharing of information is not necessarily the acquisition of knowledge, the challenge for the learner is the ability to access education that is meaningful, learner centred and that will enable a change in behaviours. If the latter does not occur, educational impact remains limited and knowledge acquisition remains *speculative*.

'Lyotard's Triangle'[4] is a way of illustrating three methods of knowledge acquisition. The three points of the triangle are labelled 'speculative', 'practice' and 'emancipatory'. These can be described as follows:

Speculative

- Knowledge for its own sake.
- Not concerned with application to practice.

Practice

- Neo-managerialism:
  - improvement
  - modernisation of management and performance.

Emancipatory

- Holism.
- Humanism.
- Development of person in the world.
- Emancipation through knowledge.

'Change agency' occurs between these three. This phrase applies to improved practitioner capacity in terms of confidence, motivation and developmental insights at practice level. It not only results in better patient care at local level but also includes a greater personal awareness and application of tactical and strategic change insights. Education and training must be directed towards promoting change agency because it will automatically underpin any capacity and capability planning cycle if this is to be delivered.

Figure 22.1 shows the capacity and capability planning cycle that must support education and training.

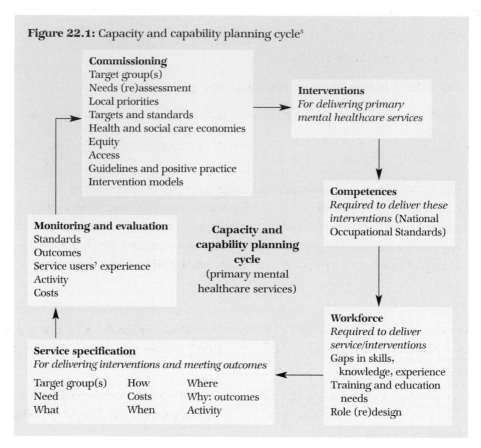

Figure 22.1: Capacity and capability planning cycle[5]

How will educational delivery meet the challenge of addressing both the individual's and organisation's developing needs?

In complex interventions, it is often difficult to establish the active ingredients of an effective strategy.

Some research around the management of depression in primary care has alluded to the fact that, even despite well-developed clinician education packages and guideline implementation, these interventions have little or no effect on either recognition rates for depression or on clinical improvement.[6,7] It is however important to note that there was no organisational support to enhance individual patient care in these studies.

A systematic review of educational and organisational interventions to improve the management of depression in primary care[8] significantly concluded that, in order for guideline implementation and educational interventions to be successful, these also needed to be accompanied by complex organisational interventions such as nurse case management, collaborative care or intensive quality improvement initiatives.

Cognitive psychological research has also shown that *deliberate practice* is a far better method to acquire expertise than simple unstructured practice.[9] Simply, *deliberate practice* is the combination of acquiring expertise with activities that help learners to become more conscious of their learning. Key elements in deliberate practice are:

- supervision and detailed feedback

- well-defined tasks to improve certain aspects of performance

- ample opportunity to improve performance gradually by performing tasks repeatedly.

Further interesting research is now emerging as to how primary care clinicians derive their individual and collective healthcare decisions and the concept of *mindlines*:

> Clinicians rarely accessed, appraised or utilised explicit formal evidence. Instead, they relied on 'Mindlines' – Collectively reinforced, internalised tacit guidelines, which were informed by brief reading, but mainly by their interactions with each other and with opinion leaders, patients and other sources of largely tacit knowledge that built on their early training and their own colleagues' experience.[10]

Further exploration as to how to maximise such approaches, and thinking at a local and individual level, may well be crucial if individual behaviours are to alter and change agency is to occur.

Clearly any training directed at the primary care workforce should attend to skills in flexible and generalist practice, core skills and primary care culture, capacity building and collaborative practice.

Recent key influences on the mental health education and learning agenda

Recently, there have been some important developments that have shaped, and will continue to shape, mental health educational development. These also have begun to address quality assurance of educational provision. The following list is not exhaustive but briefly describes some of the more important influences:

- ten essential shared capabilities

- RCGP *Care of People with Mental Health Problems* curriculum statement

- quality assurance of educational provision

- *Key Skills for Key Staff*.

Ten essential shared capabilities

The ten essential shared capabilities[11] have been compiled via the involvement of mental health service users, carers and mental health experts. They comprise the ten areas that should be considered by any persons providing mental health care. These can be roughly grouped into three sections:

Values-based practice

- Practising ethically.
- Promoting recovery.
- Respecting diversity.
- Challenging inequality.

Socially inclusive practice

- Working in partnership.
- Promoting user-centred care.

Evidence-based practice

- Promoting safety and positive risk taking.
- Identifying peoples' needs and strengths.
- Making a difference.
- Personal development and learning.

These capabilities should be used as benchmarking statements that can guide the development of any mental health training. By bearing the ten essential shared capabilities in mind when planning and delivering training the by-product should be an incremental increase in the psychological mindfulness of learners.

At first glance the statements may seem more suited to specialist mental health care but every service user receiving specialist care also is a patient in primary care. Their needs and aspirations remain the same and so should the broad values underpinning care wherever that is delivered.

Royal College of General Practitioners, *Care of People with Mental Health Problems* (curriculum statement 13)

As from 2008, in order to demonstrate the core competences in the area of mental health, a general practitioner will require knowledge, skills and appropriate attitudes in the areas defined under the new RCGP curriculum statement 13 – *Care of People with Mental Health Problems*.[1]

This is just one of a large number of statements that comprise the new RCGP curriculum for specialty training for general practice that will require implementation. The statement was based around the work of the RCGP Mental Health Task Group. It should not be looked at in isolation but in conjunction with the core statement, *Being a General Practitioner*.[12]

Although the curriculum has been designed for GP registrars, it should be viewed as providing the framework for competence for all GPs upon which further expertise can be developed. Other developments in progress include specific work around the accreditation of the practitioner with a special interest (PwSI) role in mental health. In conjunction with the charitable organisation Primary Care Mental Health and Education (www.primhe.org), the RCGP is currently designing and developing specific training courses to address this accreditation (personal communication, LA).

A detailed review of the statement is inappropriate but the authors of this chapter feel that the important content and learning outcomes relating to mental health education can easily be lost or disregarded. As such, we have listed the more important features of the statement, as follows.

Key messages of the curriculum statement

- Depression is common in general practice.
  - GPs should be able to recognise depression and assess its severity.
  - All depressed patients should be screened for suicidal intent.

- People with severe mental illness have a high prevalence of physical co-morbidity that should be looked for and treated by GPs.

- The skills to both recognise and manage somatisation will lead to considerable savings in patient suffering and healthcare costs.

- All physical illness has a psychological component; this should be taken into account in management plans.

The continuous improvement of communication skills and patient-centred practice is likely to be the single most important factor in improving recognition and effective management of mental health problems.

UK health priorities underpinning the development of the curriculum statement

Providing care for people with mental health problems and promoting mental health is a priority for the NHS in each of the four countries of the UK. A range of ideas has been influential in determining policy and practice.

The Mental Health National Service Framework, published in 1999 by the Department of Health, outlined the care that should be provided. It has formed the basis for most mental healthcare developments since then and made clear that the priority within mental health services should be the care provided for people with a severe and enduring mental illness.

Primary care is charged with providing care for 'common mental health problems' and contributing to health promotion, but there is a lack of clarity about who should lead on the care of those with chronic, complex and disabling non-psychotic problems. General practitioners require a good understanding of the healthcare needs of all these groups.

The Social Exclusion Unit's report on mental health emphasises the role of discrimination, low expectations, unemployment and lack of community engagement as both cause and consequence of mental illness. It explores new ways of working with those in marginalised groups.

Others have cautioned against the exclusive use of psychiatric models and emphasised the potential harms as well as benefits both diagnosis and treatment can bring. There is a general consensus that mental ill-health can best be tackled by a full exchange of information, by shared decision making and valuing individuals' resilience, and by drawing upon the resources within individuals (self-help) and local communities, as well as health and social care. The RCGP has endorsed a position statement on mental health and inequalities that incorporates many of these ideas.

More recently the new General Medical Service's contract of 2004 and subsequent amendments have increased the mental health agenda within the Quality and Outcomes Framework relating specifically to care for people with a severe and enduring mental illness, depression and dementia.

In December 2004 the National Institute for Health and Clinical Excellence (NICE) published guidelines for the management of depression and the management of anxiety in primary and secondary care.

The Scottish Executive's Health Department launched its National Programme for Improving Mental Health and Well-being in October 2001.

A review of mental health and learning disability was carried out in Northern Ireland in 2003. As part of the development of 'Investing for Health' a five-year strategy for promoting mental health was published in 2003.

Mental health has been made one of the Welsh Assembly Government's top three priorities. The Revised National Service Framework for Adult Mental Health Services in Wales was published in 2005.

Intended learning outcomes from the curriculum statement

The following learning objectives relate specifically to mental health. The RCGP curriculum statement should be used in conjunction with the other curriculum statements, especially the core curriculum statement 1, *Being a General Practitioner*, and those covering learning disabilities and the care of drug-using adults.

In order to demonstrate the core competences in the area of mental health, the general practitioner will require knowledge, skills and appropriate attitudes in the following areas:

Primary care management

- Manage people experiencing mental health problems in primary care, bearing in mind that several interventions may be effective for each mental health condition, including different forms of talking therapy, medication and self-help.

- Describe specific interventions and guidelines for individual conditions, using where appropriate best practice as described in the Scottish Intercollegiate Guideline Network (SIGN) or NICE guidelines.

- Describe the need to check for psychological illness whilst avoiding the habit of checking extensively for physical illness.

- Demonstrate how to screen and diagnose people experiencing mental health problems, using effective and reliable instruments where they are available.

- Describe the varied ways that young people who are developing a first episode of psychosis present.

- Describe how to access health and social care organisations, both voluntary and statutory, which are an essential component of managing people with mental health problems.

- Describe when it is appropriate to refer to and collaborate with the specialist mental health services.

- Describe early indicators of difficulty in the psychological wellbeing of children and young people.

Person-centred care

- Describe how to engage with people experiencing mental health problems; to be able to elicit a person's unedited story.

- Describe how to enable people experiencing mental health problems to fully engage in delineating their difficulties and deciding on appropriate interventions.

- Describe the special challenges of rapport building with patients with mental health problems.

- Describe the concept of concordance that is particularly important in mental health care.

- Describe the importance of continuity of care for people with mental health problems.

- Demonstrate gender-specific communication skills.

Specific problem-solving skills

- Describe the prevalence of mental health problems and needs amongst the practice population.

- Describe how to screen and diagnose people experiencing mental health problems, using effective and reliable instruments where they are available.

- Describe how to deal with uncertainty that certain patients produce.

A comprehensive approach

- Describe how to deal with the associated physical health problems of people with mental health problems.

- Describe how to screen and diagnose people with physical illness at risk of mental health problems.

- Describe the principles of mental health promotion.

Community orientation

- Describe the extent and implications of stigma and social exclusion.

- Describe how to challenge inequality.

- Demonstrate how to work in partnership with other agencies to secure appropriate social interventions for individuals.

- Describe how to work in partnership with other agencies to secure wider public health of the local population.

- Demonstrate the ability to contribute to the health improvement programme that reflects the perspective of the local population.

- Describe the importance of avoiding medicalising some mental distress.

- Describe the ethical dilemma of the use of psychotropic drugs to sedate people for social reasons.

A holistic approach

- Describe the impact that social circumstances can have on mental illness and that recovery is contingent on the effective management of those social circumstances.

- Understand that a model of mental illness that creates an artificial separation between mind and body is often unhelpful – particularly in understanding psychosomatic complaints, psychological consequences of physical illness and somatisation.

- Demonstrate an understanding that mental illness is culturally determined and depends on assumptions that may not be universal.

- Demonstrate cultural sensitivity.

Contextual aspects

- Demonstrate sufficient knowledge of the current Mental Health Act to undertake the responsibilities that this requires of general practitioners.

Attitudinal aspects

- Understand the major part that drug companies play in promoting use of psychotropic drugs.

- Understand that attitudes and feelings are important determinants of how GPs practice.

- Describe the importance of self-awareness issues for the doctor such as family-of-origin issues and personal prejudices.

- Understand the need for GPs to have personal management plans for how they manage their own mental health.

- Understand the need for reflective practice.

Scientific aspects

- Adopt a critical and research-based approach to practice. This is particularly important in mental health, where evidence on effective treatment is often of poor quality.

- Recognise the use of value judgements in psychiatric diagnosis and understand the concept of a values-based approach to mental health.

Psychomotor skills

- Mental state assessment.

- Suicide risk assessment.

The knowledge base

Symptoms

- Tired all the time, insomnia, anxiety, depression, multiple somatic complaints, dizziness, palpitations, paraesthesiae, abdominal pain (children), early signs of possible psychotic illness.

Common and/or important conditions

- The most common primary care mental health problems are depression, eating disorders and anxiety disorders, ADHD, post-traumatic stress disorder, alcohol and drug misuse.

Investigation

- Use of depression rating scales, and other aids to evaluation of possible diagnosis and severity.

Treatment

- Pharmacology, CBT and simple behavioural techniques, problem-solving therapy and basis of systemic and strength-focused therapies, self-administered therapy.

Emergency care

- Threatened or attempted suicide, delirium, psychosis, panic, aggressive or violent patients, drug overdose and alcohol withdrawal.

Resources

- The family of the patient.

- Members of the primary healthcare team, receptionist, counsellor, Citizens Advice Bureau worker.

Prevention
- Mental health promotion, especially children, families and adolescents.
- Screening of all language-delayed children for autism.
- Early intervention in psychosis.

Promoting learning about mental health problems

Work-based learning – in primary care

Primary care both inside and outside the practice is the ideal environment to learn about the care of people with mental health problems. GP registrars should take the opportunity to gain a better understanding of the practice's patients that are looked after in partnership with the specialist team. Attending clinic appointments with their patients will help GP registrars gain a better understanding of the patient's journey.

GP registrars should learn from patients and carers by offering health reviews and participating in their training practices' mental health activities. They should take the opportunity to learn how to adopt a shared-care approach to primary care mental health with their community mental health teams and intermediate-care mental health teams.

Teamwork learning resource

There is a toolkit specifically designed for primary care teams to evaluate the extent to which they and their practices promote mental health. It is available from d.p.c.tomson@ncl.ac.uk or maryanne.freer@pcpartners.org, or from NIMHE (www.nimhe.csip.org.uk).

Work-based learning – in secondary care

Learn from community mental health teams about which patients are receiving shared care, and understanding their physical health needs. There should also be opportunities to learn from graduate mental health workers (and other primary care mental health service providers) which resources are available locally, and how to create a local practice resource directory.

Quality assurance of educational provision

There have been various developments attempting to address the issues of identification of competences and quality assurance of educational provision within mental health. Although at times there has appeared to be some confusion or disagreement as to their usefulness or what needed to be provided, progress has been made through the work of the Core Skills element of the Care Services Improvement Partnership (CSIP) Primary Care Programme[13] in integrating existing developments and influencing the thinking around this area.

GPs and other primary healthcare workers undertaking mental health education and training are more likely to have their learning needs addressed if the educational provision has been guided and influenced by the following best-practice indicators.

National Continuous Quality Improvement Tool for Mental Health Education, 2003[14]

This was developed to help in the commissioning of post-qualification mental health education programmes. It was a particular response to the fact that most courses that were then currently being commissioned were not closely allied to the national policy agenda and lacked service user and carer involvement. Subsequently, a useful handbook and implementation guide have been issued.[15]

Postgraduate Medical Education and Training Board *Standards for Curriculum Development*, 2005[16]

This sets out the characteristics that curricula should display to be effective in guiding learning, teaching and experience for all specialties including general practice across the UK. The standards describe how to ensure that the curriculum can be the basis of blueprinting for the assessment system.

Skills for Health[17]

Skills for Health (SfH) works with employers and other stakeholders to ensure that those working in the sector are equipped with the right skills to support the development and delivery of healthcare services. It has developed a labour market intelligence database to help identify the health sector's workforce needs. Visit www.skillsforhealth.org.uk for more details.

One of the main functions of SfH is to develop National Occupational Standards (NOS) and National Workforce Competencies (NWC) for use within the health sector. The NOS/NWC development links, where applicable, to key government agendas across the four countries, such as National Service Frameworks, key targets, and the Knowledge and Skills Framework (KSF) as part of Agenda for Change.

SfH and the NHS National Workforce Projects (NWP) have also developed a (UK-wide) Workforce Planning Competence Framework. The framework provides a suite of competences that are necessary to carry out workforce planning to enable the delivery of safe and effective care to patients and the public. Visit www.healthcareworkforce.org.uk for more information. To complement the framework, NWP is presently exploring opportunities to use the competences in delivering development programmes for those involved in workforce planning.

The competences developed by SfH can be used by individuals, employers and education providers for a number of purposes, including:

- individual development/appraisal
- team development
- role design
- role redesign
- service design, e.g. new ways of working
- education programme/curriculum design
- evidence gathering for KSF post outlines.

Skills for Health, *Assuring and Enhancing the Quality of Healthcare Education*, 2006[18]

These recently released Interim Standards are designed to support education commissioners in their responsibility to quality assure the programmes they purchase, and can be used with the National Standard Contract Framework. Whilst not mandatory, the Interim Standards will support commissioners with the transition to future agreed national quality assurance arrangements. The Interim Standards will be reviewed and through further consultation revised if necessary, before being incorporated into the arrangements specified in the National Standard Contract Framework.

The Interim Standards should be used to support the enhancement of partnership working between academic and practice providers at all levels, and their application should be through negotiation between commissioners and education providers (academic and practice).

Key Skills for Key Staff[19]

This recent resource will provide busy staff with a framework to support individuals experiencing mental health difficulties. It will help staff to identify their existing levels of mental health knowledge skills and attitudes, and will also suggest ways in which staff can improve their competence. *Key Skills* has been designed specifically for people working in primary care such as GPs, practice nurses, receptionists, health visitors, midwives, district nurses, community matrons and primary care practice managers.

The *Key Skills* document contains a section that outlines the competences that practitioners working in primary care will need to attain in order for them to offer optimum levels of care. This document can be used to inform the curricula of a range of mental health courses.

Addressing the challenges facing the primary care mental health education and learning agenda

If change agency is to occur, educational initiatives will need to be targeted specifically at the *ideal aims and objectives* (listed previously) underpinning any mental health training aimed at GPs and other primary care mental health practitioners. Core funding and resources will need to be protected in order to implement a thought-out, integrated, educational strategy that is directly targeted to, amongst others, NICE guidance, capacity and capability cycles, and the nGMS contract/the Quality and Outcomes Framework. If there is to be a much greater chance of a fit-for-purpose workforce equipped to deliver on the mental health agenda, primary care organisations and individuals concerned will not only need to be prepared to take on and, dare we say it, risk a long-term perspective but also to invest in and see education and training as core business.

Educational delivery will need to respond to this challenge as well, with a greater shift within higher education institutes (HEIs) to provide more *workplace* (occurring at the place of work) and *work-based* (related to the nature of the work) training. They will also have to build on more opportunities with non-accredited training, to provide greater flexibility of access to such training.

Distance learning or e-learning clearly offer important educational opportunities and have their place, but it is important to remember that *judgement* is an essential component of any clinician's practice. Judgement is particularly hard to teach solely through these approaches. This problem can be alleviated to some extent by utilising other methods such as e-mail groups, web logs and telephone conferencing.

As educators, for us one of the key concepts that is as important as knowledge, skills or attitude acquisition is the process of learning about learning. The latter is the means by which the individual is enabled to develop as an adult learner. Individuals need help and support developing as learners but this is often sadly lacking. There needs to be a focus shift with a parallel emphasis on developing the learner's educational capabilities in order to maximise on any learning opportunities provided.

Enhancing and improving the knowledge base of primary care practitioners

It is known that training and education alone are unlikely to have a lasting impact on the behaviour and practice of practitioners for the reasons discussed above. In fact it is evident that learners need to be steered towards ongoing learning resources and opportunities for reinforcement of learning.

Learning strategies must impart knowledge but this requires judicious planning. The RCGP curriculum content has now been decided upon but it is crucial that the learning strategies aimed at imparting this knowledge relate directly to the working practice of the busy GP or primary healthcare (primary healthcare team [PHCT]) practitioner. The aim of training and education should be clearly to support generalists to enhance their practice but should avoid any pretensions to convert generalists into specialists. The message should be loud and clear that any developmental programmes or policy initiatives are directed at promoting specialism within generalism and not vice versa.

The planning of relevant educational sessions can be simply assisted by constantly reviewing the relevance of the knowledge content by ensuring the following questions are asked:

- will the knowledge gained in this session improve patient care?
- should/could this intervention/strategy be delivered in primary care?

If the answer to either of these questions is NO then the content should be removed from the session and learners should be given the opportunity and references to explore the knowledge should they feel the need.

Providing primary care practitioners with increased mental health skills

Most mental health problems are assessed and treated in primary care. However, GPs' or PHCT practitioners' ability to detect and manage mental disorders is variable. A recent leader in the *British Medical Journal*[20] regarding the management of depression refers directly to one major barrier to effective treatment seeming to be the clinicians' perceptions of depression. They can be trained to develop mental health clinical skills, but if such training is to become widely available in primary care then primary care educators need to learn not only how to teach such skills and impart knowledge but also how to challenge attitudes. There is evidence which shows that community mental health GP registrar innovative training placements (ITP) have added value in taking registrars, at an early stage in their career, to a higher level of personal expertise and giving them the immediate opportunity to apply new mental health skills with general practice patients – specifically, mental health assessment and risk assessment.[21]

There is a huge variety of teaching tools available but the World Psychiatric Association (www.wpanet.org) has developed a mental health skills training resource for use in primary care. The training pack utilises video to model and teaches a range of mental health skills. The pack encourages the use of role-plays to allow learners to practise the new skills they have been taught. The training pack consists of a training manual for use by trainers. The pack includes a set of videos covering a range of mental health problems seen in primary care (depression, chronic fatigue, psychosis, somatisation and dementia), a floppy disc with a set of introductory lecture slides, lecture notes and a set of role-plays.

This approach is currently utilised in both Northampton and Leicester where video, role-play and simulated patients are used to enhance skills acquisition. The use of micro-skills teaching methods, which entail workshopping distinct consultation skills, ensures that knowledge and skills are gained in a tight format that reflects the nature of the GP consultation. There are three main benefits gained from this style of learning:

- understanding of the basic principles and practice of primary care mental health and the clinical tools used

- acquisition of the basic skills to provide safe and well-managed mental health care

- increased understanding of mental health services and the resources needed in general practice to provide high-quality care.

The particular strength of such experiential teaching is that the cognitive material or evidence base can be introduced at just the point in the learners' experiential thinking when they have generated a need for information and when it will therefore be more readily assimilated.

Training can be supplemented and enhanced by developing a range of disorder-specific or topic-specific 'masterclasses'. Such a combination of presentations with skill acquisition workshops can hugely add to the learning experience. This combination of coursework and masterclasses ensures that a range of learning styles can be employed.

Increasing the psychological mindfulness of GPs and primary care practitioners

When planning mental health training and education it is worthwhile building into the curriculum space to hear firsthand from patients about their own experiences of living with mental health problems. By involving patients in the learning experience primary care staff can be encouraged to explore the values underpinning their practice. The research describing users [people suffering from mental health problems] as trainers of service providers[22,23] indicate the merits of involving service users in the training of health professionals. The research by Wood and Wilson-Barnett is of particular interest because it illustrates that exposure to service users in training can lead to increased empathy amongst students.[23]

The training should also encourage the routine use of a range of mental health tools and screening questions that, when applied, will lead to an increased awareness of the psychological ramifications of many physical illnesses, especially those of a long-term nature. Interestingly, some of these have now been incorporated into the nGMS depression QOF clinical domain (see Chapter 1).

The process of *modelling* as part of the training process can be important in increasing psychological mindfulness. Many GP training teams are comprised of GPs with a special interest in mental health and specialist mental health practitioners who have an awareness and understanding of primary care ways of working. This combination should model psychological mindedness not only in the content of the training but also in the delivery. The trainers should ensure that the wellbeing of those receiving training is also highlighted. It is only by developing one's own understanding of our personal mental health that we can better focus on the needs of others.

As doctors' spare time is constantly eroded away trying to implement new government policy and changes, the worry is that discussions take place about changes in the practice and not about the patients. 'There is an essential need for patients, their problems and emotions to be looked at outside the consulting room.'[24] Balint groups or Balint-like discussions provide such an opportunity to 'enable doctors to take a fresh look at their everyday experience and see that there are problems which because medicine has tried to ignore them, cause a great deal of unnecessary suffering and irritation'.[25] Balint groups are still thriving and have developed successfully across some vocational training schemes (VTS) with a view to improving the psychological mindfulness of the attendees. An RCGP occasional paper recently examined what happened and what were the likely benefits and outcomes when a Balint group takes place within VTS training.[26]

Reflecting on my role as a Balint group facilitator (personal communication, LA) on my local VTS, I have certainly been impressed with the rapid growth of psychological mindfulness within the group members over a few months – I have also sadly realised that something essential had been lacking from our existing curriculum delivery! With general practice undergoing such constant change and having to deliver on various targets and outcomes, it will be interesting to see with time whether the poignant thinking and ideas of Michael Balint will remain influential or become something valuable that has become neglected or lost.

Enabling primary care practitioners to feel more secure about their mental health role

By ensuring that mental health training combines both an exploration of values with an increased knowledge and skills acquisition, it is safe to assume that GPs and other primary care practitioners will feel more confident about helping people with mental health-related issues and thus feel more secure in this role. A research study by Scanlan *et al.*[27] illustrates that with such training practice nurses can develop an effective and viable mental health role. Interestingly the research supports the view that for the knowledge and skills to be sustained the training and the ongoing role must be supported by good effective clinical supervision. The issue of patient pathways needs to be constantly highlighted and explored. An understanding of referral protocols needs to be delineated but more importantly the rationale for this should be discussed and explored via interactive teaching methods. This would ensure that the recipients of the training would feel secure about where the role of the primary care practitioner begins and when it changes to being one of supporting specialist care. Once again it is perhaps significant that the structure inherent in working to clear patient pathways was a factor that enhanced the effectiveness of the practice nurses' management of depression in Scanlan *et al.*'s study.[27]

Training can play an important role in impacting positively on the wellbeing of GPs. It is known that feelings of lack of control and prolonged feelings of uncertainty can, when combined with a range of other work stressors, impact negatively on symptoms of psychological burnout and occupational stress.[28] A learning experience that has building the confidence of participants around mental health issues as one of its objectives can help to remedy any early symptoms of burnout. One such initiative that needs to be discussed in further detail is the mental health Trailblazer programme, which has been rolled out nationally (see Box 22.1).

Box 22.1: Basic Trailblazer structure

- Three residential modules of one and a half days over a six-month period.
- Recruitment of pairing of individuals from different mental health service sectors.
- Pair collaboration in a local service improvement project.
- Courses composed of 6–10 pairs run by 2–4 facilitators from different professional backgrounds with relevance to mental health.
- Course emphasis to be on primary care in an integrated system of mental health provision.

Although Trailblazer programmes tend to vary locally in their format, evidence from evaluation has shown that:[29]

- a practitioner support approach focused exclusively around worthwhile health improvement projects using *critical friendship* and *action learning set* techniques appears to have the potential to produce significant outcomes in patient health care at local level

- space and time away from the working environment make an important contribution to this professional learning approach

- a process that excludes direct teaching and concentrates on individual development can produce a significant increase in professional capacity with experienced practitioners who are not wedded to more directive learning approaches.

The Trailblazer programme approach directed at change agency fits well with the educational philosophy as espoused within Lyotard's Triangle (see p. 409).

In summary, it is apparent that the rate of change within primary care often exceeds the rate of learning within the workforce. Throughout the course of this chapter we have attempted to highlight some of the present challenges and solutions to address this imbalance. Mental health education and training will only be effective in driving through change if it is delivered through an integrated and systematic approach. This will remain a major challenge when resources and funding are limited. The heterogeneity of primary care reflects the fact that there will never be a 'one shoe fits all' approach appropriate to educational provision. The response to this challenge and the need to meet a variety of learning styles, however, offers as much of an opportunity as a threat.

Education and training providers can supply patient-led curricula that offer both skills acquisition and that also address the values and attitudes required to deliver a fit-for-purpose workforce.

References

1. Royal College of General Practitioners. *Care of People with Mental Health Problems* (curriculum statement 13), 2006, www.rcgp-curriculum.org.uk/PDF/curr_13_Mental_Health.pdf [accessed November 2007].

2. National Institute for Mental Health in England. *Making it Possible: improving mental health and well-being in England* Leeds: NIMHE, 2005.

3. New Economics Foundation. *A Well-being Manifesto for a Flourishing Society* London: New Economics Foundation, 2006.

4. Lyotard J-F. *The Postmodern Condition: a report on knowledge* Manchester: Manchester University Press, 1984.

5. Capacity and Capability Planning Cycle. CSIP SW 2005.

6. Thompson C, Kinmonth J, Stevens L, *et al.* Effects of a clinical-practice guideline and practice-based education on detection and outcome of depression in primary care: Hampshire depression project randomized controlled trial *Lancet* 2000; **355**: 50–7.

7. Kendrick T, Stevens L, Bryant A, *et al.* Hampshire depression project: changes in the process of care and cost consequences *British Journal of General Practice* 2001; **51**: 911–13.

8. Gilbody S, Whitty P, Grimshaw J, *et al.* Educational and organizational interventions to improve the management of depression in primary care: a systematic review *Journal of the American Medical Association* 2003; **289(23)**: 3145–51.

9. Lambert W, Schuwirth T, Cees P, *et al.* Medical education: challenges for educationalists *British Medical Journal* 2006; **333(7567)**: 544–6.

10. Gabbay J, Le May A. Evidence based guidelines or collectively constructed 'Mindlines'? Ethnographic study of knowledge management in primary care *British Medical Journal* 2004; **329**; 1013.

11. Department of Health. *The Ten Essential Shared Capabilities: a framework for the whole of the mental health workforce* London: NIMHE and the Sainsbury Centre for Mental Health Joint Workforce Support Unit in conjunction with NHSU, 2005.

12. Royal College of General Practitioners. *Being a General Practitioner* (curriculum statement 1), 2006, www.rcgp-curriculum.org.uk/PDF/curr_1_Curriculum_Statement_Being_a_GP.pdf [accessed November 2007].

13. National Institute for Mental Health in England. Core Skills Programme. NIMHE Primary Care Programme, www.csip.org.uk [accessed November 2007].

14. Northern Centre for Mental Health. National Continuous Quality Improvement Tool for Mental Health Education, 2003, www.lincoln.ac.uk/ccawi/publications/National%20QAT%20for%20MH.pdf [accessed November 2007].

15. Brooker C, Curran J. *National Continuous Quality Improvement Tool for Mental Health Education: handbook and implementation guide* Centre for Clinical and Academic Workforce Innovation, University of Lincoln, 2005, www.lincoln.ac.uk/ccawi/RsrchPublications.htm [accessed November 2007].

16. Postgraduate Medical Education and Training Board. *Standards for Curriculum Development: background paper*, 2005, www.pmetb.org.uk/fileadmin/user/QA/Assessment/Generic_standards_for_training_-_new_branding_Jan_2007.pdf [accessed November 2007].

17. www.skillsforhealth.org.uk [accessed November 2007].

18. Skills for Health. *Assuring and Enhancing the Quality of Healthcare Education: interim standards* Bristol: SfH, 2006.

19. Department of Health. *Key Skills for Key Staff* Cheshire: CSIP, 2006.

20. Scott J. Depression should be managed like a chronic disease *British Medical Journal* 2006; **332**: 985–6.

21. Leicestershire, Northamptonshire and Rutland Postgraduate Deanery. *Going There: an evaluation report on two community mental health GPR training posts* Leicester: University of Leicester, 2005.

22. Cook J, Jonikas J. A randomised evaluation of consumer versus nonconsumer training of state mental health service providers *Community Mental Health Journal* 1995; **31(3)**: 229–38.

23. Wood J, Wilson-Barnett J. The influence of user involvement on the learning of mental health nursing students *NT Research* 1999; **4(4)**: 257–70.

24. Zalidis S. *A General Practitioner, His Patients and Their Feelings* London: Free Association Books, 2001.

25. Balint M. *The Doctor, His Patient and the Illness* London: Pitman, 1968.

26. Pinder R, McKee A, Sackin P, *et al. Talking about My Patient: the Balint approach in GP Education* (Occasional Paper 87) London: RCGP, 2006.

27. Scanlan M, Smart D, Gregory S, *et al*. Evaluation of the effect of practice nurses on the management of depression *Primary Care Mental Health* 2007; **4(2)**: 107–13.

28. Health and Safety Executive. *Stress at Work: a guide for employers* Sudbury: HSE Books, 1995.

29. Worrall P, Ashton L. In press.

Web resources

www.dh.gov.uk
Department of Health (separate locations for NSF, *The NHS Plan*, etc.)

www.rcgp.org.uk
Royal College of General Practitioners

www.nice.org.uk
National Institute for Health and Clinical Excellence. Site for NICE guidelines

www.csip.org.uk
National Institute for Mental Health in England

www.scmh.org.uk
Sainsbury Centre for Mental Health

www.primhe.org
Primary Care Mental Health and Education. A non-profit-making organisation dedicated to developing and delivering better mental health care

www.northamptonshire.nhs.uk/Changing_Minds_Education_Centre/index.htm
The Changing Minds Education Centre

www.mhhe.heacademy.ac.uk
Mental Health in Higher Education project

www.lincoln.ac.uk/ccawi
Centre for Clinical and Academic Workforce Innovation

www.npcrdc.man.ac.uk
National Primary Care Research and Development Centre

www.pcpoh.bham.ac.uk/primarycare/research/mental_health
University of Birmingham Department of Primary Care and General Practice

www.skillsforhealth.org.uk
Skills for Health

www.sdcmh.org.uk
Scottish Development Centre for Mental Health

www.niamh.co.uk
Northern Ireland Association for Mental Health

www.wales.nhs.uk/sites/home.cfm?orgid=438
NHS Wales, Mental Health – National Service Frameworks

Further reading

Agen E, Tomson D, Tomson P, *et al. Ten Minutes for the Family: systemic interventions in primary care* London: Routledge, 2003.

Balint M. *The Doctor, His Patient and the Illness* London: Pitman, 1968.

The Centre for Economic Performance's Mental Health Policy Group. *The Depression Report: a new deal for depression and anxiety disorders* London: Centre for Economic Performance, London School of Economics and Political Science, 2006.

Davies T, Craig T. *ABC of Mental Health* (second edition) London: BMJ Books, 2006.

Dowrick C. *Beyond Depression* Oxford: Oxford University Press, 2004.

Harris EC, Barraclough B. Excess mortality of mental disorder *British Journal of Psychiatry* 1998; **173**; 11–53.

Nolan P, Badger F (eds). *Promoting Collaboration in Primary Mental Health Care* Cheltenham: Nelson Thornes, 2002.

Phelan M, Stradins L, Morrison S. Physical health of people with severe mental illness *British Medical Journal* 2001; **22**; 443–4.

Sainsbury Centre for Mental Health. *Primary Solutions* London: Sainsbury Centre for Mental Health, 2002.

Sainsbury Centre for Mental Health. *Economic and Social Costs of Mental Illness* London: Sainsbury Centre for Mental Health, 2003.

Sainsbury Centre for Mental Health. *Investing in General Practice: the new General Medical Services contract for GPs. Policy briefing 21* London: Sainsbury Centre for Mental Health, 2003.

WHO Collaborating Centre for Research and Training for Mental Health. *WHO Guide to Mental and Neurological Health in Primary Care* (2nd edn) London: RSM Press, 2004.

Appendix I: Mental health promotion fun quiz – how are you doing?

Tick the box that most fits for you on average:	Just surviving	Well done	Great
Taking part in *physical activity* that lasts for 30 minutes and is enough to make you warm and at least slightly out of breath	Less than three times a week	Three to four times a week	Five or more times a week
Doing something *creative* that you enjoy, such as music, dance, writing, painting, gardening, cooking, woodwork, etc.	Less than three times a week	Three times a week	More than three times a week
Learning a *new skill* – for pleasure, to make new friends or to improve your chances of a job	None in the last 12 months	One new skill	More than one new skill
Getting involved, such as joining a club or a faith community, or becoming a volunteer	Not a member or volunteer	Member of one or a volunteer	More than one and a volunteer
Keeping in touch with family and friends	No meetings with friends or family in an average week	At least one meeting	More than one meeting
Accepting yourself and others – everyone, including yourself, is entitled to respect and everyone has something to offer	Disagree	Agree	Agree strongly
Talking about it – it is better to share your feelings with friends, family or a helpline	Hardly ever share my feelings	Sometimes share my feelings	Usually share my feelings
Being a good listener rather than offering advice – let people work things out as they talk, avoid making judgements and check from time to time that you've understood	Never do this	Sometimes do this	Usually do this
Drinking in moderation – recommended levels are up to 21 units for women and up to 28 units for men (a unit is one small glass of wine, or half a pint of beer or a pub measure of spirits)	More than recommended levels and/or binge drinking	Less than or the same as the recommended levels	At least two alcohol-free nights a week; no more than recommended
Avoiding illegal drugs – using illegal drugs can trigger mental health problems	Use illegal drugs	Never use	Never use
Asking for help when you need it, be it from friends, family or local services	Hardly ever	Sometimes	Usually
Relaxing – try to make time for yourself to unwind, such as reading, listening to music, meditation, prayer	Less than three times a week	Manage this at least three times a week	More than three times a week

Total: How many boxes did you tick in the column?

This quiz has been adapted from Mentality's 'Twelve steps to positive mental health' and from resources originally produced for the North East London Strategic Health Authority website (which no longer exists). It was first published in the *Greenwich Mental Health Promotion Strategy* in 2004. Mentality also no longer exists but the positive steps can be found in *Making it Possible*.[1]

Scores

This is a fun quiz and aims to give an idea about 12 things we can do to ensure we get the best out of our lives. Add up how many boxes you ticked in each column.

Mostly 'just survivings'

When times are difficult, it is sometimes all we can do to survive. Take one day at a time and don't be too hard on yourself. Take time out if you need it. If you have a long-term mental health problem, try to plan the care you need with your keyworker and others for when you're less ill. If you think you need more help contact your GP.

Mostly 'well dones'

You are doing all the right things and are probably enjoying your life as a result. Be aware of the need to make more time for the things that are important in life.

Mostly 'greats'

You don't need us to tell you that life is going well and what is needed to make life the best it can be right now. To keep it that way look at the chart and see if there are any areas you are not covering and work out with a friend how to fill in the gaps.

Reference

1. Care Services Improvement Partnership. *Making it Possible: improving mental health and well-being in England* Leeds: NIMHE, CSIP, 2005.

Appendix II: Non-pharmacological sleep management techniques

Stimulus control

The main aim of stimulus control is to fall asleep quickly and maintain sleep by:

- strengthening the association of the bed and the bedroom as a cue for sleep
- weakening the association of the bed/bedroom as a cue for activities that might interfere with sleep
- developing a consistent sleep rhythm.

The client is usually given a set of instructions to follow such as those in the box.

Stimulus control instructions

- Go to bed only when you are sleepy.
- If you do not fall asleep within 15 minutes, or wake up and cannot resume sleep within 15 minutes, leave the bedroom and return only when sleepy again. Repeat as often as necessary.
- Use the bedroom only for sleep and sex. Do not read, watch TV, work or eat in bed.
- Get up at the same time every morning, irrespective of how much sleep you got during the night, including weekends.
- Avoid daytime napping.

Source: adapted from www.holistic-online.com. Reproduced by permission of Concept to Classroom © Educational Broadcasting Corporation.

One study in 1983 found that stimulus control was the most effective intervention regardless of severity of sleep onset insomnia.[1] A later study found that stimulus control was as good as sleep hygiene education and meditation at reducing wake time after sleep onset in a group of people with sleep maintenance insomnia. However, people valued the stimulus control and meditation treatments more highly.[2]

Sleep restriction or compression

The aim of sleep restriction is to maximise the time in bed spent asleep and to match this to the individual's need for sleep. By increasing this to 90 per cent it is then possible to extend the total time asleep. Some individuals need less than eight hours of sleep and feel more rested if they spend less time in bed awake.

Sleep restriction instructions

- Keep a sleep diary for two weeks to find out total time in bed and total time asleep.

- Divide the time asleep by the time in bed. This is a measure of sleep efficiency. If this is less than 85 per cent follow the next step.

- Go to bed 15 minutes later than usual in week 1.

- Maintain the same time to get up throughout, regardless of how much sleep is achieved.

- Continue to put bedtime back by 15 minutes until a sleep efficiency of 90 per cent is reached or 5 hours.

- At this point go to bed 15 minutes earlier each night to gradually extend the night's sleep (maintaining a sleep efficiency of at least 85 per cent).

Source: adapted from www.holistic-online.com and Morin *et al.*[3]

Paradoxical intention

A paradoxical intention means to take a paradoxical approach to a problem – i.e. doing the opposite of what you are trying to do. Therefore in this case the instruction would be to try to stay awake. It is not clear how paradoxical intention works, but it may be that it reduces performance anxiety. In a setting with a therapist who is resistant to advice it may break any power struggle. There is a theoretical chance that this could make things worse but in practice this has not been found to be the case.

Paradoxical intention instructions

- Step one: work out the most appropriate paradoxical instruction to maintain the problem, e.g. 'Try to stay awake as long as possible', 'Try to wake as many times as possible', 'See your sleep problems as a source of strength'.

- Step two: put the paradoxical instruction into effect with zest.

- Step three: keep following the plan until the desired outcome is reached. This is paradoxically by 'failing' to follow the instruction.

Source: adapted from www.holistic-online.com.

Biofeedback

Biofeedback techniques require special equipment available in sleep laboratories and produce relaxation through the feedback of physiological measures such as heart rate and breathing rate.

Cognitive restructuring

This is usually part of a group cognitive behavioural treatment package with one or two of stimulus control, sleep restriction or paradoxical intention. The aim is to challenge negative thoughts about sleep, such as 'It's awful, I'll never fall asleep', with evidence from the sleep diary, with evidence from the person's own experience and to reframe how awful the sleep problems are in the larger scale of things (e.g. not as bad as having cancer or losing a leg). Cognitive restructuring also focuses on dysfunctional beliefs about sleep, such as 'I must have eight hours of sleep'. Changes in these thoughts correlate with improvements in objective and subjective measures of sleep.[4] Sustained improvements over three years have been shown following short-term (six sessions) cognitive behavioural therapy consisting of stimulus control, bedtime restriction, muscle and cognitive relaxation, thought stopping and cognitive restructuring.[5] Total sleep time improved by 1 hour 20 minutes on average at three years.

Progressive muscle relaxation

Relaxation techniques promote sleep by reducing physiological tension and cognitive arousal. It is usually taught by tape or by a group leader. Muscles are tensed and then relaxed following a routine progression such as arms, head, chest, abdomen and legs. Relaxation techniques work well where there is daytime drowsiness and the aim is to maximise sleep, or where there is pain or other disturbance preventing sleep.

References

1. Lacks P, Bertelson AD, Gans L, *et al*. The effectiveness of three behavioural treatments for different degrees of sleep onset insomnia *Behaviour Therapy* 1983; **14(5)**: 593–605.

2. Schoicket SL, Bertelson AD, Lacks P. Is sleep hygiene a sufficient treatment for sleep maintenance insomnia? *Behaviour Therapy* 1988; **19(2)**: 183–90.

3. Morin CM, Hauri PJ, Espie CA, *et al*. Nonpharmacologic treatment of chronic insomnia *Sleep* 1999; **22(8)**: 1134–56.

4. Edinger JD, Wohlgemuth WK, *et al*. Does the cognitive-behavioural insomnia therapy alter dysfunctional beliefs about sleep? *Sleep* 2001; **24(5)**: 591–9.

5. Backhaus J, Hohagen F, Voderholzer U, *et al*. Long-term effectiveness of a short-term cognitive-behavioural group treatment for primary insomnia *European Archives of Psychiatry and Clinical Neuroscience* 2001; **251(1)**: 35.

Index